A CORE CURRICULUM

for

NURSE LIFE CARE PLANNING

A CORE CURRICULUM

for

NURSE LIFE CARE PLANNING

American Association of Nurse Life Care Planners

Dorajane Apuna-Grummer
BSN, MA, DHA, RN, CCM CNLCP
Clinical Editor

Wendie A. Howland
MN, RN-BC, CRRN, CCM, CNLCP, LNCP-C, LNCC
Editor

iUniverse LLC
Bloomington

A Core Curriculum for Nurse Life Care Planning

iUniverse books may be ordered through booksellers or by contacting:

iUniverse LLC
1663 Liberty Drive
Bloomington, IN 47403
www.iuniverse.com
1-800-Authors (1-800-288-4677)

Because of the dynamic nature of the Internet, any web addresses or links contained in this book may have changed since publication and may no longer be valid. The views expressed in this work are solely those of the author and do not necessarily reflect the views of the publisher, and the publisher hereby disclaims any responsibility for them.

Any people depicted in stock imagery provided by Thinkstock are models, and such images are being used for illustrative purposes only.
Certain stock imagery © Thinkstock.

ISBN: 978-1-4917-0656-5 (sc)
ISBN: 978-1-4917-0657-2 (ebk)

Library of Congress Control Number: 2013916528

Printed in the United States of America

iUniverse rev. date: 09/26/2013

Authors and Contributors

Barbara Bate, RN-BC, CCM, CNLCP, LNCC, MSCC
Jean Beaubien, BSN, RN, CRRN, CDMS, CCM, CNLCP
Nancy J. Bond, M.Ed., CCM, CLCP
Nicki Bradley, BS, RN-BC, CCM, CNLCP, MSCC
Terri Brandley, BSN, RN, CCM
Sandra Callaghan, MSN, RN, BS, NP-C, CLCP, CNLCP, MSCC
Chris Ann Daniel, BSHS, RN, CCM, CNLCP, MSCC, LNC, CHC
Glenda Evans-Shaw, BSN, RN, PHN, CCM, CNLCP
Shelene Giles, MS, BSN, BA, RN, CRC, CNLCP, CLCP, MSCC, LNCC
Barbara Greenfield, BSN, RN, CCM, CNLCP
Dorajane Apuna-Grummer BSN, MA, DHA, RN, CCM CNLCP
Liz Holakiewicz, BSN, RN, CCM, CNLCP
Wendie A. Howland, MN, RN-BC, CRRN, CCM, CNLCP, LNCP-C, LNCC
Linda Husted, MPH, RN, CNLCP, LNCC, CCM, CDMS, CRC
Shelly Kinney, MSN, RN, CCM, CNLCP
Barbara Krasa BSN, RN, CNLCP MSCC
Lyn Leake, RN, BSN, CNLC
Barbara Malloy, BSN, RN, CCM, CLCP, MSCC, LNCC
Joan K McMahon, MSA, BSN, CRRN
Jacquelyn Morris, BSN, RN, CRRN, CNLCP
Peggie Nielson, BSN, RN, CNLCP, MSCC
April Pettengill, BSN, RN, CRRN, CNLCP, MSCC
Kathy Pouch, MSN, RN-BC, CCM, CNLCP, CNCC
Anne Sambucini, RN, CCM, CDMS, CNLCP, MSC-C
Joan Schofield, BSN, MBA, RN, CNLCP
Lynne P. Trautwein, MSN, RN, CCM, CMAC, CNLCP
Kim Wages, BSN, RN, BBA, CRRN, CNLCP, MSCC
Ginger Walton, MSN, RN, FNP, CNLCP
Catherine Winslow, BSN, RN, CCM, CDMS, CNLCP
Karen Yates, RN, LNC, NLCP
Nancy Zangmeister RN, CRRN, CCM, CLCP, MSCC, CNLCP

From the Clinical Editor

Dorajane Apuna-Grummer BSN MA DHA RN CNLCP CCM

This book provides both a study guide for the credentialing exam and a reference for working nurse life care planners. It is not meant to be all-inclusive; it is a foundation for our discipline to encourage nurse life care planners to research and learn. Built on the American Nurses Association Scope and Standards of Practice definitions of nursing process and nursing diagnoses and the American Association of Nurse Life Care Planners Standards of Practice, it includes:

Section 1: Foundation of nurse life care planning.
> An overview of the book, history and evolution of our organization, critical thinking for the nurse life care planner, and the evaluation of life care plans.

Section 2: Injury and condition management
> A reference for the nurse life care planner on major injuries and conditions, using critical nursing tools such as standards of practice, nursing process, nursing diagnoses, and the development of individualist life care plans that nurses have been using since early clinical practice. Chapters include burns, chronic pain, spinal cord injuries, traumatic brain injuries, cerebral palsy, amputations and managing the natural aging process from pediatrics to seniors.

Section 3: Legal aspects
> Expert witnessing, the Daubert challenges, disability rights laws, rehabilitation act, and the litigation process.

As this Core goes to press, I want to thank each of the many members of our organization who worked so hard on this book, spending countless hours writing, writing, and then more writing. Dr. Colleen Manzetti, acting director of the Ocean County College School of Nursing, edited some of the chapters to give guidance to authors. Special thanks to Anne Sambucini for her tireless efforts to organize and keep everyone on track.

She gave many, many hours to working with the development team, the credentialing board, and the executive board to keep this project moving. I would like to thank Kelly Lance for her vision and for establishing our organization. A special thanks to NANDA-I for assistance with the nursing diagnoses sections in the chapters and for Nancy Zangmeister, who organized many of the diagnoses used. I know there are many that I cannot thank individually due to space constraints, but I truly thank everyone who participated in the development of this book. This has been both a humbling and rewarding experience. Hillary Clinton stated, "It takes a village." It took an organization to write our book.

Acknowledgements
Anne Sambucini RN, CCM, CDMS, CNLCP, MSC-C
President AANLCP 2012

This first AANLCP core curriculum has evolved over many years. During the slow and often interrupted evolution of this book, AANLCP has undergone many changes. This amazing organization is comprised of individuals with remarkable talent and professionalism, all of whom are dedicated to sharing their knowledge with others so future nurses can excel in the field of nurse life care planning.

This book would not have been possible without a great deal of help from many people. I would like to express my heartfelt gratitude to the clinical editor, the many authors, peer reviewers, researchers and all those who have helped behind the scenes, without whom this book would never have been published. They shared their knowledge, their ideas, and numerous tips all of which culminated in the completion of this book.

First, as nurse life care planners, we owe the genesis of our specialty to Kelly Lance MSN, APRN, FNP-C, CNLCP, LNCP-C, founder of AANLCP. Her vision, hard work, and organizational skills gave us direction and created the foundation for the practice of nurse life care planning.

This book was started over 6 years ago, with much of the initial preparation done by past presidents Shelene Giles MS, BSN, BA, RN, CRC, CNLCP, MSCC, CLCP and Karen Apy BSN RN, CNLCP, LNCC.

I would like to express my sincere thanks to past president Jackie Morris BSN, RN, CRRN, CNLCP for her leadership, support, and vision. This book began to develop its present form during her presidency. She trusted me with bringing it to fruition.

This book would not have been possible without the dedication, perseverance, and long hours away from her family and business by our clinical editor Dorajane Apuna DHA, BSN, MA, RN, CCM, CNLCP. We owe Dorajane a debt of gratitude that can never be repaid.

When I called for help with clinical editing, Colleen Manzetti DNP, RN, CNE, CNLCP was there and provided much needed support with the clinical editing.

Special thanks to Wendie Howland MN, RN-BC, CRRN, CCM, CNLCP, LNCP-C, LNCC for being so magnanimous with her time: authorship, professionalism, tech support, being an all around gal-Friday, and editing the entire final work and proofs. I am grateful that she always answered the phone and somehow solved any issue at hand. Thank you for obtaining approval from NANDA-I to use NANDA language extensively in this work.

As a special mention, I would like to thank Liz Holakiewicz BSN, RN, CCM, CNLCP, whose insights added immeasurably to this book.

We want to thank Brent Giles for designing our book cover. We appreciate the time you spent on this project.

The authors are recognized in their respective chapters. Each of these authors gave countless hours writing, reviewing, revising, updating, and finally validating each chapter. This book could not have been completed without their dedication.

I would like to thank many others who took time to contribute and review this book: Jean Beaubien, BSN, RN, CRRN, CDMS, CCM, CNLCP; Sandra Callaghan MSN, RN, BS, NP-C, CLCP, CNLCP, MSCC; Marianne Cosby MPA, MSN, RN, PHN, CEN, NE-BC, LNCC, CLCP, CCM, MSCC; Laura E. Fox, MSN, RN, CLCP; Liz Holakiewicz BSN, RN, CCM, CNLCP; Shelly Kinney MSN, RN, CCM, CNLCP; Marilyn Litwin MS, RN, BSN,

CDMS, CNLCP, MSCC; Joan Schofield BSN, MBA, RN, CNLCP; Ginger Walton RN, MSN, FNP, CNLCP; JoAnn White BSN, RN, CNLCP; and Lora White BSN, RN-BC, CCM, CNLCP, MSCC.

Special thanks for the 2012 executive board of AANLCP:
- Jackie Morris, for providing leadership as president and being team leader for the TBI chapter
- Joan Schofield, for coming to my rescue in developing a much-needed chapter revision
- Nancy Zangmeister, for inputting all the NANDA-I Nursing diagnoses in the chapters
- Peggie Nielson, for providing many hours of research to ensure accuracy

And to Denise Nelson, AANLCP secretary, recognition for outstanding support.

To my loving family and colleagues, thank you for your patience, support, and sacrifice with this seeming never-ending labor of love.

If you are not currently a member please consider membership and visit us at www.aanlcp.org

A Word From the Editor About Nursing Diagnosis

Wendie A. Howland MN, RN-BC, CRRN, CCM, CNLCP, LNCP-C, LNCC

As nurse life care planners we are fully aware of the centrality
of nursing diagnosis
in nurse life care planning. Registered nurses are permitted,
and in most jurisdictions mandated, to diagnose and treat
human responses to illness or injury by virtue of our
professional licensure, a privilege that we do not take lightly.
The nursing process of assessment, analysis, planning,
intervening/delegating,
and reassessment (when possible and appropriate)
is the conceptual framework of nurse life care planning.

We are grateful to NANDA-International
for their collegial collaboration and assistance
helping us incorporate nursing diagnoses in this work.
Particular thanks to Isabel Rollings at John Wiley:
"To boldly license, where no-one has licensed before . . ."

*Please note that in order to make safe and effective
judgments using NANDA-I nursing diagnoses, it is
essential that nurses refer to the definitions and defining
characteristics of the diagnosis listed.
The nursing diagnoses in this work are approved for usage
by NANDA-I in Nursing Diagnoses—
Definitions and Classification 2012-2014
© 2012, 1994-2012 NANDA International.
Used by arrangement with John Wiley and Sons Ltd.*

CONTENTS

Section II   Nurse Life Care Plans In Practice

Terri Brandley, BSN, RN, CCM
Linda Husted, MPH, RN, CNLCP, LNCC, CCM, CDMS, CRC
Shelly Kinney, MSN, RN, CCM, CNLCP
Jacquelyn Morris, BSN, RN, CRRN, CNLCP
Kathy Pouch, MSN, RN-BC, CCM, CNLCP, CNCC
Karen Yates, RN, LNC, NLCP
Jean Beaubien, BSN, RN, CRRN, CDMS, CCM, CNLCP,
contributor

Nicki Bradley, BS, RN-BC, CCM, CNLCP, MSCC
Sandra Callaghan, MSN, RN, BS, NP-C, CLCP, CNLCP, MSCC
Barbara Greenfield, BSN, RN, CCM, CNLCP
Barbara Malloy, BSN, RN, CCM, CLCP, MSCC, LNCC
Catherine Winslow, BSN, RN, CCM, CDMS, CNLCP
Peggie Nielson, BSN, RN, CNLCP, MSCC, contributor

Terri Brandley, BSN, RN, CCM
Shelly Kinney, MSN, RN, CCM, CNLCP
Karen Yates, RN, LNC, NLCP
Jean Beaubien, BSN, RN, CRRN, CDMS, CCM,
CNLCP, contributor

Chapter 5   Burns and Life Care Planning 325

Chris Ann Daniel, BSHS, RN, CCM, CNLCP, MSCC, LNC, CHC
Glenda Evans-Shaw, BSN, RN, PHN, CCM, CNLCP
Shelene Giles, MS, BSN, BA, RN, CRC, CNLCP, CLCP, MSCC, LNCC
Wendie Howland, MN, RN-BC, CRRN, CCM, CNLCP, LNCC
April Pettengill, BSN, RN, CRRN, CNLCP, MSCC
Kim Wages, BSN, RN, BBA, CRRN, CNLCP, MSCC
Barbara Bate, RN-BC, CCM, CRRN, CNLCP, LNCC, MSCC, contributor

Lynne P. Trautwein, MSN, RN, CCM, CMAC, CNLCP
Nancy J. Bond, M.Ed., CCM, CLCP

Chapter 7   Age-Related Issues in Life Care Planning...... 392
    Shelene Giles, MS, BSN, BA, RN, CRC, CNLCP, CLCP, MSCC, LNCC
    Barbara Krasa, RN, BSN, CNLCP MSCC
    Jackie Morris, BSN, RN, CRRN, CNLCP
    April Pettengill, BSN, RN, CRRN, CDMS, CNLCP, MSCC
    Anne Sambucini, RN, CCM, CDMS, CNLCP, MSC-C
    Joan Schofield, BSN, MBA, RN, CNLCP
    Nancy Zangmeister, RN, CRRN, CCM, CLCP, MSCC, CNLCP
    Ginger Walton, MSN, RN, CNLCP, contributor

Section III   Legal Considerations

Terri Brandley, BSN, RN, CCM
Lyn Leake, BSN, RN, CNLC

Barbara Bate, RN-BC, CCM, CNLCP, LNCC, MSCC

Chapter 3   Disability Rights Laws **450**
    April Pettengill, BSN, RN, CRRN, CNLCP, MSCC

Section I

Foundations of
Nurse Life Care Planning

CHAPTER 1

History and Evolution of The Nurse Life Care Planning Specialty

Anne Sambucini, RN, CCM, CDMS, CNLCP, MSC-C

Nursing continues to evolve, expanding into new roles and offering numerous opportunities for growth. Nurses pioneering new and expanded roles make nursing roles even more dynamic. Nurse life care planning, planning care for the lifetime needs of an individual, is relatively new; projecting medical needs and associated costs for a lifetime are new and exciting expansions of older concepts (Lance, 2012).

The American Nurses Association's *Nursing Scope and Standards of Practice* (ANA, 2010), builds on previous nursing development and provides the following definition of nursing:

> Nursing is the protection, promotion, and optimization of health and abilities, prevention of illness and injury, alleviation of suffering through the diagnosis and treatment of human response, and advocacy in the care of individuals, families, communities, and populations (ANA, 2010).

Definition of Nurse Life Care Planning

Expanding on the ANA's *Scope and Standards of Practice*, the American Association of Nurse Life Care Planners (AANLCP) defines nurse life care planning in this way:

> The specialty practice in which the nurse life care planner utilizes the nursing process for the collection and analysis of comprehensive client-specific data in the preparation of a dynamic document. This document provides an organized, concise plan that estimates for reasonable and necessary (and reasonably certain to be necessary) current and future healthcare needs with the associated costs

and frequencies of goods and services. The nurse life care plan is developed for individuals who have experienced an injury or have chronic healthcare issues. Nurse life care planners function within their individual professional scope of practice and, when applicable, incorporate opinions arrived upon collaboratively with various health professionals. The nurse life care plan is considered a flexible document and is evaluated and updated as needed (AANLCP, 2008).

NLCPs formulate life care plans by using the nursing process, collecting and analyzing comprehensive, client-specific data, and coordinating care in a variety of healthcare settings. Nurse life care planners function within their individual professional scopes of practice, and, when applicable, incorporate opinions arrived at by collaboration with various healthcare providers.

Actual implementation of recommended interventions in the life care plan is delegated to the nurse case manager, who also helps identify when the life care plan needs to be updated. Updated needs will trigger a referral to a nurse life care planner for re-evaluation of the life care plan (AANLCP, 2012).

The National League of Nurses defines critical thinking in nursing practice as "a discipline-specific, reflective reasoning process that guides a nurse in generating, implementing, and evaluating approaches for dealing with client care and professional concerns" (NLN, 2011). When critical thinking is used in nursing, it is called *the nursing process*. The practice role of the NLCP uses the nursing process to develop a plan of care for the injured or chronically ill person's lifetime throughout the continuum of healthcare in multiple settings.

Professional nurses' extensive education and wealth of experience are excellent preparation for nurse life care planning. Nurses complete a thorough assessment of an individual's physical, functional, emotional, and spiritual needs, and collaborate as members of the healthcare team. Nurses' extensive knowledge base includes pharmacology, rehabilitation, orthopedics, pediatrics, and medical-surgical nursing, as well as coordination of care, utilization review of costs, and medical coding. Working knowledge of all these areas is needed in nurse life care planning.

Evolution of Nurse Life Care Planning

The nurse's role in coordinating care and services began in the early 1900s with the advent of privately funded home nursing for the poor. In the early 1900s, Lillian Wald promoted the term "public health nurse," expanding nursing practice to encompass employment, recreation, health education, and sanitation. Visiting nurses used community-based coordination, which was further developed by publicly funded health nursing in the 1930s. By the 1940s, the insurance industry was using case management as a method of cost containment (CMSA, 2008). During World War II, industry used case management nurses to help maintain a healthy workforce for the war effort.

Care planning in nursing advanced further in 1961 with the identification of the nursing process by Ida Jean Orlando. As care planning has evolved, so have its purpose and tools. Case management roles expanded as early as 1966, when nurses began adding budget planning to coordinating care and services.

In the mid-1970s, Paul Deutsch first identified the term "Life Care Planning," referring to future needs, to describe a tool to project the costs of medical care in the litigation environment. In *Damage in Tort Action* (1981), Deutsch referenced case management, catastrophic disability case management, and catastrophic disability research as means to project future medical care (Deutsch, 2011). This was introduced to the healthcare industry in 1985 in his *Guide to Rehabilitation* in short seminars and, later, a defined curriculum. Numerous professionals, including nurses, continue to learn and adapt this methodology.

In 1997, the discipline of nurse life care planning (NLCP) began when Kelly Lance, MSN, RN, CNLCP, LNCP-C, FNP-BC, recognized that a registered nurse's multidimensional healthcare education combined with nursing's own professional standards and scope of practice were ideal preparatory foundations for life care planning. She identified the nursing process as the methodology by which a registered nurse develops a life care plan. Nurse life care planning held that the ANA's scope and standards of practice were the defining conceptual base for future care planning; therefore, nurse life care planners use the critical thinking skills of the nursing process to assess, diagnose, and formulate a plan of care for the lifetime of an individual. Following the nursing process, the NLCP develops the life care plan estimating the costs and resources necessary for future medical and nonmedical needs and expenses.

In 1997, Lance founded a nonprofit, professional nursing association for nurses who develop life care plans: the American Association of Nurse Life Care Planners (AANLCP). She developed a NLCP curriculum with the nursing process methodology at its core, including concepts and skills pertaining to LCP application in the medical-legal arena. This included specialized formal educational training addressing the use of the nursing process and professional nursing scope and practice concepts as the foundation for life care planning and its application. The AANLCP continues to represent and support all nurses engaged in or interested in life care planning.

Professional Journal
The Journal of Nurse Life Care Planning (JNLCP) is the official, peer-reviewed publication of the American Association of Nurse Life Care Planners. Read by nurse life care planners, other specialty nurses, and professionals as a source for

education pertinent to nurse life care planning, it is the only peer-reviewed life care planning journal presented from the perspective of the nursing process.

Initially published in 1998, the *Journal* has evolved from a few articles shared by AANLCP members to meet educational needs of their peers to the AANLCP's sole journal, peer-reviewed and published quarterly to meet criteria for ANA and American Board of Nursing Specialties (ABNS) standards. The JNLCP has been published electronically since 2009.

Nurse Practice Act

Nurse life care planners must maintain active registered nurse licensure to become and remain certified as nurse life care planners. They must also adhere to the nurse practice acts (NPA) and common law for the state(s) in which they are licensed and practice. These laws define the scope of nursing practice for a state and are designed to protect public health, safety, and welfare. This protection includes shielding the public from unqualified and unsafe nurses. In each state, statutory law regulates entry into nursing practice, defines the scope of practice, and establishes disciplinary procedures. State boards of nursing oversee this statutory law. They have the responsibility and authority to protect the public by determining who is competent to practice nursing

Legal and Regulatory Issues

When providing nurse life care planning services, each NLCP adheres to a professional registered nurse scope and standard of practice, as specified by a state, province, or territorial nurse practice act. Each governing body outlines the RN's scope of practice, which may or may not include each of the nursing process components of assessing, diagnosing (construed differently than medical diagnosis), identifying outcomes, planning, implementing, and evaluating. Each NLCP must also know the applicable nurse practice act when testifying as an expert.

Each NLCP must follow the applicable law when handling, using, transmitting, and communicating personal information in the process of preparing the LCP.

- **The Health Insurance Portability and Accountability Act (HIPAA) Privacy Rule** must be followed when handling all private health information. This includes the proper destruction of all medical and confidential records when the case has been completed. The full text of HIPAA, summaries, and FAQs are available in the Office of Civil Rights (OCR) section of the Department of Health and Human Services website at http://www.hhs.gov/ocr/privacy/hipaa/faq/index.html

- **The Family Educational Rights and Privacy Act (FERPA, the Buckley Amendment)** applies to access to data concerning student enrollment, grades, behavioral issues, and other school information, at all levels of institutions and agencies that receive U.S. Department of Education funding. It also applies to states transmitting information to federal agencies. General information about the legislation and policies can be found at http://www2.ed.gov/policy/gen/guid/fpco/ferpa/index.html

- **Health Information Technology for Economic and Clinical Health (HITECH)** Act is concerned with, among other provisions, information technology and electronic health records. It also extends the privacy and security provisions of HIPAA to business associates of covered entities. Information on this can be obtained at http://www.hhs.gov/ocr/privacy/hipaa/administrative/enforcementrule/hitechenforcementifr.html

Each NCLP should be knowledgeable of current federal and state laws pertaining to testifying, as well as worker's compensation laws for the jurisdiction. If a case will require trial or deposition testimony, the NLCP should consult with the retained attorney for advice and specifics. However, NLCPs should be familiar with two important regulations: Rule 702 in the Federal Rules of Evidence, which concerns testimony by experts and outlines the requirements for a person to be qualified as an expert for the purposes of testimony; and Rule 703, which establishes the bases of opinion testimony by experts. These Rules may be reviewed at the Cornell Law School website, http://www.law.cornell.edu/rules/fre/

Practice Roles

The primary role of the nurse life care planner is to provide a life care plan applying the nursing process: assessment, diagnosis, outcome identification, planning, implementation, and evaluation. While specific individual practice environments, settings, and experience may differ, the nursing process methodology is common to all registered nurses. The nurse life care planner:

- Reviews available data, requesting additional records when needed as part of the assessment process for the LCP.
- Completes a comprehensive assessment of the injured or chronically ill person when able, using a comprehensive assessment tool that identifies current and probable future care needs, durable medical equipment, medical care providers, laboratory and diagnostic tests, personal care assistance, supplies, therapies, activity/exercise needs, educational/leisure/ vocational needs, and environmental modifications as indicated.
- Collaborates as necessary with healthcare providers for current and probable future healthcare treatment plans.
- Uses critical thinking to analyze and categorize assessment data to identify human responses to the injury or chronic illness; makes nursing diagnoses for the life care plan.
- Considers associated risks, benefits, costs, current scientific evidence, medical guidelines and literature, and cultural and ethical considerations, to achieve the identified outcomes.
- Plans for identified reasonable and essential needs, including frequency of caregiver follow-up and

maintenance and replacement of equipment, including the annual cost of each item and possible alternatives.

- Considers promotion and restoration to health and injury/illness/disease prevention to achieve the desired outcome.
- Provides for implementation of the plan within an appropriate, reasonable timeline.
- Uses scientific evidence-based guidelines, nursing research, and other guidelines.
- Identifies community resources and systems; identifies and delegates the different sections of the life care plan to an appropriate provider to coordinate the care in the plan.
- Provides for health teaching and promotion and safety and prevention strategies from an appropriate, delegated provider.
- Provides life care plan consultation using analysis, summarization, research, evidence-based guidelines, and literature; communicates appropriate recommendations to the injured or chronically ill person to facilitate learning.
- Evaluates the life care plan to ensure a systematic approach for the completion of the LCP and the effectiveness of planned strategies.
- Completes an ongoing data assessment with appropriate revisions of the nursing diagnoses, outcomes, plan and implementation as needed.
- Demonstrates quality of practice, delivering life care planning consultation services as a NLCP and demonstrating the application of the nursing process in a responsible, accountable, and ethical manner.
- Testifies as an expert witness, educating the court including attorneys, jury, and judges, concerning facts regarding the identified care needs and costs pertaining to those needs within the life care plan.
- Practices following current statutes, rules, regulations and guidelines.

Practice Environments and Settings

The nurse life care planner may practice in any of a variety of environments, such as legal practices, government entities, insurance companies, or banks, or in private practice as a self-employed consultant. Whenever possible, the nurse life care planner consults with the injured or chronically ill person and associated support system, legal entities, healthcare providers, insurance companies, employers, Centers for Medicare and Medicaid Services, other civil agencies, and the community at large.

The nurse life care planner may serve as testifying expert, providing testimony about the facts of the nursing care needs, reasonable and necessary future care needs, and costs for the injured or chronically ill person. In this role, the nurse life care planner educates the court (attorneys, jury, and judge) about the needs identified via the nursing process and provides evidence regarding the life care plan data within the nurse life care plan.

The nurse life care planner collaborates with other healthcare providers in order to address recommendations outside the scope of nursing. Within the various practice roles, the mechanism of collaboration may include on-site meetings, review of medical records, one-on-one meetings with any member of the healthcare team, teleconferences, and written letters and questionnaires, with such written documents becoming part of the life care plan document or file.

Special Areas of Practice

In nurse life care planning, there are several areas of specialization. However, the specific ability to assess the catastrophically injured or chronically ill, throughout the continuum of healthcare, in multiple settings over the lifetime, remains constant. With this assessment, the NLCP can create a plan that not only addresses medical care, diagnostic testing, and laboratory tests, but the basic protection and safety needs for the person and caregivers. NLCPs who serve as testifying experts must be familiar and comfortable with the various rules and procedures inherent to this role. They should also be knowledgeable about their own specialized foundational knowledge, experience, skill and training, so that they can provide their opinions to the court.

Scope and Standards

Each member of the AANLCP receives a complimentary copy of the *Scope and Standards* used by nurse life care planners.

Educational Preparation

The specialty role of the nurse life care planner is independent, autonomous, and self-motivated, requiring excellent assessment, critical thinking and communication skills. Additional qualifications include proficiency in computer research methodology, literature and medical record reviews, technical writing, and mathematical concepts in order to complete a comprehensive life care plan, as well as a situational, fundamental understanding of applicable laws. Educational preparation can be obtained through continuing education and other formal education methods

The nurse life care planner is a professional registered nurse (RN) with several years of general nursing experience in such areas as medical/surgical, orthopedic, intensive care, pediatric, or rehabilitation nursing in a variety of settings. The RN builds experience by working as a nurse case manager (CM) within the hospital setting, home healthcare, and long-term facilities, as well as working with worker's compensation insurance or in the health insurance field. The CM will often seek out and demonstrate expanded expertise by meeting the requirements to achieve related specialty certifications, e.g., Certified Registered Rehabilitation Nurse (CRRN), Certified Case Manager (CCM or other designation), or Certified Disability Medical Specialist (CDMS). The nurse CM is eligible to participate in the nurse life care planning formal education process after two years of experience in case management within the rehabilitation, insurance, or home health care settings. Having the aforementioned certifications is not mandatory, but it is beneficial and may enhance credibility.

Different options are available for obtaining course work for nurse life care planning, each with a different focus. Independent nurse life care planners in a traditional classroom or online via webinars instruct formal NLCP courses. These courses closely follow the American Association of Nurse Life Care Planning's *Core Curriculum* and the Certified Nurse Life Care Planner Certification Board's *Certification Examination for Nurse Life Care Planners Handbook for Candidates.* This includes the standards of practice, scope of practice, code of ethics of the organization, state nursing practice acts, ANA's Scope and Standards of Practice, and ANA's Code of Ethics. Many programs will include a business section that assists a nurse in developing and marketing a business. Life care planning course work may also be offered in a university or online setting; however, in these programs, it is generally taught without the nursing process as a foundation.

Certification

A passing score on the certification exam allows a RN to use the designation of Certified Nurse Life Care Planner (CNLCP). The current examination is specific to the specialty of nurse life care planning, as it evaluates the core knowledge base required for certification in nurse life care planning. This includes, but is not limited to, the nursing process (with special expanded knowledge of the rehabilitative and the lifetime needs of the catastrophically injured or chronically ill person) and the ability to conduct appropriate and specific research related to the individual's specific current and future needs.

Since 2003, the CNLCP Certification Board has provided oversight of the certification exam for NLCPs. Both AANLCP and the CNLCP Certification Board adhere to the Code of Professional Ethics Mission/Vision Statement. The Professional Testing Corporation (PTC) currently administers the certification examination for NLCPs for the CNLCP Certification Board. The CNLCP credential must be renewed every five years demonstrating continuing education credits. Details regarding credentialing and renewal may be found on the CNLCP website at www.cnlcp.org.

Continuing Education

The commitment to lifelong learning is a NLCP core value. The NLCP seeks additional education in areas such as regulatory issues, reimbursement, medical coding changes, adaptive technology, and research relevant to items in the LCP. Continuing education programs are offered through the AANLCP and other providers. Educational offerings focus on current trends and research pertaining especially to persons with catastrophic injuries or conditions: traumatic brain injury, spinal cord injury, amputation, burns, and chronic pain. This includes disease entities such as cancer, chronic illnesses, Guillain-Barré syndrome, and psychiatric conditions; effects of toxic substances; organ or other tissue transplants; and pediatric conditions like autism, cerebral palsy, and other developmental conditions; and muscular dystrophy.

AANLCP supports and encourages nurse life care planners to be lifelong learners and to strive to integrate new knowledge into practice whenever possible. To that end, the NLCP embraces evidence-based practice as a part of the methodology and looks for ways to improve critical reasoning skills. Lifelong learning can be attained through networking with colleagues, participation in small group programs in nurse life care planning, self-study via medical and nursing journals, the JNLCP, and other relevant literature, and certifications and advanced degrees. AANLCP offers annual educational conferences that incorporate nursing concepts and process throughout the conference programming and are approved for recertification.

AANLCP Code of Ethics and Conduct

The AANLCP Code of Ethics and Conduct committee was created in 2011 to explore the current and evolving issues that might be encountered by the nurse life care planner. The committee developed the following *Code of Ethics and Conduct* as a guide to the core values and obligations of nurse life care planning. In aligning with the ANA's Code of Ethics, the AANLCP's code affirms that all nurse life care planners have an ethical obligation to practice with integrity, demonstrate competency, and have accountability.

AANLCP Code of Ethics and Conduct

1. *The nurse life care planner does not discriminate against any person based on age, gender, ethnic background, religious beliefs or practices, social or economic status, functional status, health status, or disability.*

NLCP Explanation:

- An individual's differences or beliefs are respected. Personal attitudes do not negatively influence or interfere with professional performance.
- Each individual's inherent worth, dignity, and human rights are respected by the nurse life care planner without prejudice, regardless of whether the nurse agrees with or condones certain individual practices.
- The nurse life care planner performs in a nonjudgmental and nondiscriminatory manner.

NLCP Examples:

- A nurse life care planner whose religious beliefs prohibit her from accepting blood transfusions plans for platelet and red blood cells transfusions for a patient with chronic malignancy.

2. *The nurse life care planner maintains competency in nursing practice and nurse life care planning practice.*

NLCP Explanation:

- The nurse life care planner maintains an active registered nurse license in good standing.
- The nurse life care planner practices within the nurse practice act and AANLCP scope of practice.
- The nurse life care planner pursues professional growth through personal study; attendance at educational

programs, national nursing conferences, seminars, and professional meetings; reading the *AANLCP Journal* and other relevant professional journal articles; and collegial collaboration.

NLCP Examples:

- A CNLCP earned credits towards recertification by attending the AANLCP annual conference and a continuing education seminar on spinal cord injury and by presenting an offering on nurse life care planning to other nurses.

3. *The nurse life care planner demonstrates high standards of professional conduct in delivering nurse life care planning services.*

NLCP Explanation:

- The nurse life care planner demonstrates honesty, integrity, responsibility, accountability, timeliness and respect for human dignity.
- The nurse life care planner practices ethically and lawfully.
- The nurse life care planner accurately represents professional background and credentials.
- The nurse life care planner does not promote personal interests for personal gain.
- The nurse life care planner remains objective and does not impose individual values on others.

NLCP Examples:

- The nurse life care planner positively exemplifies nursing to individuals, the community, the legal field, and the media.
- The nurse life care planner seeks consultation as necessary.
- The nurse life care planner remains respectful and open in the exchange of views with all individuals with relevant interests.

4. *The nurse life care planner safeguards privacy rights.*
NLCP Explanation:
- The nurse life care planner exercises responsibility, discretion, and respect in handling and use of all protected or sensitive information and materials.
- The nurse life care planner considers that the rights, well-being, and safety of the individual should be the primary factors in arriving at any professional judgment concerning the disposition of confidential information.

NLCP Examples:
- The NLCP shares relevant data only with those with a need to know.
- The NLCP is aware of and complies with local, state, and federal privacy and security regulations.
- The NLCP recognizes that in some circumstances private information must be disclosed in compliance with federal or state law or regulations.
- The NLCP uses appropriate technology to maintain data security with electronic communication.

5. *The nurse life care planner assumes responsibility and accountability for professional actions, opinions, recommendations, and commitments.*
NLCP Explanation:
- The NLCP assumes accountability for life care plan and actions, opinions, and decisions.
- The NLCP accepts, declines, or refers cases in good faith based upon personal competence, education, experience, and capabilities.
- The NLCP's professional services are delivered in a competent, concise, and timely manner.

NCLP Examples:
- The NLCP accepts responsibility for initiating consultation with other health care providers when necessary.
- The NLCP questions incorrect or inappropriate collaborative suggestions.

- The NLCP seeks opportunities for improvement based on feedback from clients and colleagues concerning professional work.

6. *The nurse life care planner provides professional services with objectivity.*

NLCP Explanation:

- The NLCP demonstrates critical thinking in decisions, recommendations, and opinions.
- The NLCP actively seeks to eliminate personal opinion, prejudice, conflict of interest, consideration, or appearance of any of these that could interfere with objectivity, performance, or outcome, or that tend to create the appearance of bias.

NLCP Examples:

- The NLCP applies standards of nursing practice (the nursing process) consistently in all life care plans, thereby not confusing bias with advocacy.
- The NCLP identifies and resolves any potential conflict of interest as soon as possible.

7. *The nurse life care planner participates in the advancement of the profession through participating in and promoting mentorship, collegiality, education, and ongoing knowledge development.*

NLCP Explanation:

- The NLCP maintains active involvement in the professional association's ongoing development and revisions of standards, policies, and guidelines for nursing and nurse life care planning.
- The NLCP collaborates with mentors, peers, colleagues, and others.
- The NLCP shares materials and information designed to advance the practice of nursing and nurse life care planning with peers, colleagues, clients, and others.

NLCP Examples:
- The NLCP stays current with trends and decisions regarding healthcare delivery dynamics and expanding scopes of practice at the local, state, and national levels.
- The NLCP maintains an active membership in a national nursing organization.
- The NLCP collaborates with members of other professional organizations at international, national, state, and community levels.
- The NLCP facilitates and participates in critical self-reflection and evaluation within the profession.
- The NLCP serves as a leader, mentor, or committee member in professional associations.

Trends and Issues

Healthcare costs and healthcare reforms continue to make headlines. As the ANA states, "Registered nurses must proactively deal with constant change and must be prepared for an evolving healthcare environment" (2010). The healthcare, litigation, and insurance issues surrounding tort reform, worker's compensation, Medicare, and an aging baby boomer generation all point to long-term need for certified nurse life care planners.

Nurse life care planning has its historical roots in the day-to-day, month-to-month, and year-to-year ongoing nursing plans created, implemented, and evaluated by visiting nurses and home care nurses. Case management nurses and rehabilitation nurses were likely among the first nurse life care planners, especially in the litigation arena. That said, life care planning as a nursing specialty is still at a relatively early stage in its evolution.

Many NLCPs first learn and practice long-term care coordination as case managers in the insurance industry, notably in workers' compensation. The experienced case manager often moves into the role of NLCP with the realization that nursing expertise is invaluable both in establishing

17

reserves for an injured worker' lifetime healthcare needs in the insurance world, and in settlement negotiations. This need will continue as long as there are injured persons who fall under the current workers' compensation system.

The Medicare Modernization Act, enacted in 2003, requires that Medicare remain the secondary payer whenever possible. As a result, nurse life care planners with an expertise in Medicare guidelines are in high demand to assess expected care needs in workers' compensation cases and to develop plans that protect Medicare's interests (Medicare set-asides, MSAs) in settlements. The Center for Medicare and Medicaid (CMS) has considered expanding the requirements for MSAs to civil litigated case settlements to expand protection of CMS' interests. This could possibly result in an increased demand for NLCP expertise.

The potential for across-the-board tort reform could lead to capping the damages in medical malpractice, liability, and personal injury cases. This will warrant the need for nurse life care planners to provide appropriate lifetime healthcare dollar amounts to care for injured persons and give direction to their future care needs. Attorneys will likely come to depend on nurse life care planners to provide direction as to what the injured person *needs* so that cases can be resolved appropriately.

The United States is about to see the baby boomer generation shift into retirement, creating the largest population of older adults in our history. This will pose a challenge for Medicare and Medicaid that could potentially lead to tighter controls on healthcare funding. The NLCP can assist the Medicare system and the baby boomers in planning for their healthcare needs; the expanded need will open the door for more experienced nurses to become Certified Nurse Life Care Planners.

References

American Association of Nurse Life Care Planners (AANLCP). (2012). Code of professional ethics and conduct for nurse life care planners with interpretive statements. *AANLCP Membership Guide.* Retrieved from:www.aanlcp.org/homepage

American Association of Nurse Life Care Planners (AANLCP). (2012).Nurse life care planners standards of practice with interpretive statements. *AANLCP Membership Guide.* Retrieved from:www.aanlcp.org/homepage

American Association of Nurse Life Care Planners (AANLCP). (2012). Position statement on the definition of the nurse life care planning. *AANLCP Membership Guide.* Retrieved from: www.aanlcp.org/homepage

American Nurses Association (ANA).(2010). *Code of ethics for nurses with interpretive statements.* Washington, DC: American Nurses Publishing.

American Nurses Association (ANA). (2010). *Nursing: Scope and Standards of Practice* (2nd ed.). American Nurses Association. Silver Springs, Md.

American Nurses Association (ANA). (2010). *Nursing's social policy statement* (3rd ed.). Washington, DC: retrieved from www.Nursesbooks.org.

The ARC. (2011). Retrieved from: http://www.thearc.org/page.aspx?pid=2414

Brock, P. (2010). From clinical nurse to entrepreneur: becoming a life care planner. *American Journal of Nurse Life Care Planning,* X(4), 285-291. Retrieved from: http://www.aanlcp.org/resources/journal.htm

Centers for Medicare and Medicaid: Workers Compensation Medicare Set-aside Arrangements (WCMSAs). Retrieved from: https://www.cms.gov/WorkersCompAgencyServices/04_wcsetaside.asp

Cornell University Law School: Legal Institute. Federal Rules of Evidence. Article VII, Opinions and Expert Testimony, Rules 701-706. (amended December 1, 2011). Retrieved from: http://www.law.cornell.edu/rules/fre/

Deutsch. P. M. (2011). Life care planning. Retrieved from:
    http://www.paulmdeutsch.com/LCP-introduction.htm

Deutsch, Paul M.; Raffa, Frederick(2011): *Damages in Tort
    Actions*, **9,10,11: Ahab Press**.

Howland, W. (2010) NANDI-I. *Journal of Nurse Life Care
    Planning*, X(4), 292-294. Retrieved from: http://www.
    aanlcp.org/resources/journal.htm

LaGasse, N., and McDaniel, H. (2010). The Life Care Planning
    Expert. In A. Peterson and L. Kopishke (Eds.), *Legal
    Nurse Consulting Practices* (3rd ed. vol. 2, pp. 273-303).
    Boca Raton, FL: CRC Press.

National League of Nursing. (2011). *Critical Thinking in Clinical
    Nursing Practice/RN Examination*. Retrieved from:
    http://dev.nln.org/testproducts/pdf/CTinfobulletin.pdf

The Student Nurse Forum. (2012) Nurse Practice Act. Retrieved
    from: http://kcsun3.tripod.com/id110.htm

U. S. Department of Education. (2011). Family Educational
    Rights and Privacy Act (FERPA) Retrieved from: http://
    www2.ed.gov/policy/gen/guid/fpco/ferpa/index.html

U. S. Department of Health and Human Services. (2011) Health
    information privacy: HIPAA Frequently asked questions.
    Retrieved from: http://www.hhs.gov/ocr/privacy/
    hipaa/faq/index.html

U. S. Department of Health and Human Services. (2011) Health
    information privacy: HITECH Act enforcement interim
    final rule. Retrieved from: http://www.hhs.gov/ocr/
    privacy/hipaa/administrative/enforcementrule/
    hitechenforcementifr.html

CHAPTER 2

Critical Thinking, Nursing Process, and Standards

Liz Holakiewicz, BSN, RN, CCM, CNLCP

Introduction

Nurses have "been educated and socialized to focus on our virtues rather than our knowledge and our concrete everyday practice," according to Gordon and Nelson (2005) However, it is the nurse life care planner's knowledge and thought process that becomes particularly relevant as the life care plan is supported in court. The Federal Rules of Evidence Rule 702, also known as the Daubert Decision, indicates the following:

> If scientific, technical, or other specialized knowledge will assist the Trier of fact to understand the evidence or to determine a fact in issue, a witness qualified as an expert by knowledge, skill, experience, training, or education, may testify thereto in the form of an opinion or otherwise, if 1) the testimony is based upon sufficient facts or data, 2) the testimony is the product of reliable principles and methods, and 3) the witness has applied the principles and methods reliably to the facts of the case.

Critical thinking and the nursing process support these requirements and serve as the foundation for our opinions as nurse life care planners. This chapter defines critical thinking as it relates to nursing practice, identifies the characteristics of a critically thinking nurse, demonstrates how the nursing process and the American Nurses Association's *Scope and Standards of Practice* (ANA, 2010) establish the mechanism for critical thinking in nurse life care planning, and identifies ways to integrate critical thinking into an individual's life care planning practice.

Critical Thinking

Although the concept is centuries old, the modern term *critical thinking* came into use in the early 1900s in American education. They defined the process as "the art of thinking about your thinking while you're thinking so as to make your thinking more clear, precise, accurate, relevant, consistent, and fair." (Paul et al., 1989) Clearly, self-reflection is integral to the critical thinking process, which results in accuracy, precision, and relevance.

Paul et al. (1989) defined universal intellectual standards for critical thinking with corresponding questions to elucidate the standard, as follows:

Clarity
- Can the point be further elaborated upon?
- Could you express that point in a different way?
- Is there an illustration or example that would give better understanding?

Accuracy
- Is it that statement true?
- Can we check the facts?

Precision
- Can you give more details?
- Can you be more specific?

Relevance
- How does your point connect to the question at hand?
- How does your point bear on the issue?

Depth
- How does your answer address the complexities in the question?
- Are you taking into account the problems in the question?
- Is that dealing with the most significant factors?

Breadth
- Do we need to consider another point of view?
- Is there another way to look at the question at hand?
- What would this point look like from a conservative/ liberal standpoint?
- What would this point look like from the point of view of the opposing life care planner

Logic
- Does the point really make sense?
- Does that follow from what you said?
- How does that follow?
- Before you implied this but now you are saying that; how can both be true?

Fairness
- Do I have a vested interest in this issue?
- Am I sympathetically representing the viewpoints of others?

Facione and Facione (2008) describe critical thinking as relates to clinical judgment as "the process we use to make a judgment about what to believe and what to do about the symptoms our patient is presenting for diagnosis and treatment." Here the clinician is involved in a process that considers the evidence (symptoms) in context of the patient's health and life circumstances. The clinician's knowledge, skills, and experience are used to anticipate the treatment and the consequences of care.

Critical Thinking in Nursing

The nursing definition of critical thinking is both behavioral and descriptive in nature. Specific habits of mind and cognitive skills of the critical thinker are described. In a research study of 55 nurse experts, Rubenfeld and Scheffer (2000) developed the following definition:

> Critical thinking in nursing is an essential component of professional accountability and quality in nursing care. Critical thinkers in nursing exhibit these

habits of mind: confidence, contextual perspective, creativity, flexibility, inquisitiveness, intellectual integrity, intuition, open mindedness, perseverance, and reflection. Critical thinkers in nursing practice the cognitive skills of analyzing, applying standards, discriminating, information seeking, logical reasoning, predicting, and transforming knowledge.

Characteristics of the Critical Thinking Nurse

Alfaro-Le Fevre (2009) developed a model of critical thinking comprised of four intersecting circles further elaborating the habits of mind in Rubbenfeld's and Sheffer's definition. In her model, the four factors affecting critical thinking are knowledge, critical thinking attitudes or characteristics, interpersonal skills, and practice-related technical skills.

Critical Thinking Attitudes or Dispositions

The critically thinking nurse wants to attain the best knowledge, even if it fails to support or undermines his or her preconceptions, beliefs, or self-interest. Open-mindedness is inherent and characterized by a tolerance for views or values with which one may or may not agree.

These values are kept in mind when making decisions and planning care for an individual. Self-monitoring and reflection for identification of personal bias are integral to this attitude. The critically thinking nurse analyzes and applies standards that are evidence based. There is alertness to problematic situations and an inclination to anticipate consequences. Gaps in information or data are identified, and additional data are researched and acquired. In using this process, decision-making becomes more precise and accurate. Differences and similarities are distinguished, categorized, and prioritized by the critically thinking nurse.

The analytical process used for problem solving is systematic, organized, and focused. Diligence is applied to problem solving at all levels of complexity. Concurrently, the critically thinking nurse is inquisitive in nature, observing, questioning, and probing for new information and better explanations in order to develop creative solutions.

Confidence, or trust in one's own reasoning skills also characterizes the critical thinker, as does maturity or caution in making, suspending, or revising judgment. There is an awareness of the necessity of multiple solutions in some situations and an appreciation of the need to reach closure even in the absence of complete knowledge.

Knowledge and Intellectual Skills

Knowledge and intellectual skills are another influence on the critical thinker in Alfaro-Le Fevre's (2009) model. Four intellectual traits include:

- *Intellectual humility:* willingness to admit what is not known or when mistakes are made. Mistakes are valuable stepping-stones to refining one's thinking ability, but only if they are acknowledged and the lessons learned are assimilated.

- *Intellectual integrity*: a continual evaluation of one's own thinking while looking at the consistency in the standards held for one's self in comparison to those held for others. There is a propensity to question one's own reasoning as quickly and thoroughly as the reasoning of others.

- *Intellectual courage*: awareness of the need to face and fairly address ideas beliefs or viewpoints about which one has negative feelings and has not given serious hearing.

- *Intellectual empathy*: a conscious effort to understand others by putting one's own feelings aside and imagining oneself in their place.

The knowledge required of the critical thinker falls into two main categories: 1) that which is obtained by learning and 2) that which is obtained by experience. Intuition is an assimilation of learning and experience. In a study of skill acquisition and clinical judgment in nursing practice, Benner (2009) found that "intuitive grasp is based on experience and not on extrasensory powers or wild hunches." Inexperienced nurses start problem-solving in their clinical practice using textbook strategies. Initially, changes in plans or strategies are made in response to new and expanded information. As an intuitive grasp of situations comes with experience, the expert nurse responds in a fluid manner. When changes occur in the patient or the surrounding context, and the relevance of actions taken change, the expert nurse is anticipating and responding fluidly. Not everyone is able to achieve this level of expertise or intuition. The ability to engage with others on a moral and emotional level further characterizes the expertise of the nurse, as well as his or her ability to comfort or assist the patient in coping with the demands of injury or illness (Benner, 2009).

Interpersonal Skills

Interpersonal skills comprise the third area impacting critical thinking skills. Those conducive to critical thinking include trustworthiness, collegiality, collaboration, and emotional intelligence (Alfaro-Le Fevre, 2009). The latter concept requires further exploration.

Emotional intelligence is defined as "the ability to monitor one's own and others' feelings and emotions, to discriminate among them and to use this information to guide one's thinking and actions" (Salovey, Brackett and Mayer, 2004). Recognition of emotions includes reading an angry response as demonstration of some other emotion such as fear, disappointment, and grief.

Making the appropriate determination or diagnosis of the underlying emotion results in intervention that is more effective. Recognition of emotions in one's self is just

26

as important as recognizing them in others. The person who recognizes his or her own anger and deals with it in an appropriate manner will likely not act out inappropriately, such as belittling a store clerk because he or she argued with his or her spouse.

Contrary to the belief that effective reasoning is emotion-free, Salovey et al. (2004) found that using emotions to facilitate reasoning integrates thinking and feeling. Dealing with someone who is defensive and dismissive is frustrating; however, the recognition that this individual may be fatigued will likely eliminate the emotional charge of the situation, alter the response, and ultimately result in more effective interaction.

Understanding emotion involves appreciating its depth, diversity, and complexity. Emotions evolve, change, and blend with other emotions, and these evolutions must be appreciated. Doing so enables nurses to assess and intervene creatively and constructively (Codier, Muneno, and Freitas, 2011).

Once emotions are correctly identified and understood, they are more effectively managed in patient and family settings and in interdisciplinary relationships. This includes recognizing the necessity for a time out in an emotional or stressful situation, giving more time to an interaction because of emotions involved, or requiring attention to self in order to function at optimum. Emotional intelligence is a valuable characteristic of the nurse life care planner not only in situations with colleagues and injured individuals, but also in the courtroom. Attorneys are adept in the tactical use of emotion in the courtroom. Discernment in these emotionally charged situations comes from preparation and care for oneself in the period leading to trial.

A calm demeanor in the face of emotional tactics may effectively defuse vigorous and emotional cross-examination. Finally, technical skills or habits affect critical thinking abilities.

Again, Benner's (2004) findings demonstrate that the mastery of technical skills and knowledge base of nursing frees the nurse to access higher level functioning.

The Nursing Process: A Critical Thinking Tool

The ANA's *Scope and Standards of Practice* (2010) indicates, "The science of nursing is based on an analytical framework of critical thinking known as the nursing process, comprised of assessment, diagnosis, outcome identification, planning, implementation, and evaluation. These steps serve as the foundation of clinical decision making and are used to provide evidence based practice." This scientific method and these same integral steps are used throughout life care plan development.

The nurse life care planner provides for the needs of an individual throughout the health care continuum, across multiple settings, and throughout the lifetime. The individualized assessment and diagnoses of that particular person's response to disability or illness as well as the potential health risks stemming from that disability or illness is the foundation for the care plan. It is designed to minimize risk and promote function over the lifetime, while anticipating the effect of aging and the evolution of the disability or illness itself on that individual's future needs. The nurse life care planner may identify community, public, and insurance resources and define access to those resources in the life care plan while documenting the costs necessary to implement the care plan. Case management within the care plan provides for implementation of the recommended interventions and evaluation of the process. According to the *American Association of Nurse Life Care Planners Handbook* (2007), the result of the process is a life care plan document that "provides an organized, concise plan of estimated reasonable and necessary (and reasonably certain to be necessary) current and future healthcare needs with the associated costs and frequencies of goods and services."

The nursing process provides a framework for organizing and prioritizing patient care. It formalizes critical thinking, assuring that nursing judgments, decisions, and actions are not based on guesswork, but solid evidence-based information. The life care plan is the end product of this process. The nursing process is not linear. Evaluation and assessment occur throughout the life care planning process as new data and symptoms arise and the care plan evolves.

The life care plan addresses specific categories of care recommendations, including but not limited to physician care and evaluations, nursing or facility care, therapy and counseling services, and other professional services such as advocacy or tutoring, diagnostic testing, equipment, adaptive aids, and supplies for mobility, hygiene and bathing, feeding, incontinence, dressing, respiratory procedures, hospitalizations, transportation needs, and home modifications. Each care need is explored in terms of timing, frequency, cost, and cost source.

Assessment

Assessment is the first standard in both the American Nurses Association's *Scope and Standards of Practice* (2010) and the AANLCP's *Scope and Standards of Practice* (2012) The assessment process for the life care plan is extensive and includes three phases:

- Review of medical and billing records; reports and depositions of experts; depositions of the injured person, family members, and acquaintances; and review of interrogatory responses;
- On-site and in-person assessment or interview of the injured party when possible; and
- Collaboration with treating providers and experts either by phone or in person.

Record Review

Upon receipt of referral, medical and billing records are requested. Once records are obtained, they are reviewed in a systematic fashion. Records may include those from the acute care setting, physician offices, therapy providers, counselors, neuropsychologists or psycho-educational providers, and home care providers as well as from laboratories, radiology centers, surgery centers, pharmacies, schools, and community services.

When pertinent, academic and employment records, day-in-the-life videos, or client journals may be reviewed and considered. The life care planner chronicles medical diagnoses and events, while simultaneously assessing the record for treatment trends, efficacy, and future care recommendations. Documentation may detail, for example, frequent emergency room visits over a 10-year period for treatment that could be delivered in the primary care setting, or frequent Botox injections with no demonstrated functional improvement. Very few care providers have the benefit of this type of perspective in treatment planning. This information becomes relevant and invaluable in later stages of the assessment process when collaborating with treating physicians, therapists, and other providers.

Throughout the record review the nurse life care planner assesses for additional records that might be pertinent, validates and verifies information between data sources, organizes and clusters data and symptoms for potential patterns, identifies cues, and makes inferences from the data for consideration during the onsite assessment and collaboration with the healthcare providers and experts. This continues throughout the life care planning process as additional data become available, necessitating the need to clarify and adjust care recommendations.

For instance, the records might reference recurrent hand tremors that started after an individual had kidney transplant surgery. During the assessment visit with the individual, that information can be further explored and clarified by asking the following questions:

- When do the tremors occur?
- Are they constant?
- Are they related to intentional movement only?
- When did they start?
- What makes them worse?

With the additional data gleaned and clarified through the assessment interview, this information can then be presented for dialogue with the physician to explore cause and possible treatment. Anti-rejection medication doses may be adjusted in the care plan as a result of this dialogue and a system for evaluation of this side effect on an ongoing basis included in the care plan. The issue can also be raised for dialogue with the occupational therapist or vocational counselor if the patient has trouble with fine motor activities in work or home activities, with adaptive aids proposed for the care plan.

Onsite Interview

Onsite, in-person assessment is the next step in the assessment phase. In a legal context, the plaintiff attorney may not allow access for an in-person assessment. It is wise to request this opportunity of the referring attorney regardless of who retains you. When not allowed to complete the in-person assessment by the opposing party, documentation of this decision in the file is valuable to support testimony. In this case, it is also helpful to inquire about attending an expert independent medical examination (IME) as an alternative.

The onsite, in-person assessment follows a consistent pattern and process for the nurse life care planner. In a study of 293 life care planners (47% registered nurses, 45% rehabilitation or mental health counselors), Neulicht et al. (2010) found that a majority of life care planners used structured interview forms, standardized questionnaires, or standardized checklists to document information obtained from clients, families, and health professionals. They also used standardized questionnaires and checklists in their management of the life care planning processes, obtained consent forms compliant with the Health Insurance Portability and Accountability Act (HIPAA), and reviewed medical records in their process. No specific information is available on the content of the referenced checklists. However, while checklists may be valuable tools to assure nothing is missed, they are not a substitute for the nursing process or critical thinking.

Upon meeting the injured or disabled individual to be evaluated, the nurse life care planner discusses his or her role and the intended use of the care plan. A signed HIPAA-compliant authorization for medical records and for collaboration with providers is obtained during this initial visit. The injured or disabled individual should be advised that the information provided in the course of the interview may not necessarily be private and will be used for the purposes of life care planning. If one decides to function as case manager and life care planner, this dual role should be explored with the referring attorney, as well as the injured or disabled individual. Conflict of interest is a risk in this arrangement and this risk could jeopardize the perception of objectivity of the life care planner's opinions.

Although the nurse life care planner is typically not a treatment provider, the life care plan can also be acquired from the attorney for use as a health educational tool for the interested individual or family.

The following basic demographic, financial, and social information is collected during the interview process:

- Family members in the household and their involvement in the individual's care and treatment.
- Names of treating physicians, therapists, prosthetist, pharmacists, dentists, and counselors

- Frequency the individual sees each provider
- Treatment provided by each provider
- Contact information for each provider
- Medications currently taken, as evidenced from the prescription bottles
- Inventory of equipment, supplies, adaptive aids, and over-the-counter supplements,
- Photographs, if helpful, (Obtain a photograph release from photographed individuals)
- Assessment of the daily living skills and routine, in home and community
- Detailed nursing review of systems
- Functionality within the family and community
- Caregiving resources, patterns, cost, and duration

Areas of focused assessment may then occur based on review of records, if available prior to assessment. This is an opportunity to clarify and define the symptom pattern, while exploring their relationships. Preliminary nursing diagnoses are developed in anticipation of the collaborative phase to follow and may be discussed with the family and injured or disabled individual during the interview to verify and clarify accuracy.

Collaboration

Collaboration is the final phase of assessment. The nurse life care planner identifies abnormal findings from the assessment data and communicates these with care providers and experts. The current diagnoses and treatment of the individual are reviewed, long-term goals and prognosis are discussed, and future care recommendations are detailed and refined. Paul's standards of critical thinking and the related questioning particularly apply here (Paul et al., 1989). Creative solutions are often needed to complete this phase of the process as providers may not be familiar with the role and function of a life care planner and have some reluctance to participate in the planning process. Ideally conference calls can be set up allowing time to thoroughly discuss needs of the injured or disabled individual. However, this is not always possible. Fax or email communication with questions and answers back and forth are also effective, although this can be arduous when attempting to clarify responses. Education of the providers on the goal of the care plan and their integral role in the process to establish a budget for care needed is usually helpful.

Nursing Diagnosis

Lunney (2009, 2001) notes that nurses are diagnosticians. They analyze data from the nursing assessment, and draw conclusions to address actual and potential health problems and identify risk factors, resources, and strengths. Nursing diagnosis is the second Standard of Practice as defined by the ANA and AANLCP. It is helpful to look at data collected from the assessment stage in several different ways using different models, such as Gordon's model or the North American Nursing Diagnosis Association International (NANDA-I) taxonomy (Table 1), a review of systems model, or Maslow's hierarchy of needs (Table 2). Considering the assessment data from multiple perspectives gives greater depth to nursing diagnoses and ultimately further substantiates recommendations outlined in the life care plan. Prioritizing nursing diagnoses is important to the care planning process as relates to the goal or expected outcome of the care plan. Interventions are geared to addressing prioritized nursing diagnoses.

Nursing diagnoses are broad and holistic, assessing mind, body, and spirit. Medical diagnoses are focused on anatomy and pathophysiology with a goal of treating a disease or correcting a trauma-based injury. The medical model is a problem-focused system developing diagnoses that focus on organ or system dysfunction. Nursing diagnoses consider how *people* are affected by medical problems. "Nursing is the protection, promotion and optimization of health and abilities, prevention of illness and injury, alleviation of suffering through diagnosis and treatment of human response, and advocacy in the care of individuals, families, communities and populations" (ANA, 2010).

For example, the nursing diagnoses listed below provide data to substantiate recommendations for walker, physical therapy, occupational and speech therapy, glasses, educational services and advocacy and provide a clear sense of how this child's function is assessed through the diagnostic process:

- Delayed development and risk for further delay secondary to communication disorder and diagnosed autism spectrum disorder.
- Impaired physical mobility and walking as defined by gait disturbance, fine motor limitations, uncoordinated movement and postural instability requiring supervision, adaptive aids and occasional assistance of another individual.
- Impaired verbal and written communication, as defined by need for keyboard for functional written communication
- Disturbed sensory perception: visual and kinesthetic

How nurse life care planners incorporate nursing diagnoses into their care planning process is individualized. The nursing diagnoses can be part of the case file, narrative documentation of the assessment or as rationale within the tables that detail recommendations and costs of future care.

Table 1. Gordon's Model and NANDA-I Taxonomy   Adapted from Nursing
Diagnoses- Definitions and Classifications 2012-2014. Copyright 2012, 1994-2012 by
NANDA International. Used by arrangement with Blackwell Publishing Limited, a
company of John Wiley & Sons, Inc.

Health Perception/ Health Management	Perception of general health status and well-being; adherence to preventative practices
Nutritional/Metabolic	Patterns of food and fluid intake; fluid and electrolyte balance
Elimination	Bowel, bladder, and skin patterns and their perceptions about the pattern
Activity/Exercise	Exercise, leisure activities, recreation and activities of daily life; factors that interfere with desire activities or patterns
Cognitive/Perceptual	Adequacy of sensory modes: vision, hearing, taste, touch smell, pain, cognitive function
Sleep/Rest	Pattern, quality, and quantity of sleep rest and relaxation in a 24-hour period
Self-Perception/ Self-Concept	Attitudes about self, perception of abilities, body image, identity, sense of worth, and emotional patterns
Role Relationship	Perception of major roles and responsibilities in current life situation
Sexual/Reproductive	Satisfaction or dissatisfaction with sexuality; reproductive stage and pattern
Coping/Stress/Tolerance	General coping, stress tolerance support system; perceived ability to control and manage life situations
Life Principles	Values, beliefs, goals that guide choices or decisions
Safety/Protection	Freedom from danger, physical injury, or immune system damage
Comfort	Sense of mental, physical, or social well-being or ease
Growth/Development	Age-appropriate increases in physical dimension, organ systems, and attainment of milestones

Table 2. Maslow's Hierarchy of Human Needs

Maslow's Hierarchy of Human Needs
Physiologic
Safety and Security
Love and Belonging
Self Esteem
Self-Actualization

Outcomes Identification

The American Nurses Association's *Scope and Standards of Practice* (2010) and the AANLCP's *Scope and Standards of Practice (*2012) provide measurement criteria that are specific to the third Standard of Practice, outcomes identification. The nurse life care planner's recommendations are placed in the care plan based on the nursing diagnosis, but once part of the care plan they need to have a purpose, beginning, and end considered. Outcomes are measured by using the following principles in the care planning process:

- *The nurse life care planner involves the individual, and others when possible and appropriate in formulating expected outcomes.* Inclusion of the family and consideration of community and home environment are integral to life care plan development. During the assessment phase, individuals and their families are approached on their goals and concerns for ongoing their health as relates to an injury or disease process. These same issues are raised with the care providers and experts in the collaborative process of life care planning. For instance, an autistic child with mild mental retardation should be able to live semi-independently based on the neuropsychologist's prognosis. Services in the care plan are then focused to that goal.

- *The nurse life care planner considers associated risks, benefits, costs, scientific evidence, and clinical expertise in formulating outcomes.* For instance, recommendation for hydrophilic catheters for a child with recurrent bladder infections with an intermittent catheterization program will likely affect the frequency of emergency room visits and recurrent visits with the urologist. Though the price for the catheter is more per unit, the benefit to the health and wellbeing of the child is evident. Similarly, a percussion vest used in the home care setting to move secretions in combination with respiratory treatments may prevent recurrent admissions for pneumonia and ultimately improve life expectancy.

- *The nurse life care planner identifies time estimates for attainment of expected outcomes.* Specific time periods are identified in the life care plan for each recommendation. This measurement criterion is pertinent for instance, when considering the need for an intervention such as a pain management program. Upon completion of a pain management program, it is reasonable to assume an outcome of reduced pain medication usage or improvement in function. The time periods and recommendations identified in the care plan should reflect achievement of that outcome. This applies for the next principle as well.

- *The nurse life care planner documents expected outcomes as measurable goals*: see above.

- *The nurse life care planner provides for continuity of care within the plan.* Continuity and practicality of goal accomplishment are considered. Multiple therapy services by multiple providers, often in varied locations, make care planning complex. Overlap and practicality of the schedule should be considered. For instance, a child may require speech therapy three times a week, as well as occupational therapy, a social skills group, individual counseling, and physical therapy weekly. Factors such as time spent in school, time spent traveling to and from school, and the need to play impact time available for therapeutic services. When nursing diagnoses are prioritized, it benefits the planning phase. High priority services are implemented first and secondary interventions are packaged over time frames such as weekends or school breaks or clustered during certain developmental periods.

Planning and Intervention

Planning and Intervention, Standard 5, in the life care plan are designed to detect, prevent, and manage health problems, promote optimum function and wellness, and achieve desired outcomes safely and efficiently. Current research and trends affecting care are incorporated into the planning process. For instance, this may include consideration for disc replacement in a younger patient rather than spinal fusion or use of vagal nerve stimulation for the child who experiences sedating effects from a seizure protocol that is not controlling the seizures.

The care plan should also be consistent with statutes and laws within the individual's state of residence. This relates specifically to recommendations for home care. Some states have delegation options for skilled care needs. If the Nurse Practice Act for that state does not have this option, then skilled care cannot be delegated. The care plan should reflect priorities in the nursing diagnoses and be a fluid and dynamic process resulting in evaluation and re assessment as outcomes are or are not attained.

Relevant treatment guidelines and literature searches for evidence-based recommendations can be a source of support for recommendations and a source of discussion with providers when recommendations are unusual. For instance, the Medical Disability Advisor and MDGuidelines. com provide evidenced-based guidelines for therapy following shoulder arthroscopy as well as estimated period of disability. A literature search on cardiac transplant can show that use of a left ventricular assist device at home has evolved to provide a bridge to transplant so the patient can leave the hospital while waiting for a heart or even live with the device in place.

Once the outline of care needs is developed using the nursing process and collaborating with other healthcare professionals, cost research begins. The price for each service or item in the care plan is researched either by phone calls with providers, Internet research, review of current billing records, by the use of various databases, or a combination of these methods.

A majority of respondents to one survey do not use negotiated fees or an established fee schedule (Neulicht, Riddick-Grisham and Goodrich, 2010). This same survey indicates most respondents do not use cost information older than one year. The number of cost estimates varied based on the availability of a current vendor or provider of service, nature of the time or service, recent experience, cost of the item, period required, and the availability of a database. In other words, market rates for services are obtained, not discounted rates. Geographic specificity to the client is important in plan development. A national price quote (from insurance or other national databases) for a service rendered in New York City negatively skews the price for that service downward and will result in insufficient funding for the service when it needs to be delivered. Alternatively, it may be necessary for complex procedures to be provided out of a local area in order to access quality and experienced providers.

Implementation and Evaluation

The nurse life care planner collaborates with the patient and family to determine the ability of the injured or disabled individual for effective self-maintenance. If the care plan is complex or the individual is unable because of age, physical, cultural, cognitive, or economic difficulties to implement the recommendations in the care plan, the planner identifies a case manager as a recommended provider to facilitate health maintenance, coordination of care and reevaluation of the care plan. There is divided thought on the appropriateness of case management and life care planning being provided by the same individual. As mentioned earlier, it is a dual role and that role should be clearly explained to all parties in terms of benefits and risks at the outset of services.

Reviewing an Opposing Life Care Plan

The same principles of critical thinking and nursing process apply to the review of the opposing life care planner or development of a care plan for the defense. The credentials of the opposing planner should be evaluated and verified. Medical record review will often become the primary source of information in these situations unless the opposing counsel allows a home visit or attendance at an IME appointment.

Collaborating experts are often the source of divergence in life care plans. It is not the role of the nurse life care planner to define which expert to believe but to provide the data for those on whom they have relied. This allows the trier of fact to decide which opinions are the most accurate. Defense physician experts may recommend that no medical care is needed for the future. In these instances, it may be prudent to discuss with the referral source whether alternatively researched prices for the submitted life care plan are desired based on opposing experts' opinions for treatment.

In review of the opposing expert's life care plan, the process and methodology used to develop the life care plan are assessed and commented upon if appropriate (i.e. assessment data are missing or do not support recommended services). The data source for the plan is checked and verified for accuracy. Prices are checked with the listed source data through phone calls or reproduction of the research. If no costs sources are noted in the submitted plan, this should be identified as a deficiency in the care planning process. Using the opposing planner's format, with comments directly adjacent to those recommendations, can be helpful to the trier of fact, as it requires familiarity with only one format. See Chapter 3, *Reviewing a Life Care Plan,* for a more detailed discussion on this process.

The Business of Life Care Planning

Upon receipt of the referral, it is important to obtain details of the case (name, opposing counsel, and venue) in order to check for conflict. It may be that one party will contact the care planner and many months may pass before the opposing side will call about the same matter. Having a system in place to manage this eventuality is helpful and can prevent issues with conflict. The venue becomes important because the reporting requirement for federal court is more comprehensive. A Rule 26 report includes all opinions, a list of the last four years of the nurse's testimony, and details about the nurse's qualifications to testify in the matter at hand. At the time of the initial call, it is also wise to discuss the timelines involved in the requested matter to assure it is congruent with one's ability to accomplish the work product on time. The nurse life care planner's caseload should be assessed on a regular basis to assure enough time is allotted to complete all work in a quality manner.

Neulicht et al. (2010) found that 65% of the life care planners surveyed required a signed retainer agreement or letter of engagement prior to accepting a case and 72% required a retainer. A case file typically comprises assessment/ interview data, medical record review, billing/ time sheets, correspondence, and the cost research data materials. The majority of life care planners in this survey retain their files for 7 years. The average life care plan required about 40 hours to complete with a range of 10 to 120 hours based on those surveyed. Upon closure of case, all records should be shredded and removed from computer hard drive and other storage media used by the nurse life care planner (Neulicht, Riddick-Grisham and Goodrich, 2010).

Promote Critical Thinking in Your Life Care Planning Practice

The first step to integrating critical thinking into practice is to familiarize oneself with the principles of critical thinking and to absorb the qualities of a critical thinker explored in this chapter. For the nurse life care planner this means understanding the remaining standards in the *ANA Scope and Standards of Practice* (2010) as well as the *AANLCP Scope and Standards of Practice* (2012) that follow the logic of critical thinking principles. Several standards are reviewed here with a description of ways to integrate critical thinking principles to your nurse life care planning practice.

Standard 7. Ethics: The nurse life care planner practices ethically.

- Ethical thought requires a mastery of basic ethical concepts and principles, learning to distinguish between ethics and other domains of thinking with which ethics is commonly confused (law, religion, social norms), and learning to identify when egocentrism and socio-centrism impedes ethical judgment (Paul and Elder, 2002).
- The *ANA's Code of Ethics for Nurses with Interpretive Statements* (2010) should guide nursing practice. The fundamental principle is a respect for human dignity. This applies to all relationships: with injured individuals, with colleagues, and in the greater community. Protection of an individual's privacy and delivery of service in a nonjudgmental and nondiscriminatory manner, with sensitivity to diversity, is mandatory to critical thinking and effective practice as a nurse life care planner.

Standard 8. Education: The nurse life care planner attains knowledge and competence that reflects current nursing practice.

As discussed earlier, knowledge is attained in two ways: 1) through acquisition of information in nursing, medicine, health care, reimbursement, and community resources and 2) through experience as a nurse life care planner.

Consider the following principles in the pursuit of learning:

- Strive for an intellectual curiosity that has no bounds or biases.
- Become a lifelong learner.
- Take the "I'll find out" approach instead of the "I don't know" approach.
- Ask clarifying questions and anticipate questions that others might ask. What if and what else? What if something goes wrong? What else do we need to do?
- Hone strategies that promote critical thinking and turn them into habits and ultimately a fluid flow of thought results in the intuition mentioned by Benner (2004).
- Think aloud or on paper. Diagram, cluster, list, paraphrase, and mind map your ideas.
- Compare and contrast, organize and reorganize the information, clustering, and thoughts. Prioritize symptom patterns and diagnostic impressions.
- Develop good habits of inquiry and habits that aid in the search for truth.
- Keep an open mind and verify information.
- Take your time. Do not hurry or procrastinate, forcing you to complete your work at the last minute. Strategize your caseload to manage for the eventuality of last minute attorney requests, as this is typical.
- Educate yourself on the way you think. How does that differ from the way that others think? Do you reach the same end point? Are there places for agreement?

Standard 9. Evidence-based practice and research: The nurse life care planner integrates research findings and evidence into practice.

- The critically thinking nurse life care planner develops the care plan based not only on collaboration but also on evidence-based guidelines. Upon receipt of referral, the nurse life care planner considers and explores literature based on questions raised out of the record review, on-site, in-person interview or the collaborative process with other health professionals. The information obtained from a literature review provides a framework to discuss potential treatment options with other health care professionals and further substantiates the life care plan in the process.
- Participation in the research process further advances the profession of nurse life care planning.
- Sharing knowledge and skills with others fosters an environment of mutual respect, creativity, and better practice.
- Difference of opinion can be identified with respect and professionalism. Criticizing an opposing planner's report or opinions should not involve personal attacks.
- Effective networking and cooperation in business can also become an excellent source of growth of the nurse's professional practice and experience.

Standard 13. Collegiality: The nurse life care planner collaborates with healthcare consumers, health care providers, and others, when possible and appropriate in the conduct of practice.

- Collaborative effort yields wonderful benefits to the life care plan.
  - o Collaboration with the client in the assessment process makes the care plan more specific to the client's particular needs. This can mean, for example, using a disabled child's love for basketball to motivate him/her to exercise, work on balance,

strength, and muscle coordination in physical therapy through basketball-related activities.

o Collaborating with family. For example, consider the needs of the aging parents of a disabled child by providing for counseling services during the transition of the adult child into a group home living environment, and respecting the family's timing for this transition. Collaboration with family members fosters understanding. For example, a young mother of five small children may need help caregiving for a disabled child to avoid jeopardizing the growth and development of her other children. Family collaboration could also reveal a husband who is reluctant to return to work because his wife with chronic pain is falling at home while under the influence of her pain medications. An open mind throughout the assessment process facilitates an environment where family concerns can be heard and collaborative goals set for care planning.

- The nurse life care planner's interpersonal ability to recognize discomfort, confusion and other emotions and agendas is integral to effective collaboration with other professionals. It is a challenge for healthcare providers to anticipate an individual's acute needs and, particularly, lifelong needs. Being respectful of this challenge and being supportive by conveying the importance of their contribution results in a quality life care plan.

- The collaborative mindset and one's ability to keep an open mind are integral to fostering professional relationships, interdisciplinary teamwork and respect. Life care planning is a multidisciplinary profession.

Standard 14. Professional practice evaluation: The nurse life care planner self-evaluates nursing practice in relation to professional practice standards and guidelines, relevant statutes, rules, and regulations.

- This standard mandates the nurse life care planner evaluate his or her own nursing practice in relation to the professional practice standards and relevant local statutes and regulations. Become familiar with the Nurse Practice Act in your state and know the nursing scope of practice and its limits.
- The characteristic of self-reflection and intellectual humility is critical to one's growth in this area.
- Peer review of a care plan for thinking flaws can be invaluable. Often we may be too close to our own work to be objective. Having an outside party review the life care plan may identify inconsistencies or biases that may not be seen without direction. This means looking at one's mistakes and turning them into learning opportunities. Sharing mistakes with colleagues, although it feels risky, provides an opportunity for discussion and growth.

Standards 15. Resource utilization: The nurse life care planner recommends appropriate resources for safe, effective, and financially-responsible healthcare services.

- Factors such as safety, effectiveness, availability, cost, and benefits are evaluated when considering care options resulting in the same outcome.
- The care plan provides a tool by which the patient and family will be able to identify care needs and resources for their health care needs and will help them to become informed consumers of services when shared with them.

Critical Thinking Errors in Life Care Planning

Avoid these errors in critical thinking specific to life care planning.

- Using an inconsistent approach to the life care planning process based on the referral source, i.e., defense, plaintiff, trust, or private. Always use the same methodology.
- Incomplete assessment. Questions left unasked do not result in an accurate plan.
- Using preconceived opinions are preconceived that are not based on findings from assessment or evidence. All opinions and recommendations must be supported.
- Ignoring assessment data or not integrating them into the plan. Account for all assessment data collected.
- Generating recommendations outside the scope of one's experience or practice without appropriate collaboration or basis in literature
- Taking dictation from collaborators without asking questions. The plan is your work product; take responsibility for its recommendations.
- Outsourcing work on your care plan without proper evaluation and supervision of the work product. Your name is on the work product; be sure any subcontractor's work is acceptable.
- Manipulating data or collaboration to say what you want, i.e., ignoring literature that substantiates alternate opinions or taking data out of context. Transparency is a basic concept in life care planning.
- Putting redundant recommendations in the plan. If two similar or identical items are not needed achieve the same goal, consider removing one.
- Recommending items that are not be practical to accomplish (for example, too many therapies)
- Recommending items that do not reflect plan goals (e.g., intensive therapy without any indication that outcomes are accomplished from therapy)

- Failing to individualize recommendations. Formulaic plans or extensive use of cut and paste from other sources do not give evidence of individual assessment.

Summary

The concept of critical thinking has recently come to the forefront in the educational literature and has become an integral concept in nursing. In fact, the nursing process itself is a critical thinking tool used by the nurse life care planner as the foundation for the life care plan. Not only is the process itself integral to a quality life care plan, but the nurse life care planner's habits of mind or characteristics ultimately provide the scientific foundation required of a testifying or supporting expert in litigation.

The litigation environment requires a scientific basis for the life care plan. The nurse life care planner creates an effective tool using assessment, diagnosis, outcome identification, planning, implementation, and evaluation. Outside the litigation environment, the life care plan may be used as a tool for case management, health education, trust administration, care for those injured by vaccines, and elder care management. Additional uses are inevitable as the practice of nurse life care planning evolves and grows.

References

Alfaro-Le Fevre R. (2009). Critical thinking and clinical judgment: A practical approach to outcome focused thinking (4th ed.). St. Louis, MO: Saunders Elsevier.

American Association of Nurse Life Care Planners. (2012). AANLCP standards of practice / Code of professional ethics for nurse life care planners with interpretive statements. Salt Lake City, UT.

AANLCP. Definition of Nurse Life Care Planning, AANLCP Executive Board 2007.

American Nurses Association. (2010). Code of Ethics for Nurses with Interpretive Statements. Silver Spring, MD: Nursingbooks.org.

American Nurses Association. (2010). Nursing: Scope and standards of practice (2nd ed.). Silver Spring, MD: Nursesbooks.org.

American Nurses Association. (2010). Nursing's social policy statement: The essence of the profession (3rd ed.). Silver Spring, MD: Nursesbooks.org.

Benner P. (2004). Using the Dreyfus Model of skill acquisition to describe and interpret skill acquisition and clinical judgment in nursing practice and educations. Bulletin of Science, Technology, and Society, 24(3), 188-199. Retrieved from http://bst.sagepub.com/cgi/ content/ abstract/24/3/188

Codier E, Muneno L, and Freitas E. (2011). Emotional intelligence abilities in oncology and palliative care. Journal of Hospice and Palliative Nursing, 13(3) 183-188

Elder L. and Paul R. (2010, October). Universal intellectual standards. Retrieved from http:// www.criticalthinking. org/pages/universal-intellectual-standards/527

Facione NC and Facione PA. (2008). Critical thinking and clinical judgment. In Critical thinking and clinical reasoning in the health sciences: A teaching anthology (pp. 1-14) Millbrae, CA: California Academic Press.

Federal Rules of Evidence. Rule 702. Testimony by Expert Witnesses, Pub. L. No. 93 595 §1, 88 St. 1937 (1975).

Finkelman A and Kenner C. (2010). Professional nursing concepts: Competencies for quality leadership. Sudbury, MA: Jones and Bartlett Publishers.

Gordon S and Nelson S. (2005). An end to angels. American Journal of Nursing, 105(5), 62-69.

Lunney M (2012). Assessment, clinical judgment, and nursing diagnoses: How to determine accurate diagnoses. In NANDA International, Nursing Diagnoses 2012-2014: Definitions and classification (pp. 70-83). West Sussex, United Kingdom, John Wiley and Sons.

Lunney M. (2001). Critical thinking and nursing diagnoses: Case studies and analyses. Philadelphia, PA: NANDA International.

Neulicht A, Riddick-Grisham S, and Goodrich W (2010). Life care plan survey 2009: Process, methods, and protocols. Journal of Life Care Planning, 9(4), 129-161.

Paul R, Binker AJA, Martin D, and Adamson K. (1989). Critical thinking handbook: High school (A guide for redesigning instruction). Dillon Beach, CA: Foundation for Critical Thinking.

Paul RW andd Elder L (2002). Critical thinking: Tools for taking charge of your professional and personal life. Upper Saddle River, NJ: Financial Times Prentice Hall.

Salovey P, Brackett MA and Mayer JD (2004). Emotional intelligence: Key readings on the Mayer and Salovey model. Port Chester, NY: Dude Publishing.

Scheffer B K and Rubenfeld MG (2000). A consensus statement on critical thinking. Journal of Nursing Education, 39(8), 352-359.

Wilkinson J (2006). Nursing process and critical thinking (4th ed.). Upper Saddle River, NJ: Prentice Hall

CHAPTER 3

Critiquing a Life Care Plan

Dorajane Apuna-Grummer, BSN, MA, DHA, RN, CCM, CNLCP

Introduction

Each nurse life care planner has a different perspective on how to approach a life care plan, based on the individual's training and knowledge level. Most nurse life care planners format plans using the nursing process and diagnoses; consistency of practice is paramount. Clarity, organization, and comprehensive methodology are essential in both the planning and the reviewing process.

In litigation, information concerning costs and medical needs forms a large part of a personal injury case. Because life care planners' knowledge and educational backgrounds vary, marked differences in life care figures and perceived needs can be presented in the same case. Attorneys, insurance adjusters, and trust officers are aware of these variations and seek to discover problems in a life care plan prior to settlement or trial. An insurance company or trust company requests a life care plan review to ensure that reasonable amounts of monies will be set aside to cover future needs.

The main goal of reviewing a life care plan submitted by another life care planner is to evaluate whether the plan is reasonable, necessary, and complete with respect to needs related to the injury or illness at issue. This is achieved by using knowledge of life care plan development, construction, and nursing analytical and critical thinking skills. In Figure 1, the components are similar to the process for editing a plan prior to giving it to the client. The process outlined in this chapter will focus on critical thinking and reflective evaluations.

Nurse life care planners (NLCPs) will experience times when a client will request a review of a life care plan completed by another life care planner. The type or focus of the review depends on needs of the referral. Reviews may be requested by many sources, such as defense counsel, plaintiff's attorney, a trust company, or an insurance company. The focus of this chapter is to examine the background necessary to complete this task, the components of a review for a life care plan, and the steps an NLCP should take to finish the review opinion.

Referral

When receiving a referral for a life care plan review, the NLCP should identify the client's purpose prior to assessing the merits of the plan. Is the review to be used as a work product to understand the pitfalls of the life care plan, or will the review be used to support expert witness testimony? If it is to be used as work product, the NLCP follows the same process as litigation opinion reports; following the presentation of the opinions, NLCP services may no longer be needed on the file. This is often the case when the NLCP is developing the analysis for trust or insurance companies.

In preparing opinions for litigation, the NLCP develops the report using standard formatting for opinion reports. This includes credential identification, background information for the plan, identification of medical records and documents used for the opinions, differences of opinions about the life care plan, and the foundation for the opinions. The client may ask to have a second life care plan prepared to counter the original life care plan. The discussion of the original or reviewed life care plan and the new life care plan is either incorporated into the expert's written opinion or presented as a stand-alone document.

A well-written report reflects the planner's credibility. The report becomes part of the expert's record; a poorly prepared report can be used in the future to impeach the expert's credibility. All reports are legally required to include a complete statement of all opinions expressed, along with the foundations and support for those opinions. Exhibits or documents supporting the opinions are required to be disclosed with the report. A federal case requires additional information, including a list of all publications previously published by the life care planner, a closing bill documenting the LCP's compensation for the report, and a list of other cases in which the life care planner has testified either by deposition or trial testimony. The presence of substantive mistakes, bad grammar, typographical errors, or misspelled words may give the opposing side reason to suspect the report and have it discharged from the case.

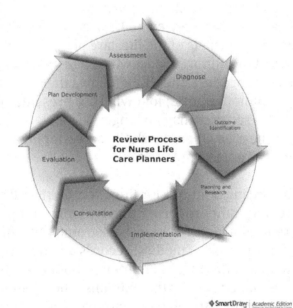

Fig. 1. Review Process for Nurse Life Care Planners.
Illustration courtesy of D. Apuna-Grummer

The Standards of Practice for Nurse Life Care Planners and the Standards of Practice for the American Nurses Association form the foundation for the review process. This foundation recognizes that NLCPs follow a consistent organized methodology in the development of life care plans and in life care plan reviews. George and Hagg-Heitman (2011) stated,

"Peer review is one of the essential components of professional nursing practice that helps ensure the quality and safety of both the care provided and the care provider." The AANLCP's Standards of Practice supports the review process, not only for the nurse life care planner, but also for plans developed by other disciplines.

Preparation for the Analysis

When a client makes a referral for a life care plan analysis, typically there has been a clear effort to obtain the patient's medical records, including records from all treating entities: hospital, clinic, physician's office, physical therapist, occupational therapist, and other providers. Additional records needed include medical and pharmacy billing, depositions, treatment records, and other related documentation. All the documents discussed or reviewed by the developer of the life care plan should be requested.

If foundation support or research is mentioned in the plan, those items should be available to the analyzer. It is important to establish a reliable system for tracking important facts in each case. Whether using sticky notes, highlighters, or proprietary software, the NLCP should have a methodology to efficiently track the key facts needed to write the review or prepare to testify.

At the time of this writing, there are two major life care planning organizations, the American Association of Nurse Life Care Planners (AANLCP) and the International Association of Rehabilitation Professionals (IARP). The NLCP will need copies of both organizations' standards to complete the review process. The NLCP reviewer will ensure that the submitting life care planner based the plan using the standards of the applicable organization. The rebuttal life care plan, if requested, is formulated on the standards of the AANLCP as outlined in the core curriculum.

One of the more challenging problems with reviewing defense life care plans is that often the plaintiff's attorney can block access to the injured party or treating team members (depending on jurisdiction). The NLCP should always request access to the injured party and document if this is not granted. If so, the NLCP should complete the assessment using medical records or interviews with the medical providers (if permitted).

If the plaintiff's attorney, a trust company, or an insurance company has requested the review, the reviewer should have access to the client and should ask to complete an assessment of daily living activities for the individual in addition to reviewing the records and collaborating with the treating team, as above.

Credentialing Review

The following are critical in evaluating the submitting life care planner's credentials:

- What is the educational and professional background of the life care planner?
- Did the planner receive training and credentialing in life care planning standards and process?
- Does the developer have the background to render opinions concerning costs of treatment?
- Has the developer stayed within credentialed scope of practice related to making recommendations concerning medical treatments, supplies, equipment, or home care?
- Were life care planning standards followed, a home assessment completed, and other medical providers contacted for their expertise with the client or the client's medical needs?

One of the key factors of a nurse life care planner's education is the development of a consistent model for the life care planning process. Attending educational classes in life care planning and annual life care planning and case management conferences, combined with the experience and knowledge base of the life care planner, enables the NLCP's professional development to grow within the model.

The NLCP often has years of experience in patient care and an understanding of what patients need for treatments and safety. A minimum of two years of case management experience across the continuum of care is required before obtaining life care planning credentials. This experience provides the NLCP with a strong foundation of specialized skills to help determine what is necessary for the injured party. Registered nurse licensure gives credibility to the nurse performing assessments and developing nursing diagnoses related to function and daily needs, the basis for care planning. Registered nurses have intense extensive education in developing plans of care based on specific nursing diagnoses using the nursing process. Life care planning is an extension of care planning that focuses on specific diagnoses over a longer period, often life expectancy.

Daubert v. Merrell Dow Pharmaceuticals (1993) established that expert testimony was based on the credentials (degrees, certifications, etc.), skills (work experience and special knowledge), and reputation of the witness in the area of expertise. This formed the basis for the acceptance of an expert's opinions. A nurse life care planner has expert witness knowledge as a registered nurse and through patient care experience. In addition, each NLCP derives authority as an expert witness based individual experience, professional certifications, and advanced education levels. As noted above, a certified nurse life care planner must have a minimum of two years of active case management experience across the continuum of care to sit for the national certification examination for nurse life care planning.

The Nurse Practice Act regulates the nursing practice in each individual state, mandating the registered nurse's ability to complete nursing assessments and develop nursing diagnoses, thus providing the foundation for nurse life care planning. Each state has its own nurse practice act delineating nursing practice in that state. Case management and nurse life care planning standards work within the nurse practice act to form the foundation of practice for the NLCP.

As a registered nurse, the NLCP has legal ability to assess human response to injury and ability to function in daily living activities, and to prescribe, delegate, and recommend interventions to other health care providers involved with patient care. This includes care in a home, hospital, or rehabilitation setting.

Although some variation between states does exist, for the most part, the SOPs are similar. The California Nursing Practice Act (2012), Scope of Practice, Section 2725(b) defines the practice:

> A broad, all-inclusive definition states that the practice of nursing means these functions, including basic health care, which help people cope with difficulties in daily living which are associated with their actual or potential health or illness problems, or the treatment thereof, which require a substantial amount of scientific knowledge or technical skill.

Subsection (b) (1) of section 2725 (2012) states that this includes "direct and indirect patient care services that ensure the safety, comfort, personal hygiene, and protection of patients; and the performance of disease prevention and restorative measures."

In New York, the State Education Law, Article 139 (Nurse Practice Act, 2012) states:
The practice of the profession of nursing as a registered professional nurse is defined as diagnosing and treating human responses to actual or potential health problems through such

services as case finding, health teaching, health counseling, and provision of care supportive to or restorative of life and well-being, and executing medical regimens prescribed by a licensed physician, dentist or other licensed health care provider legally authorized under this title and in accordance with the commissioner's regulations.

If the submitting life care planner is not certified in life care planning, it is important to know what legal scope of practice defines the planner's practice. It is important to note deviations from practice limitations defined by that scope. Regardless of profession, the planner must have life care planning credentials and follows the life care planning methodology. Has the submitting planner

- Conferred with other medical providers on areas outside his expertise?
- Conferred with physical therapists, rehabilitation therapists, psychologists, or neuropsychologists if needed?
- Followed guidelines for obtaining local pricing?
- Supported his opinions with research or appropriate resources?
- Had specialized training in life care planning?

Assessment
Reviewing Medical Records
In preparation for reviewing life care plans, it is important to ensure the reviewer has the same records that the submitting life care planner used to develop the life care plan. The medical records needed are clarified not only by reading the list of medical records used to develop the life care plan, but also through the data analysis or medical record review and by direct requests to the client. The reviewing NLCP will also need depositions and any related medical records to prepare a rebuttal plan. The reviewer may reference the medical records, and often cite the source for the information in the review, whether directly in the report or in footnotes or

endnotes. This provides the medical basis for the life care plan review.

Few, if any, medical disciplines practice without using specialty guidelines. They have written standards of practice, participate in evidenced-based practice, or use guidelines for diagnosis and treatment. Each specialty develops these standards by researching the latest techniques supporting good patient outcomes and determining what the majority of practitioners in that specialty use to attain good outcomes. The life care plan foundation uses nursing diagnoses; medical records; physician prescriptions; recommendations from physical therapists, occupational therapists, speech therapists; and information and notes from any other involved disciplines.

This documentation and collaboration provides support for plan conclusions and opinions. The foundation for the life care plan can also be supplemented by applicable standards of care, evidence-practice research, and clinical practice guidelines developed through national associations, such as the American Pain Association, American Pediatric Association, American Spinal Injury Association, Association of Rehabilitation Nurses, Home Health Nurses Association, and many other national medical and nursing associations. The Joint Commission, a medical care accreditation organization, rates facilities on their ability to provide good healthcare by applying evidence-based practice standards. Because this organization has supported the use of standards and evidence-based medicine, many healthcare disciplines have implemented these standards and practices into their fields.

Audit Tool for Life Care Plan Reviews
The following checklist, or a similar checklist, assists the nurse life care planner in organizing the approach to reviewing a life care plan. It also serves as an audit tool for the life care plan produced for a case.

- Is there a clear understanding what the retaining client wants from this assignment?

- Documentation check:
  o Was a life care plan developed by the opposing party included?
  o Are tables and the narrative part of the report included in the records?
  o Are there depositions of the injured party, the family of the injured person, and treatment providers? Has the opposing life care planner been deposed? If so, was that deposition included?
  o Are there videos of activity in the patient's daily life or functional assessments?
  o Are copies of the medical records, records of the healthcare providers, and diagnostics included?
  o Are copies of all medical records used by the opposing life care planner included?

- Credentials check for life care planner:
  o Does the planner have professional training as a life care planner?
  o Does the planner have background experience with patients who have similar diagnoses as the subject of the life care plan?
  o Does the opposing life care planner meet the Federal Rules of Evidence, Rule 702 criteria for an expert witness (knowledge, skill, experience, training, or education)?

- Plan validity
  o Are copies of the standards, policy and procedures, and ethical considerations for the life care planner included? (www.aanlcp.org and www.rehabpro.org)
  o Is the foundation for the life care plan supported by
    - Medical records
    - Treatment records?

- Evidenced-based practice, as in the standards of practice used by the medical providers treating the injury?
  o Is the life care plan appropriate for the injury?
  o Do any overlaps or duplication of care exist in home care versus facility care for pediatric or adult rehabilitation?
  o What research was used? Was it identified either through footnotes or in the appendix?

- Cost validation
  o Are the calculations correct?
  o Is there supportive documentation of cost sources?
  o Are necessary items omitted from the plan? Are excessive items included?
  o Are the costs appropriate to the locality for the injured person? Or were they taken from the Internet or discount prices, such as private insurance rates or private buying groups?
  o What are the cost reductions of equipment and supplies for general expenses as compared to those related to the injury?

- Plan reliability
  o Is the plan a formulaic "cookie cutter" plan, or is it individualized to the injured person?
  o Is there evidence of the collaboration of treating team?
  o Are the appropriate medical equipment, supplies, treatments, and medical providers identified for the injury described?
  o Are similar services listed in different areas more than once?
  o Are there duplicate services (e.g. physical therapy, chiropractic, and a personal trainer) provided for the injured person? Are they provided separately rather than from one general provider?
  o Are the timeframes overlapping or definitive?

o   Are the rationales for the entries clear and
        supported by medical records, medical provider
        records, or by medical provider reviewers?

There are many ways to approach report preparation.
This chapter provides suggestions regarding formatting and
content, but ultimately the reviewer can decide what to use.
There are specific components that should be included in the
life care plan review. The main goals are to provide clarity,
assess reliability, and facilitate understanding of the complete
life care plan. See the example at the end of this chapter.

The NLCP's approach to building a life care plan uses
the nursing process and critical thinking to assess the patient's
needs, providing the necessities within the plan. These tools
assist the NLCP to arrive at an organized, concise plan for
future needs for the patient associated with reasonable local
determined costs. Statements identifying the purpose of the
opinions, clarifying the goals, and providing the conclusions
can be placed in an abstract or in the first few pages of the
report.

Abstract or opening paragraph examples:
- "This report is a review of the life care plan for (name)
  presented to (attorney) for the purpose of clarification.
  It is **INTERNAL ATTORNEY WORK PRODUCT and not
  to be presented in evidence."**
- "The goal of the life care review is to provide
  information concerning validity, clarity, and reliability of
  the life care plan for (name). The review was requested
  by (attorney's name) for the purpose of (purpose)."
- "This report is a review of the (name) life care plan for
  establishing a trust following settlement or litigation.
  The goal is to provide validity, clarity, and reliability of
  the life care plan for (name). The review was requested
  by (attorney/trust name) for the purpose of validity,
  clarity, and reliability of the life care plan for (name)."

- "The following review is presented in rebuttal of the life care plan for (name). It is the opinion of (your name) for the purpose of litigation. The goal of this opinion is to provide validity, clarity, and reliability for the life care plan for (name). In this plan the following opinions were made: (summary of main points of the plan)"

The presentation of the review can be set up as a comparison report (see end of chapter) or a stand-alone report. A comparison report is easier to read if it is consistent with the format established by the opposing life care planner to make the differences evident to the reader. In litigation and possible trial, the jury does not have the training of the nurse life care planner or have medical terminology knowledge, so clarity is critical.

Key Factors

Knowing your audience is important when deciding on the specificity of the information or the rationales presented in a critique of another's life care plan. Professionals may be familiar with terminology, but a judge or jury may not. Define terms in the body of the report and in a list provided in the appendix. Include rationales for all opinions, either listed as each opinion occurs in the body of the report or listed in an appendix with supporting references.

Life Expectancy

Sample language to address life expectancy information used in different sections of the report:

- Narrative section: "On page X of this report, Dr. Smith determined life expectancy for the client while discussing future needs. He used the client's current medical status, the calculations for the National Data Center, the CDC expectations, and the advancement or sequence of the disease processes related to the injuries. The life expectancy is 32 more years. Costs and projections related to frequency and replacement of services, equipment, and supplies use the life expectancy provided by Dr. Jones."

- Footnote: "Dr. Smith determined life expectancy based on the client's current medical status, the calculations of the National Data Center and the CDC, and the sequence or development of the disease processes related to the injuries."
- Appendix: "The life expectancy figure used in this report was developed by Dr. Smith, who assessed the client's current medical status utilizing the life expectation calculations from the National Data Center, the CDC mortality rates, and his knowledge of disease process sequence to establish a life expectancy of 32 years."
- Rationale: "Using Dr. Smith's life expectancy figure of 32 years, the above costs were determined to include $446,000 for future medications."

If no current physician opinions for life expectancy are available, the sources for the figures, such as the *National Vital Statistics Reports*, should be identified clearly. (See http://www.cdc.gov/nchs/products/nvsr.htm)

Cost Clarity Examples

Other examples of definitions needed in a life care plan include the terms *real dollars, annual cost, local pricing,* or *medical providers.* The main point of this section is to provide clarity for the readers. There should be no misunderstanding concerning these points in the life care plan.

Costs are a large factor in a life care plan. The reviewer should define the difference between the costs in the original life care plan and appropriate costs in the opinion of the reviewer. These differences should be highlighted and defined for the reader to ensure clarity and consistency. (*See example of review at the end of the chapter.*)

The need for specific items, whether services or equipment, is identified through the medical records review, interviews or documents from medical providers, and patient interviews.

Research on costs for locally-available items are important and should be completed using the nursing process, nursing diagnoses, and standards of care. Other factors may determine whether the costs are one-time, annual, or periodic (needed at specific times or intervals during life expectancy). If local companies cannot provide the service or equipment, then out-of-region prices should be identified as such to provide transparency.

When reviewing a plan, the NLCP may discover the following types of errors:
- Calculation errors
- Inappropriate, unrelated items and costs
- Insufficient services or equipment needed
- Duplicated costs, services, or items.

Local prices should be obtained and averaged for services, equipment, and supplies. If the medical team recommends a specialty item, then the cost may be sought through the vendors. When the NLCP determines pricing, no discounted sale price or costs involving some type of membership are to be used, as the client may not have or access to the discounted vendor or the funding to buy the membership. Three or more costs should be obtained from vendors if possible.

When costing out large items with known replacement intervals, it is often not appropriate to give an annual cost when working with life expectancy. For example, a wheelchair that costs $6000 and must be replaced every five years for a person with a life expectancy of 12 years from now should be costed thus:

- First purchase, year 0 (now)
- Second purchase, beginning of year 5

- Third purchase, beginning of year 10 (last purchase, will outlast life expectancy)
- Total cost for life expectancy, 3 purchases x $6000 = $18,000

If one were to calculate this item by dividing $6000 / 5 years = $1200/year and multiply that times 12 years, the total of $14,400 would not cover the required time period.

However, if the item were already in use, having been bought two years before today (year-2), costing hence is properly done thus:

- First purchase, beginning of year 3
- Second purchase, beginning of year 8 (last purchase, as life expectancy ends at end of year 12)
- Total cost for life expectancy, 2 purchases x $6000 = $12,000

In this situation, if one were to calculate this item at $1200/year and multiply that times 12 years, the total of $14,400 would be excessive for the required time period.

Durable medical equipment comes in discrete units. One cannot purchase three-fifths of a wheelchair and it is meaningless to budget for it in that manner. If item replacement or a service unit (e.g., MRI) comes due at one year before life expectancy, cost in full is indicated and should be so noted in the plan.

The reviewer should ensure that all aspects of the cost calculations are done correctly. Factors to consider include:

- Are all calculations correct?
- Are the formulas for the calculations correct (e.g. using 365.25 for yearly calculations)?
- Are the cost sources identified in either the report or the appendix?
- Is economic factoring used? If costs are increased for inflation, was this done by a qualified economist?

- Are potential complications identified, such as estimated costs that were not included in the plan?
- When cost calculations are put into the life care plan, has the life care planner identified the source for the numbers? These should be located in footnotes, an appendix, or the body of the cost tables.

Relationships

Implied or identified relationships between the life care planner and the vendors, suppliers, or providers should be identified in the report. The planner should include statements such as *"The attending physician owns the medical supply company that provides the splints, equipment, etc. for the client"* or *"The medications are provided through the physician's office"* as needed to clarify why alternatives were not used (e.g., buying equipment from other suppliers or medications from an independent pharmacy). Potential conflict of interest should be noted.

Overlapping Services

Review of a life care plan should identify potential overlaps in services. Factors to consider include:

- Are there several specialists that provide similar services? Could a single provider, such as a physiatrist, perform the same functions an attending physician, pain management physician, and neurologist, of whom each may address pain issues?

- Is the same item repeated in several sections?

- Are a physical therapist, chiropractor, and massage therapist all scheduled for the same period?

- One way to determine if the number of medical providers is overwhelming for the client is to do an analysis of the number of appointments scheduled for one month. Is this schedule practical for the client or overwhelming?

- Are the providers licensed for the care that they perform? Provider qualifications should be checked against the standards of care for the state in which the life care plan is implemented.

- Are appropriate levels of caregivers provided to meet the patient's needs: registered nurse, licensed vocational/practical nurse, certified nursing assistant, or home health aide? Can a lower level or unlicensed person perform the same service?

Home Care Issues

Home care is an important aspect of the life care plan. Consider the following:

- Are the identified home care needs supported by nursing documentation, the home assessment, and notes or prescription from medical providers?

- The patient or family are expected to pay for some goods and services; if an item would normally be purchased if the person were not injured, then the individual is expected to pay for that item, e.g., an automobile, which would normally be purchased by a person without injuries.

If the person becomes injured and needs a van with special modifications, then the price of the van should be borne by the patient, as it is expected for each person to provide his own vehicle. Some life care planners plan a deduction for the cost of an average vehicle and allow for the excess cost of a van if needed.

The cost for modifications and special equipment, such as lowering the van base, electronics, a ramp, and seat locks would be necessary for the plan.

- Is there evidence in the plan that the home care is based on the client's current medical needs and situation as opposed to the standard for the injury level?

- Can the service be offered more inexpensively with a more basic caregiver, or is the task or need mandated in that state to be performed by a specific provider level?

- Are enough caregiver hours included to ensure the safety of the client?

- Does the caregiver need supervision? How is the supervision provided?

Many issues concerning the levels of care should be considered. If the client is without family or lives in a home alone, the current consensus is the caregivers is best provided by an agency, as the agencies can complete background checks, assess abilities to provide care, provide bonding or insurance as required, cover absences and vacation time, and handle federal and state taxes, workers' compensation, and other tax liabilities.

When evaluating the need for home care or home services, the NLCP should evaluate the severity of the injury, the ability of the client to function in daily activities, and the client's ability to be independent, recognizing that the less functionality the client has, the more care the client will need. For patients with brain injuries, cognitive ability determines the range for the need of care and safety.

- What are the standards of care for diagnostics or testing for the specific condition?

- Are the tests appropriate?

- Is the equipment appropriate for the injury?
For example, the Paralyzed Veterans of America (www. pva.org) website recommends ranges of different levels of care by level of spinal cord injury.

- If the plan's provision is different, does the planner explain why the difference exists?

Durable Medical Equipment
The nurse life care planner can analyze necessary equipment replacement and supplies by looking at patterns of activities or billing records. Information can also be found in reports of evidence-based practice and from vendors and medical providers.

The replacement assessment takes place during the on-site assessment with the patient. During the assessment, DME should be evaluated for the client's functional needs and ability to use it. This allows the nurse life care planner to compare actual equipment needs with elements proposed in the submitted plan.

The NLCP should consider different methods for obtaining equipment, such as lease versus purchase. For example, equipment for pediatric patients is often outgrown quickly, so leasing may be more cost-effective until the patient reaches full growth. After that, purchasing is considered standard. Any equipment in the plan should have documented rationales for the need and usage by the patient.

Home Modifications
Provisions for home modifications, home additions, and remodeling to accommodate patient needs are often necessary in life care plans. A person with a catastrophic illness or injury often needs adaptive changes to the home to assist with activities of daily living, equipment storage, and exercise

equipment to promote independence or health maintenance. If a lump sum or single price for these modifications appears in the life care plan, further breakdown is needed. This should be clarified in the rationale or the appendix. Home designs, modification architectural drawings, and specification drawings supporting the need for changes are essential. The sources for pricing should be included.

Collateral Sources

The collateral source rule is a law that allows for punitive or other damages awarded to a plaintiff for an injury, illness, or disability. This rule states that damages awarded in court cannot be reduced because the plaintiff has received other sources of income, insurance benefits, or awards prior to the hearing of the case. This also includes resources in schools and disability funding. These amounts are considered to be separate and cannot be counted when the damages in the case are calculated. The collateral source rule is used to prevent admission of evidence showing the plaintiff is being compensated twice for the same injury (i.e. first by insurance, then by court-determined awards). Note that there are a few very specific exceptions to this rule, e.g., the Federal vaccine injury compensation cases; the reviewing NLCP should consult with the attorney client for guidance on any individual case.

The nurse life care planner critiquing a plan should be aware of current processes, equipment, supplies, evidence-based practice standards, and treatments, and proactively seek out information regarding these. This information is available through subscriptions to journals, attending conferences, the Internet, and news sources. After determining whether the life care plan is reasonable, necessary, and appropriate, the nurse life care planner will be prepared to move to testimony preparation or the generation of a new life care plan.

The following review of a life care plan is presented to demonstrated formatting, and formulating a model for reference. The format for a plan review is a personal choice for the life care planner. Regardless of the format used, the nurse life care planner should strive for consistency, clarity, and a comprehensive methodology.

Sample Life Care Plan Review
Review of Life Care Plan for Susan Doe by Suki Smith CLCP
Marrisa Jones, MN, RN, CNLCP
Date

Cost Summary

Item	Page	Life Expectancy	Annual Costs: Smith	Life Expectancy Costs: Smith	Annual Costs: Jones	Life Expectancy Costs: Jones
Medical services	4	65	$2345.27	$152,442.55	$2345.27	$152,44.55
Medications	6	65	120.53	3445.00	120.53	3445.20
Diagnostics/ procedures	7	65	91.96	5977.40	91.96	5977.40
Supplies and equipment	8	65	249.23	16,199.95	249.23	16,199.95
Recreation	9	65	145.00	9425.00	145.00	9425.00
Miscellaneous	11	65	481.00	30,000.00	481.00	30,000.00
Vocational needs	12	65	0.00	0.00	0.00	0.00
Scenario 1, Home/facility care	13	65	41,982.85	2,728,885.20	0.00	0.00
Scenario 2, Group home care	14	65	0.00	0.00	22,162.03	1,440.531.90
Totals			$45,415.84	$2,946,375.10	$25,595.02	$1,658,021.80

PROJECTED WORK OPTIONS

It is expected for Ms. Doe to work a normal work span of 20 years, over a 45 year program, following her leaving school at age 22.[1]

In addition to the above numbers, there are two projected future work options to be considered:

Option 1: Sheltered employment (Low supervision, constant supervision)

$7382.00—$8,182.00 per first year (includes evaluation and placement)

$3,840.00 per year during work years

Total: $84,182.80—$84,982.80

Option 2: Supportive Employment

$5,220.00—$7,000.00 per first year (includes evaluation and placement)

$3,472.00 each year during work years

Total: $74,660—$76,440.00

[1] Angel California Regional Center, Carry Curr CRC

Medical Services

Item	Suki Smith CLCP Frequency	Cost	Note	Marrisa Jones, MN, RN, CNLCP Cost	Notes
Neurology	Twice only / Annually / Every 5 years	$125-315	Annually to monitor seizures, meds, referrals	$250	Dr. Patty recommends annual visits. Dr. Man recommends 2 visits per lifetime. No support for frequency given by Smith.
Orthopedics	Annually	$125-315		$250	Dr. Man recommends annual to evaluate orthopedic problems and rule out scoliosis
Physiatry	Annually	$125-315	"Periodic evaluation by physiatrist or orthopedist because of asymmetry in her gait and persistent abnormal neurological signs."	0	Physiatry not needed with annual neurology and orthopedics visits. Neurology more appropriate to provide care as they specialize in brain injuries.
Neuropsychology	20-30 sessions over lifetime	$250		0	No medical evidence for this recommendation
Neuropsychology evaluation	0-2 times over lifetime	$1850 each	To check progress of condition	$1850 for each eval.	Will need 1 to 2 more neuropsychological evaluations over life expectancy

Comprehensive brain injury treatment center	3-6 hours per day, 3-5 days per week, 3-6 months	$1600 – 2000 per day	$1446 per day	This is appropriate. In the brain injury center the patient is evaluated and taught independent living skills appropriate for her level of injury. They assist the patient to achieve a higher level of independence and give support for community needs and resources. Local pricing.
Neuropsychology		$258	0	This a duplicate service, see above.
Occupational therapy		$315	0	These services are provided by the Center for Neuro Skills and are not needed further.
Physical therapy		$272	0	
Speech therapy		$283	0	

Neuropsychological evaluations x 2 = $5000 / 65 years life expectancy = $76.92

Center for NeuroSkills : 45 days = $81,000.00 / 65 years life expectancy = $ 1,446.15

Neuropsychology (45 days = 3 visits weekly = 21 visits x $258.00 = 5,418.00 / 65 years life expectancy = $ 83.35

Medications

Medications	Suki Smith CLCP			Marrisa Jones, MN, RN, CNLCP	
	Propranolol 40 mg daily	$29.84 / 30 tabs $363.20 / year	Agreed [1]	$0.13 / tab $47.48 / year	These prices were per local pharmacies, Walgreens, SaveMart, and CVS. It is not known if Mr.
	Ibuprofen 600mg 2x daily, 3-5 days each week	$33.37 per 60 (.55 per unit) or 173.52 - $289.21 per year	Agreed	$0.20 per unit item or $73.05 annually	Smith's medications were over the counter, but these prices are for prescriptions.

[1] Agreed means agreement with item, not necessarily costs provided by Smith

Diagnostics / Procedures

	Suki Smith CLCP		Marrisa Jones, MN, RN, CNLCP	
CT Brain	Twice	$1200	Agree	$48.61	This is appropriate for monitoring. Includes reading and interpretation.
CT reading and interpretation		$400			
EEG	Seven over lifetime	$709	Dr. Man recommends twice over lifetime	$36.92	No seizures in last five years, not on antiseizure medications. Reduce to twice, includes interpretation.
Spine x-ray	Twice	$250-300	Dr. Man prescribed this for spinal injury	$6.43	Reading and interpretation included
Xray reading and interpretation		$250-			
MRI brain w/o contrast	0-3	$939	Not recommended by Dr. Patty	0	Has CT scans ordered for this purpose
MRI reading and interpretation	0-3	$366.50	Agree	0	This is appropriate for monitoring

CT Scan =$ 1580 x 2 = $3160.00/65 years life expectancy = $48.61

EEG = $1200 x 2 =$ 2400/65 years life expectancy = $36.92

X-ray ST = $209.00 x 2 = $418.00/65 years life expectancy = $6.43

References

AANLCP Standards of Practice (2012) retrieved
     from http://www.aanlcp.org//Code_
     ofProfessionalEthicsandConduct
     11-1-11.pdf

Babitsky S and Mangraviti J (2004). Writing and defending
     your expert report, the step-by-step guide with models.
     Falmouth, Massachusets: SEAK, Inc.

Cornell University Law School. (2011, December 1). Federal
     rules of evidence. Retrieved from http://www.law.
     cornell.edu/rules/fre/

Fogelholm M. (2010). Peer review reviewed by a peer.
     International Association for the Study of Obesity. 11.
     P.169-170

George V, Haag-Heitman B. (2011) Nursing peer review: The
     manager's role. Journal of Nursing Management. 19. P.
     254-259

Scope of Regulation: California Nursing Practice Act (2010)
     retrieved from http://www.rn.ca.gov/pdfs/regulations/
     npr-i-15.pdf

Ware, M. (2011) Peer review: Recent experience and future
     directions. New Review of Information Networking.
     16:23 p. 23-53 (2012)

State Education Law, Article 139. Nursing Practice. Retrieved
     from http://www.nysna.org/practice/main.htm

Section II

Nurse Life Care Plans
In Practice

CHAPTER 1

Spinal Cord Injury

Wendie A. Howland, MN, RN-BC, CRRN, CCM, CNLCP,
LNCP-C, LNCC
Joan K. McMahon, MSA, BSN, CRRN

Introduction

Spinal Cord Injury (SCI) is a life-changing event with broad physical, emotional, social and spiritual effects for both injured person and family. SCI alters both motor and sensory function below the level of injury and affects every body system. Other effects may include changes in family dynamics, identity, coping, work, and spirituality.

The Model SCI Centers contribute information concerning traumatic SCI to a national database maintained by the National SCI Statistical Center at the University of Alabama-Birmingham (https:www.nscisc.uab.edu). These are the most complete SCI statistical data available, despite excluding nontraumatic SCI and including only patients seen in the Model SCI Centers. This information is analyzed and presented every 1-2 years; data are also summarized at the website and in special issues of the Archives of PMandR. The following statistics are from the March 2011 issue (SCI facts and statistics, Feb. 2011).

Incidence and Prevalence: Approximately 12,000 persons survive a new SCI in the United States each year. Between 232,000 to 316,000 persons were living with SCI in the United States.

Age at Injury: SCI is thought of as an injury of young adults. However, the number of older adults experiencing SCI is increasing. Possible contributing factors to this trend are:

- Healthier older persons
- Change in the median age of the population
- Survival of older persons at the scene of the accident
- Increased referral to Model SCI Centers

From 1973-1979 the average age of a person with new SCI was 28.7 years; most injuries occurred between ages 16-30. Between 2005-2010, the average age at injury was 40.7 years.

Gender: Males accounted for 80.7% of SCI reported to the database, unchanged over the years.

Race/Ethnicity: Between 2005-2010, 66.5% of persons with new SCI were Caucasian, 26.8% are African American, 2.0% Asian and 8.3% Hispanic.

Etiology: Between 2005-2010, 40.4% of reported SCI were attributed to motor vehicle accidents (MVA), 27.9% were a result of falls, 15% were violence-related, and 8% occurred in sports. Causes of the remaining are reported as either other or unknown.

Neurological Level of Injury: An injury to the spine without cord involvement will most likely produce no significant signs and symptoms. Only injury to the spinal cord causes neurologic deficits. Since 2005, the most common level of injury at discharge is incomplete tetraplegia (39.5%), followed by complete paraplegia (21.1%), incomplete paraplegia (21.7%) and complete tetraplegia (16.3%) Over the last fifteen years, the number of persons with incomplete tetraplegia has increased, while the number of complete paraplegia and tetraplegia cases has decreased.

Length of Stay in Hospital and Rehabilitation: The average length of stay (ALOS) in acute care has decreased by half since 1979, when the average time in acute care was 24 days. Since 2005, the acute ALOS has been 12 days. Trends in inpatient rehabilitation are similar: prior to 1979, ALOS was 98 days; since 2005, the new SCI patient has an ALOS in rehabilitation of only 37 days. This presents several challenges to the patient, family, and care team, as many complications or management problems may not arise until after discharge.

Lifetime Cost: The cost of health and living expenses after a SCI depends on injury level and severity, age at time of injury, education and employment history, and comorbidities. First year costs are generally 5-8 times more than subsequent yearly expenses and can be very high; cost of care for the first year post high tetraplegic injury can be close to one million dollars.

Life Expectancy: Survival in the first two years after SCI have had improved since the 1970s. However, since that time overall improvements in mortality have been modest to absent, with some increase in mortality rates after the initial 2-year post injury period (Strauss et al., 2006). The National Spinal Cord Injury Center publishes charts for life expectancy by level, i.e., no SCI, any level of function, paraplegia, C1-4 and C5-8 tetraplegias, and ventilator-dependent, both for all SCI patients and for those surviving at least one year post injury (NSCIC 2010).

Cause of Death: Renal failure as a leading cause of death in a person with a SCI has declined in recent decades. Since 1973, the leading causes of death in the SCI population are pneumonia and septicemia.

Anatomy
The spinal column is made up of 33 vertebrae (7 cervical, 12 thoracic, 5 lumbar, 5 sacral, 4 coccygeal). Each vertebra has a vertebral body, an intervertebral disc; a vertebral arch, spinous processes, transverse processes, articulating facets, and a vertebral foramen enclosing the spinal cord. See Figure 1, Neurological levels; Figure 2, Vertebral body.

Effects of Nerve Damage along the Spinal Cord

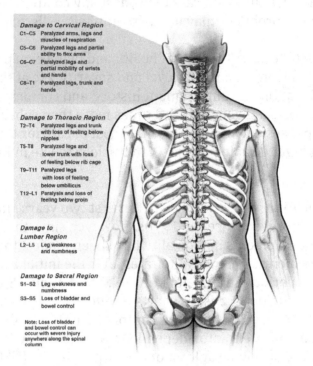

Damage to Cervical Region

C1–C5 Paralyzed arms, legs and muscles of respiration

C5–C6 Paralyzed legs and partial ability to flex arms

C6–C7 Paralyzed legs and partial mobility of wrists and hands

C8–T1 Paralyzed legs, trunk and hands

Damage to Thoracic Region

T2–T4 Paralyzed legs and trunk with loss of feeling below nipples

T5–T8 Paralyzed legs and lower trunk with loss of feeling below rib cage

T9–T11 Paralyzed legs with loss of feeling below umbilicus

T12–L1 Paralysis and loss of feeling below groin

Damage to Lumbar Region

L2–L5 Leg weakness and numbness

Damage to Sacral Region

S1–S2 Leg weakness and numbness

S3–S5 Loss of bladder and bowel control

Note: Loss of bladder and bowel control can occur with severe injury anywhere along the spinal column

Figure 1. Spinal cord levels.
Medical Illustration Copyright © 2013 Nucleus Medical
Media. All rights reserved. www.nucleusinc.com

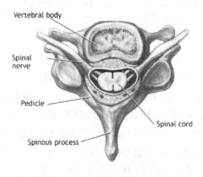

Vertebral body

Spinal nerve

Pedicle

Spinal cord

Spinous process

Figure 2. Vertebral body. Used with permission from
http://www.sci-recovery.org/sci.htm

Ligaments: The ligaments create a supportive structure around the spine and its components. The 2 major longitudinal ligaments run the entire length of the vertebral column. The anterior longitudinal ligament runs anteriorly for the entire length of the vertebral column; the posterior longitudinal ligament runs posteriorly. The vertebral arches are joined to each other by short dense ligaments. There are also the ligamenti flava and intertransverse ligaments. The spinal cord extends from the base of the medulla to the conus medullaris. It is surrounded by the same meninges that covers the brain and by cerebrospinal fluid (CSF) formed in the subarachnoid space. The pia is thicker and firmer in the spine than in the brain and contains vascular supply; the dural sac extends to S2. The dura, arachnoid and pia extend along each nerve root.

Nerves: Each cervical nerve above C8 exits the spinal cord to the upper extremities above its respective vertebral body. The thoracic nerves exit below their respective thoracic vertebrae. Lumbar nerves also exit below their respective lumbar vertebrae to the lower extremities. Sacral nerves exit from the conus and innervate bladder, bowel, and sexual function. Nerves that exit from the coccygeal portion of the cord are called the cauda equina.

Vascular supply: The vascular supply of the spinal cord comes from branches of the vertebral arteries and small radicular arteries to form the anterior spinal artery. This runs along full length of the cord anteriorly. The posterior spinal arteries run the full length of the cord along the dorsal roots.

SCI Causes Primary and Secondary Damage

Primary damage: Traumatic spinal cord injury begins with trauma that fractures or dislocates vertebrae, bruising or disrupting the cord with displaced bone, disc material, or ligaments. Axons are sheared off or damaged; neural cell membranes are broken. Blood vessels may rupture in the grey matter, with bleeding often spreading to adjacent areas of the spinal cord over the next few hours.

Secondary damage: The mechanisms of secondary damage enlarge the damaged area. The cord swells to fill the entire cavity of the spinal canal at the level of injury. Swelling cuts off blood flow to spinal cord tissue; this affects the interior grey matter of the spinal cord more than the outlying white matter. Blood vessels in the grey matter begin to leak. Cells lining the uninjured blood vessels in the spinal cord begin to swell.

The combination of leaking, swelling, and sluggish blood flow causes ischemic damage and cell death. As the reduction of blood flow becomes more widespread, self-regulation begins to turn off; blood pressure and heart rate drop.

Glutamate, an excitatory neurotransmitter that stimulates activity in neurons, is released in large amounts. The resulting excitotoxicity disrupts normal processes, killing neurons and oligodendrocytes that surround and protect axons. The axons lose their myelin insulation. Inflammation accelerates the overproduction of free radicals; these attack and disable molecules crucial for cell membrane function. Free radicals also change how cells respond to natural growth and survival factors, and turn these protective factors into agents of destruction; nerve cells self-destruct. Cells in the injured spinal cord also die from apoptosis, a normal cellular event that helps the body get rid of old and unhealthy cells by causing them to shrink and implode. Nearby scavenger cells then clear away the debris.

Diagnosis and Classification of SCI

Diagnosis is dependent on both good physical assessment of motor and sensory function and on multiple diagnostic imaging studies. Different examinations show different aspects of injury: X-rays (plain films, usually AP/ lateral/ flexion/ extension) outline the spine's bony and perispinal structures. Computerized axial tomography (CT scan) visualizes the spinal column, neural canal impingement, and soft tissue damage. Magnetic resonance imaging (MRI) shows imaging of the spinal cord, ligaments and intervertebral discs. Notice the differences in these 3 images of the same injury. (Figure 3, C-spine diagnostic images)

Figure 3: Multiple imaging of cervical spine with injury at C4-5. Images courtesy of J. McMahon

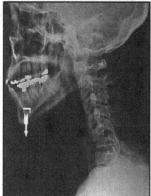

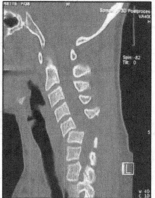

Lateral plain film   CT Scan

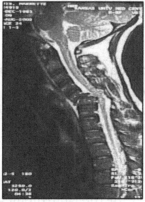

MRI Scan

Physical Assessment

A detailed motor and sensory examination is necessary to determine the extent and completeness of the SCI. The motor examination evaluates motor function in all functional units. Motor function is scored on a scale from 5-0. (See Table 1)

Table 1. Motor Examination Scale

Score	Explanation
5	Normal motor function
4	Active movement through full range of motion (AROM) with moderate resistance
3	AROM against gravity
2	AROM with gravity eliminated
1	Palpable muscle contraction- no visualized movement
0	Absent muscle function

The sensory examination evaluates sensory function in each dermatome level. A basic examination will evaluate the presence of the sensation of pain (posterior column sensory tract) and light touch (spinothalamic sensory tract). A more detailed examination looks at proprioception and vibratory sense.

The International Standards for Neurological Classification of Spinal Cord Injury
The journey to find a tool that will precisely diagnose SCI and help predict outcomes has traveled from the Frankel classification (1969) to the ASIA Standards (1982) with revisions in 1989, 1992, 1996, 2000, including a name change to the *International Standards*. The 2011 revision of the International Standards for the Neurological Classification of Spinal Cord Injury (ISNCSCI) was published in the November 2011 issue of the Journal of Spinal Cord Medicine (Kirshblum et al., 2011).

The neurologic level of injury is determined to be the lowest point on the spinal cord below which there is a decrease or absence of feeling (sensory level) and movement (motor level). This tool identifies neurological level, whether the injury is complete, ASIA Impairment Score (AIS), and zone of partial preservation by measuring motor and sensory function at each dermatome level. Each level is scored and a total is determined. This tool, if accurately administered, can help predict outcome after SCI most accurately if completed at 72 hours post injury. (See Figure 4, ASIA form)

ASIA IMPAIRMENT SCALE

☐ **A = Complete:** No motor or sensory function is preserved in the sacral segments S4-S5.

☐ **B = Incomplete:** Sensory but not motor function is preserved below the neurological level and includes the sacral segments S4-S5.

☐ **C = Incomplete:** Motor function is preserved below the neurological level, and more than half of key muscles below the neurological level have a muscle grade less than 3.

☐ **D = Incomplete:** Motor function is preserved below the neurological level, and at least half of key muscles below the neurological level have a muscle grade of 3 or more.

☐ **E = Normal:** motor and sensory function are normal

CLINICAL SYNDROMES

☐ Central Cord
☐ Brown-Sequard
☐ Anterior Cord
☐ Conus Medullaris
☐ Cauda Equina

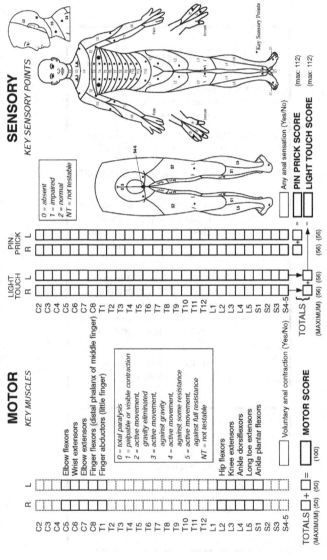

Patterns of Spinal Cord Injury:

Complete SCI No motor or sensory sensation. A complete SCI does not require complete cord transection: neural transmission can be interrupted by neuron damage due to stretching or shearing inside an intact dura or ischemia.

Incomplete SCI Some motor or sensory sensation in the lowest sacral segment (S4-5). The patient can sense light touch, deep anal pressure, and pinprick at the S-4-5 segment, and voluntarily contract the anal sphincter. Incomplete injury can occur at any level of the spine. Some specific incomplete syndromes with specific descriptors include the following:

Central cord syndrome Caused by injury to the central cervical cord. The patient demonstrates sensory sacral sparing and weakness greater in the upper extremities than the lower extremities. It is usually the result of severe cervical hyperextension injury or spinal cord tumors. (9% of all SCI)

Anterior spinal cord syndrome Caused by a lesion of the anterior two-thirds of the cord. Thereis paralysis and loss of pain and temperature sensation below the injury; however, proprioception is preserved. It is usually the result of cervical flexion and dislocation injuries or vascular insufficiency. (2% of all SCI)

Brown-Sequard syndrome Caused by injury to one side of the spinal cord, usually a result of stabbings, motor vehicle crashes, or gunshot injuries. The patient has ipsilateral motor paralysis and loss of proprioception, and contralateral loss of sensation of pain and temperature. Prognosis for ambulation is good. (2-3% of SCI)

Cauda equina syndrome is not a true SCI but an injury to lumbosacral nerve roots in the neural canal. This results in an areflexic bowel and bladder and lower extremities at an ASIA C level.

Conus medullaris syndrome is an injury to sacral cord and lumbar roots at the end of the spinal cord, usually as a result of tumor or local trauma. Pain is uncommon; there is sensory abnormality in saddle distribution, areflexic bladder and bowel. Leg examination may be normal. L1 fractures are usually conus lesions and result in upper motor neuron injury while L2 fractures usually are cauda equina injuries resulting in lower motor neuron injury.

Nursing Diagnoses To Consider:

- *Impaired Physical / Bed / Wheelchair / Transfer Mobility:* Limitation of independent movement (specify)
- *Self-Care Deficit:* A constellation of culturally framed behaviors involving one or more self-care activities in which there is a failure to maintain a socially accepted standard of health and well-being (Givens, Lauder, and Ludwick, 2006)
- *Post Trauma Syndrome / Risk for Post Trauma Syndrome:* Sustained maladaptive response / At risk for sustained maladaptive response to a traumatic, overwhelming event
- *Ineffective Self-Health Management:* Pattern of regulating and integrating into daily living a therapeutic regimen for treatment of illness and its sequelae that is unsatisfactory for meeting specific health goals

Selected Life Care Planning Considerations:

- Follow up care from all involved specialties
- Primary care
- Nurse case management
- Level of care
- Home modifications, access, safety
- Transportation
- Family support and involvement

Autonomic Dysreflexia (AD)

Autonomic dysreflexia (AD), also referred to as hyperreflexia, is a life-threatening condition that occurs in patients with a SCI at T6 and above. There are rare reports of AD in patients with lower thoracic injuries (SCIRE 2011). AD cannot occur until spinal shock is over and the reflexes return, possibly weeks post injury.

AD occurs after a noxious event causes stimulation below the level of injury. Sympathetic outflow is unopposed because the sympathetic inhibitory impulses are blocked at the level of the SCI. The patient is not aware of the problem. Reflex reaction and chemical release then cause vasoconstriction, resulting in sudden elevation in blood pressure. When baroreceptors in the carotid artery and aorta are alerted, they prompt parasympathetic nervous system attempts to help by slowly lowering the pulse. However, since these messages cannot get through to the sympathetic nervous system, this pattern continues, increasing vasoconstriction and bradycardia.

In addition to hypertension and bradycardia, symptoms of AD include:
- pounding headache
- nasal congestion
- bronchospasm
- blurred vision
- seizures
- chills without fever
- sweating and flushing above level of injury
- horripilation (goose bumps) above level of injury
- apprehension

An AD episode is a medical emergency; the cause must be identified and resolved immediately. More than 90% of AD episodes are precipitated by a noxious genitourinary (GU) stimulus. The gastrointestinal (GI) tract is implicated in about 5% of cases. When looking for the cause of AD, the following order of investigation is recommended (Consortium for Spinal Cord Medicine, 2001):

- *Bladder* The major cause is an overfilled bladder, as from a kinked or blocked catheter or overdue intermittent catheterization. If catheterization is needed (intermittent, replacement of Foley, or suprapubic), use 2% lidocaine jelly to prevent further irritation. If a catheter is plugged, try to irrigate with 10cc of normal saline. If this is not successful, remove it and recatheterize using lidocaine jelly. Other GU precipitators are urinary tract infections, (UTI) and bladder or kidney stones.

- *Gastrointestinal* Bowel distention or impaction are the most common offenders. Apply lidocaine jelly, wait five minutes, and check for impaction. Remove if needed. Other GI issues could be appendicitis, gallstones, gastric ulcers, hemorrhoids, GI instrumentation, and tube feeding (too cold; too fast; too hot; too much)

- *Others*:
  - *Skin* Constricting clothes, shoes, orthotics, or assistive devices should be removed; assess for contact with hard or sharp objects (check pockets, cushion, bed, chair); look for pressure ulcers, ingrown toenails, blisters, burns, or frostbite
  - *Reproductive system* Sexual intercourse, sexually-transmitted disease (STD), scrotal compression, infections, menstruation, and labor and delivery
  - Deep vein thrombosis, pulmonary embolus
  - Excessive alcohol, caffeine, other diuretic intake
  - Substance abuse
  - Fractures
  - Functional electric stimulation (FES)
  - Surgical or invasive diagnostic procedures

Initially blood pressure should be taken in both arms and should be rechecked after each step. Sitting the patient up and removing TED hose and abdominal binder should help to lower the BP. Once BP returns to baseline, there is no longer a need to continue looking for the causative stimulus (unless medication has been given). Antihypertensive treatment (Consortium for Spinal Cord Medicine, 2001):

- If cause of AD is not quickly identified and BP remains elevated, treat until the cause if found.
- Nitroglycerine paste. Apply 1-2 inches to skin above the level of injury. May repeat every two hours. May wipe off if BP is stable and reapply if needed.
- Nifedipine 10mg immediate-release capsule. May repeat in 2-30 min if needed.
- Do not use above medications if patient has used sildenafil (Revatio, Viagra) within 24 hours; need to use another non-nitrate, quick-acting antihypertensive.

Because of shorter length of stay in acute rehabilitation, many persons with SCI experience their first episode of AD after discharge home. Education should be provided before discharge and information sent home with the patient. This is a problem that is frequently not identified in a physician office or emergency department. Any patient who has experienced an episode of AD should create a AD kit with blood pressure apparatus, a catheter, lidocaine gel and Nitropaste (and other needed items) that is always available.

Nursing Diagnoses To Consider:
- *Autonomic Dysreflexia / Risk for Autonomic Dysreflexia*: Life-threatening, uninhibited sympathetic response /Risk for life-threatening, uninhibited sympathetic response to a noxious stimulus after a spinal cord injury at T7 or above (has been demonstrated in patients with injuries at T7 and T8).

Selected Life Care Planning Considerations:
- AD "kit" and replacements
- Medications
- Hospitalizations for acute episodes
- Patient and family education

Respiratory Considerations Following SCI

Respiratory effects after SCI depend on level of injury, age, comorbidity, associated injuries, and smoking history. Muscles needed for respiration are innervated at various levels of the spinal cord. The higher the level of injury, the higher the level of dysfunction as fewer of the muscles of respiration are innervated. (Table 2, muscles of respiration)

Table 2. Muscles of Respiration (Nelson, 2001), (Jacelon, 2011) (Sheel, 2010)

Muscle group	Spinal level innervated	Respiratory function	Anticipated long term dysfunction
	Injury above C3		Apneic Anticipate ventilator dependence
Diaphragm	C3-C5	Inspiration	Nonfunctional cough May require a ventilator at least part time VC 50% of normal
External Intercostal	T1-T7	Inspiration	Weak cough, absent chest and abdominal muscle movement VC 70% of normal
Scalene	C2-C7	Inspiration	Accessory muscles
Sternomastoid	C2-C3	Inspiration	Accessory muscles
Abdominal	T6-T12	Expiration	Fair cough VC nearly normal
Internal intercostal	T1-T11	Expiration	Fair cough VC nearly normal
	Injury below T12		Strong cough VC normal

VC, vital capacity

Noninvasive ventilation, phrenic nerve stimulation, and diaphragmatic stimulation (DiMarco and Onders, 2005) are potential alternatives to traditional mechanical ventilation. Complication rates, cost, and quality of life should be considered for each individual. Phrenic or diaphragmatic stimulation may be a long-term alternative to mechanical ventilation for subjects with injuries at C2 or above. Some evidence suggests higher survival rate, better power wheelchair management, phonation success, and patient satisfaction in phrenic paced subjects compared to mechanically ventilated subjects (SCIRE, 2010).

Atelectasis, pneumonia or bronchitis complicate many common conditions. Deep breathing and voluntary coughing are the normal intervention; however, there is no research showing their effectiveness in SCI. Insufflation-exsufflation treatment with a "coughalator" or an "in-exsufflator" machine with or without assisted cough is effective in increasing the rate of airflow (Consortium for Spinal Cord Medicine, Respiratory, 2005). Intermittent positive pressure breathing treatments (IPPB), usually with a bronchodilator, glossopharyngeal breathing to help obtain a deeper breath, and incentive spirometry are all helpful with the newly-injured patient (Consortium for Spinal Cord Medicine, Respiratory, 2005). Assisted cough (also called "quad cough") should be taught to persons with a cervical or high thoracic injury and has been shown to result in a statistically significant increase in expiratory peak airflow (Consortium for Spinal Cord Medicine, 2005). High-frequency chest wall oscillation (HFCWO) can improve secretion mobilization in the setting of a weak or absent cough (Kaufman, 2011).

Continuous positive airway pressure (CPAP) and bilevel or variable positive airway pressure (BPAP or VPAP, often erroneously called BiPAP®, the trade name of a portable ventilator) can be used to rest a nonintubated patient and to give deep breaths to help mobilize secretions (Consortium for Spinal Cord Medicine, Respiratory 2005). CPAP is also recommended for obstructive sleep apnea, common especially with cervical injuries; weight loss is also often recommended. Sleep apnea may not be recognized initially in SCI, but appropriate patients should be evaluated with sleep studies (SCIRE, 2010).

Abdominal binders can be used in an attempt to achieve immediate improvements in respiratory function, but long-term effects have not been established (SCIRE, 2010) and studies are not definitive (Wadsworth et al., 2009). They prevent the abdominal contents from falling forward when in a sitting position in the presence of slackened muscles, increase inspiratory capacity, and improve vocal strength. They also help to maintain blood pressure in an upright position by increasing intra-abdominal pressure.

Ventilator Dependence

Adjustment to ventilator-dependent tetraplegia is different for every affected person and family. Both need education, support, and new coping skills to help accommodate to a radically-changed life style (Consortium for Spinal Cord Medicine, 2005).

Durable medical equipment for home use should be based on the evaluations of therapy staff and patient preference. Consider emergency provisions (i.e., backup generator, compressed air / oxygen source if needed, alarms, suction) and assistive technology as part of a safe and effective environment (Consortium for Spinal Cord Medicine, Respiratory 2005). A small portable ventilator that can accompany the patient for travel should be considered. Other equipment to provide includes

- Replacement circuits and humidifier (check with therapist for replacement frequency, usually weekly unless soiled)
- Sterile water for humidification
- Suction and supplies
- Nebulizer and supplies
- Tracheostomy tubes, dressings and ties

Ventilator-dependent individuals can use a van equipped with a lift and tie-downs or accessible public transportation (Consortium for Spinal Cord Medicine,

Respiratory 2005). An attendant trained in personal and respiratory care, including use of the portable ventilator, portable suction, and bag-valve ventilation, should accompany them.

Pulmonary problems are one of the leading causes of hospitalization, morbidity, and mortality in persons with spinal cord injury (Smith, 2007), especially among cervical and higher thoracic injuries. Clinicians should take steps to assist the SCI injured person to prevent respiratory infections. The CDC recommends annual flu vaccine for persons with SCI. Pneumonia vaccine should also be given once with potential revaccination after 5-10 years.

Nursing Diagnosis To Consider:
- *Impaired Gas Exchange:* Excess or deficit in oxygenation and/or carbon dioxide elimination at the alveolar-capillary membrane

Selected Life Care Planning Considerations:
- Primary care for screening, immunizations
- Ventilator, circuits, humidification; consider portable vent for travel
  - back-up electrical supply/batteries/generator
  - bag-valve for manual ventilation
  - oxygen if prescribed
  - nebulizer and medications
  - respiratory therapist
- Suction and supplies; consider portable suction for travel
- High-frequency chest wall oscillation for secretion mobilization

Skin Integrity
Skin integrity is a major concern with SCI. Initial breakdown can often occur in the first few hours of the injury while the injured person waits for EMS extrication and transport. Pressure ulcers are common, costly, and potentially life-threatening. They interfere with rehabilitation

and can prevent participation in activities that contribute to independent, productive, and satisfying lives. Pressure ulcers result in long hospitalization, delayed community reintegration, reduced quality of life, and loss of self-esteem (Consortium for Spinal Cord Medicine, 2000). Cost of managing a single full-thickness pressure ulcer is as estimated to be as high as $70,000, and total cost for treating pressure ulcers in the United States is estimated at $11 billion/year (Lynch, 2010).

Incidence: According to the 2005 National Spinal Cord Injury Statistical Report, pressure ulcers are the most common medical complication (14.9%-26.7%) and the second most common (33.6%) reason for hospital readmission in the first year after initial injury (Makhsous, 2009). Of those who develop pressure ulcers, 7-8% will die from related complications (Richards et al., 2004). The cumulative risk of developing pressure ulcers over the life expectancy makes prevention a priority and daily concern for those who sustain SCI (Regan et al., 2010).

Causation: Factors that have been identified as most likely potential contributing factors are (Krause, 2001):
- limitation in activity and mobility
- injury completeness
- moisture from bowel and bladder incontinence
- lack of sensation
- muscle atrophy
- poor nutritional status, protein malnutrition
- being underweight

Other risk factors include (but are not limited to) (SCIRE, 2010):
- smoking
- comorbidities, especially renal, cardiovascular, pulmonary disease and diabetes
- residing in a nursing home/hospital
- spasticity and a history of previous ulcers

External forces, such as braces (Techer et al., 2007), splints, other orthotic devices, seating surfaces, and tight or wrinkled clothing also create risk in the setting of altered sensation.

Prevention A pressure-relieving mattress and wheel chair cushion are important. They should be prescribed, evaluated for pressure-relief characteristics, and fitted for the individual by a therapist or other clinician with expertise with persons with SCI, not a vendor. The patient and care providers must understand the importance of maintaining skin integrity and preventing accidents to the skin, and practice the following:

- skin exam, daily and after any activity that may have caused trauma
- moisture reduction
- seating system optimization
- adequate hydration / nutrition
- avoiding alcohol and smoking
- proper pressure relief / weight shifts

Recent research suggests that a forward-leaning position is the most effective pressure relief technique, if sustained for an appropriate period. Leaning side to side, having the wheelchair tipped back by 65° or more, or doing a pressure relief lift for 2 minutes also were effective. The traditional pressure relief lift (15-30 sec) was ineffective at increasing tissue oxygen levels to unloaded levels (Makhsous et al 2007). Level 4 evidence (Table 3) supports forward-leaning position as the most effective position for pressure relief, and shows that the traditional 15-30 second vertical lift is not effective (Regan et al., 2009).

Pressure ulcer treatments range widely. The most important commonality is preventing pressure on an affected area; this may mean extended bed rest. Evidence-based treatment interventions should be incorporated into treatment plans. Several are currently supported by Level 1 evidence: Electrical stimulation, US/UVC and pulsed electromagnetic energy as adjunctive therapies; and hydrocolloid dressings for healing stage I and II pressure ulcers.

Enhanced education and structured follow-up have been shown to reduce recurrence of pressure ulcers post SCI (SCIRE, 2010). Recent studies suggest that surgery for stages III and IV pressure ulcers offers the greatest benefit for improvement in general health and quality of life (Singh et al., 2010).

Table 3. **Levels of Evidence** in order of significance. (Bernstein, 2004)

Level 1
   Randomized controlled trial (RCT): A study in which patients are randomly assigned to the treatment or control group and are followed prospectively
Level 2
   Prospective cohort study: A study in which patient groups are separated non-randomly by exposure or treatment, with exposure occurring after the initiation of the study
Level 3
   Retrospective cohort study A study in which patient groups are separated non-randomly by exposure or treatment, with exposure occurring before the initiation of the study
   Case-control study A study in which patient groups are separated by the current presence or absence of disease and examined for the prior exposure of interest
Level 4
   Case Series A report of multiple patients with the same treatment, but no control group or comparison group
Level 5
   Case report (a report of a single case)
   Expert opinion
   Personal observation

Nursing Diagnoses To Consider:
- *Impaired Skin Integrity / Risk for Impaired Skin Integrity*: Altered /Risk for altered epidermis and/or dermis

Selected Life Care Planning Considerations:
- Sleep surface: low-shear, low-airloss mattress or overlay
- Orthotics, braces, wheelchair, other materials to be professionally fitted
- Nutrition and hydration
- Laboratory studies to monitor nutrition and healing ability: albumin, prealbumin, vitamin levels, testosterone level
- Invasive devices
- Skin care products
- Moisture management
- Incontinence management
- WOCN consult, plastic surgery consult

Bladder Function

During World War I, 39% of those with spinal cord injury died from acute urinary tract infections (UTI). During World War II, this dropped to 10 percent, and the most common cause of death from SCI was renal failure, likely related to UTI. Currently, less than 3 percent of deaths following SCI are now attributable to chronic renal failure (Consortium for Spinal Cord Medicine, 2006).

Normal bladder emptying requires a coordinated set of conditions and actions. First, relaxation in the proximal urethra and striated urethral sphincter decreases resistance to urinary outflow. Next, adequate contraction by the bladder smooth muscle increases intravesical pressure, resulting in urine flow (in the absence of anatomic obstruction).

The pons micturition center coordinates these actions, and the frontal cortex controls the timing. The ability to empty the bladder completely, regularly, and at low pressures is important to maintain renal health and prevent urinary tract infections. The main goals of a bladder program following a S CI include (Wolfe, 2010):

- achieving regular bladder emptying while avoiding stasis
- avoiding high filling and voiding pressures
- maintaining continence while avoiding frequency and urgency
- preventing and treating complications, e.g., UTI, stones, strictures, and autonomi c dysreflexia (which see).

Spinal cord injury can affect any part of the micturition process, depending on the location and extent of neurological damage. Tracts to and from the pons and cortex are disrupted, resulting in loss of coordinate d bladder filling and emptying (Wolfe, 2010). Most individuals with SCI are diagnosed with neurogenic bladder.

Main Types of Bladder Dysfunction in SCI

Detrusor overactivity associated with sphincter dyssynergia (DESD) is seen in persons with upper motor neuron SCI (injuries at or above L1). Also called a reflex or spastic bladder, it is characterized by the bladder automatically triggering to empty, high urine residuals, decreased bladder capacity, and sphincter dyssynergy.

Detrusor areflexia, also called flaccid bladder, is seen in patients with a lower motor neuron SCI (injuries L1 or below). Loss of detrusor muscle tone prevents bladder emptying, with bladder wall damage from over-filling, urine reflux, and an increase in infection risk due to stasis (SCIRE bladder management, 2010).

The bladder management program for each depends largely on its associated diagnosed neurological dysfunction. Since bladder function often changes over time, diagnostic studies should be planned every twelve to twenty-four months, or more often if clinically indicated (Blackwell et al., 2001, and others as cited).

Diagnostic Studies:
- *Renal sonogram/ultrasound* is a noninvasive test to evaluate the health of the kidney.

    Cystoscopy is the use of a scope to examine the bladder visually. This is done either to look at the bladder for abmormalities or to help with surgery being performed on the inside of the urinary tract (transurethral surgery (Emedicine 2001)

    Most often done after ten years of indwelling catheter use or with any other elevated risk for bladder cancer, e.g., smokers, frequent UTI, and over age 40 (Blackwell et al., 2001)
- *Urodynamics* to assess how the bladder and urethra are performing their job of storing and releasing urine in cases of voluntary or spontaneous voiding (Blackwell et al., 2001)
- *Abdominal radiography of the kidneys, ureters, and bladder (KUB)*
- *24-hour urine for creatinine clearance*
- *Urinalysis*
- *Post-void residual*
- *Other tests* as needed, e.g., renal radionucleotide scan
- *Comprehensive gynecological examination* for females

Medications for treating neurogenic bladder can be divided into two categories. For facilitating emptying in detrusor areflexia, bethanecol (Duvoid, Urecholine) is usually used. For facilitating storage in DESD, current choices are:
- propiverine (Detrunorm)
- oxybutynin (Ditropan, Lyrinel)
- tolterodine (Detrol)
- trospium chloride (Sanctura)

Tolterodine, propiverine, or transdermal oxybutynin may result in less dry mouth but are as good as oral oxybutynin in improving neurogenic detrusor overactivity (SCIRE Bladder Management, 2010).

Catheterization Options

Intermittent catheterization is the bladder management program of choice for those with sufficient cognition and hand skills. Abnormal urethral anatomy, stricture, false passages, bladder neck obstruction, bladder capacity less than 200 ml or adverse reaction to passing a catheter are contraindications (Consortium for Spinal Cord Medicine for Spinal Cord Medicine, 2006). Clean intermittent catheterization is taught to persons with SCI; however, consider sterile catheterization for individuals with recurrent symptomatic infections occurring with clean intermittent catheterization (Consortium for Spinal Cord Medicine, 2006).

Credé and Valsalva maneuvers to facilitate voiding are successful for some persons with lower motor neuron injuries with low outlet resistance, and for males who use an external catheter after sphincterotomy. Credé and Valsalva maneuvers should not be the primary method of bladder emptying because of the potential for incomplete emptying, hydronephrosis, ureteral damage, and other complications (Consortium for Spinal Cord Medicine, 2006).

Indwelling catheterization is recommended for those who are unable to perform intermittent catheterization due to physical, cognitive, or lifestyle issues. The familiar Foley urethral catheter is a usual first step. A suprapubic catheter should be considered for individuals with urethral abnormalities, such as stricture, false passages, bladder neck obstruction, or urethral fistula. Because of issues with urethral discomfort and erosion, suprapubic catheterization is recommended for any patient needing long-term indwelling catheterization. Complications associated with long term indwelling catheterization include:

- bladder and kidney stones
- recurrent symptomatic urinary tract
- incontinence; pyelonephritis
- hydronephrosis from bladder wall thickening
- fibrosis
- bladder cancer

Additionally, if the indwelling catheter pierces the urethra the additional problems of urethral erosions and epididymitis occur (Consortium for Spinal Cord Medicine, 2006).

External (condom) catheters are an option for males after spinal shock with reflex bladder contractions, if they have sufficient hand skills to put on a condom catheter and empty the leg bag, or a willing caregiver. Potential complications with reflex voiding include:

- condom catheter leakage and/or failure
- penile skin breakdown from external condom catheter
- urethral fistula
- UTI
- poor bladder emptying
- high intravesical voiding pressures
- autonomic dysreflexia (AD) (with injuries at T6 and above) (Consortium for Spinal Cord Medicine, 2006)

Individuals who use reflex voiding as their method of bladder management have two options to help decrease detrusor sphincter dyssynergia. Alpha-blockers and botulinum toxin injection into the urinary sphincter mechanism are nonsurgical. Surgical approaches are transurethral sphincterotomy and endourethral stenting. Electrical stimulation and posterior sacral rhizotomy are recommended for some individuals with problems that are unable to be addressed by other means.

For individuals with high SCI, bladder augmentation, continent urinary diversion, urinary diversion and cutaneous ileovesicostomy can afford independence and can be an alternative to other methods when side effects occur. These all involve major surgery. Detailed information for these strategies can be found in *Bladder Management for Adults with Spinal Cord Injury*, Consortium for Spinal Cord Medicine (2006).

Urinary Tract Infections

UTI is common following SCI. Signs and symptoms include:

- leukocytes in the urine generated by the mucosal lining
- discomfort or pain over the kidneys or bladder or during urination
- onset of urinary incontinence
- fever
- increased spasticity
- AD
- cloudy urine with increased odor
- malaise, lethargy, or sense of unease

Significant bacteriuria varies according to the method of urinary drainage and is defined as:
- *any* detectable concentration of uropathogens in urine specimens from indwelling or suprapubic catheters
- ≥ 102 colony-forming units of uropathogens per milliliter (cfu/mL) in catheter specimens from persons on intermittent catheterization
- ≥ 104 cfu/mL in clean-voided specimens from catheter-free men using condom catheters
- ≥ 105 cfu/mL for spontaneous management (SCIRE, Bladder Management, 2011)

Both limited and full microbial investigation may result in adequate clinical response to UTI treatment with antibiotics. Indwelling or suprapubic catheters should be changed just prior to urine collection to limit false positives. Urinalysis and urine culture results are not likely to be affected by sample refrigeration (up to 24 hours). It is uncertain if dipstick testing for nitrates or leukocyte esterase is useful in screening for bacteriuria to assist treatment decision-making (SCIRE, Bladder Management, 2011).

Any bladder management regimen should minimize foreign body access to the urinary system and reduce potential for continued bacterial presence by draining the bladder effectively. Sterile and clean approaches to intermittent catheterization seem equally effective in minimizing UTIs in inpatient rehabilitation. Although the standard for intermittent clean catheter replacement used to be weekly, effective in 2008 Medicare guidelines now provide for 200 sterile one-time use catheters per month to decrease incidence of UTI (Table 4).

Portable bladder scanners can be used to measure urinary retention, and may reduce the number of intermittent catheterizations; they also are effective in reducing unnecessary irrigation by confirming whether a decrease in urine output is due to a blockage or reduced urine in the bladder, thereby minimizing breaks in a closed drainage system (Moore and Edwards, 1997).

It is generally recommended that persons with SCI be treated for bacteriuria only if they have symptoms, as many individuals especially with indwelling or suprapubic catheters typically have asymptomatic bacteriuria (Biering-Sorensen et al., 2001). Use of pre-lubricated or hydrophilic catheters vs. non-hydrophilic; intermittent catheterization vs. indwelling or suprapubic catheters, and use of the Statlock device to secure indwelling and suprapubic catheters appear to decrease UTI incidence. Vesico-ureteral reflux likely has a greater influence on significant infection development than choice of bladder management (SCIRE 2010).

The most common antibiotics chosen for UTI treatment include fluoroquinolones (e.g. ciprofloxacin), trimethoprim, sulfamethoxazole, amoxicillin, nitrofurantoin and ampicillin. Fluoroquinolones are often chosen because of their effectiveness over a wide spectrum of bacterial strains (Garcia Leoni and Esclarin De Ruz, 2003). SCIRE (2010) reviewed a number of studies of antibiotics for UTI in SCI. These are reported at http://www.scireproject. com/rehabilitation-evidence/bladder-management/ urinary-tract-infections/pharmacological-treatment-of-uti

Nursing Diagnoses To Consider:
- *Impaired Urinary Elimination:* Dysfunction in urine elimination
- *Ineffective Self-Health Management:* Pattern of regulating and integrating into daily living a therapeutic regimen for treatment of illness and its sequelae that is unsatisfactory for meeting specific health goals
- *Risk for Compromised Human Dignity:* At risk for perceived loss of respect and honor
- *Caregiver Role Strain/Risk for Caregiver Role Strain*: Difficulty in performing family caregiver role/caregiver is vulnerable for felt difficulty in performing the family caregiver role

Selected Life Care Planning Considerations:
- Incontinence supplies, skin protection, odor control
- Catheters (see Table 4), drainage systems, gloves, lubrication
- Periodic laboratory studies: urine CandS, creatinine clearance, creatinine, BUN
- Bladder scanner
- Primary care for minor UTIs
- Urodynamics, renal system US
- Cystoscopy to check for bladder cancer if indwelling catheter >10 years, smoker >age 40, or frequent UTI
- Medications
- Periodic retraining if self-catheterizing
- Bathroom modifications
- Inpatient care for UTI
- Surgical approaches

Table 4. Medicare sterile technique catheterization guidelines, 2011. www.cms.gov

Medicare will cover sterile single-use intermittent catheters in quantities up to 200 per month with individual packets of lubricant.

- The basic coverage criteria of permanent urinary incontinence or retention must be met. Medicare members may receive quantities of catheters as ordered by their physicians to meet their specific needs.
- The prescription must clearly state the frequency of catheterization, as well as the quantity of catheters required on a monthly basis.
- Clinical documentation is required to support quantity or frequency of use that is greater than 200 per month or 6 per times per day.
- The number of times per day that an individual performs self-catheterization should be clearly documented in the medical record.

Medicare will cover closed system intermittent catheters or sterile intermittent catheters with insertion kits when the member has permanent urinary incontinence, and there is documentation that individuals meet one of the following criteria:

- The Medicare member has 2 distinct, recurrent UTI's while on a program of sterile intermittent catheterization (sterile intermittent catheters with sterile lubricant) within 12 months of each other; or
- The Medicare member resides in a nursing facility; or
- The patient is immunosuppressed; or
- The patient has a radiologically documented vesico-ureteral reflux while on a program of intermittent catheterization; or
- The patient is a spinal-cord injured pregnant female with a neurogenic bladder.

How does Medicare define UTI documentation?
- Urine culture with > 10,000 cfu (colony forming units) of a urinary pathogen AND concurrent documented presence in the urine culture of only one (1) of the following:
- Fever (oral temperature > 100.4 Degrees F)
- Pyuria; elevated white blood cell count (wbc) > 5
- Change in urinary urgency, frequency or incontinence
- Appearance of new or increase in autonomic dysreflexia (sweating, low heart rate, elevated blood pressure)
- Physical signs of prostatitis, epididymitis, orchiitis
- Increased muscle spasms

Neurogenic Bowel

Coping with bowel or bladder/bowel dysfunctions were rated among the highest priorities among individuals with SCI in numerous studies (Anderson 2004). Neurogenic bowel has the potential to influence social, emotional, and physical wellbeing. Fear of bowel accidents is common and deters persons with SCI from participating in social and other outside activities (Correa and Rotter, 2000). Chronic gastrointestinal problems that alter lifestyle and may require treatment affect 27 - 41% of patients with neurogenic bowel. As with bladder function, the type of neurogenic bowel is defined by spinal cord injury level and is also influenced by whether or not the injury is complete (Nelson, 2001).

Reflex neurogenic bowel (upper motor neuron injury) occurs with injury at or above the conus. The bowel is capable of reflexive emptying without cortical awareness of the need to defecate (Jacelon, 2011). Reflex stool evacuation is initiated by rectal stimulus, such as an irritant suppository or digital stimulation with a gloved, lubricated finger (SCIRE, 2010; Shafik et al. 2000). Achieving soft, firm stools (via medications, hydration, and diet) is optimal for this approach (Nelson, 2001).

Areflexive or flaccid bowel (lower motor neuron injury) occurs with injury below the conus. There is no reflex defecation or internal and external sphincter tone (Jacelon, 2011). Manual evacuation with gloved lubricated fingers is often needed for the lower motor neuron injured bowel program and is the method of choice for patients with areflexive bowel. Firm stool is optimal for this approach.

Persons with an incomplete injury may retain the sensation of rectal fullness and ability to evacuate bowels; no specific bowel program may be required (SCIRE, 2010). Establishing an individualized, workable bowel program is imperative. This process must involve the individual and the care team to succeed. A well-developed protocol for designing a bowel program is available from the Paralyzed Veterans Association (PVA) and can be downloaded without charge (Consortium for Spinal Cord Medicine, 1998).

The following items should be taken into consideration in developing a SCI bowel program (Consortium for Spinal Cord Medicine, 1998):

- thorough assessment to determine type of neurogenic bowel dysfunction
- thorough history of past and present bowel problems, diet, nutrition, and medications with bowel affects or side effects

- functional assessment:
  - o ability to learn
  - o ability to direct others
  - o sitting tolerance and angle
  - o sitting balance
  - o upper extremity strength and proprioception
  - o hand and arm function
  - o spasticity
  - o transfer skills

o   actual and potential risks to skin
o   anthropometric characteristics

- home accessibility

- equipment needed

Potential complications of a bowel program are delayed evacuation, unplanned bowel movements, and individual or caregiver dissatisfaction. Potential complications related to bowel programs include:

- diarrhea or constipation
- impaction
- hemorrhoids
- increased pain
- spasticity
- AD
- falls during transport or while carrying out the procedure
- pressure ulcers. (Nelson, 2001)

Establishing a good bowel program can take a longer than expected (Nelson, 2001). Taking advantage of the gastrocolic reflex and sitting on a commode, vs. lying in bed for bowel program, can assist the person with a SCI have faster results.

Medications, e.g., fiber and stool softeners, will be needed to maintain stool consistency. Stimulants such as mild laxatives, suppositories, and mini-enemas are active ingredients in many bowel programs. Bisacodyl (Dulcolax) and glycerin are the most common active ingredients (SCIRE 2010). Medications take longer to work in the neurogenic bowel than the normal bowel (Nelson, 2001). Opioids are constipating and should be avoided if at all possible.

Some individuals with SCI have a more difficult time developing an effective bowel program that results in regular bowel movements and few accidents. More complex bowel treatment /surgical strategies may be necessary, e.g., colostomy or the Malone antegrade continence enema (MACE) (Christensen et al. 2000). There has been some recent research on bowel evacuation technologies. Examples of these are pulsed water irrigation systems (Christensen et al. 2006, Puet et al. 1997), sacral anterior root stimulation (Valles, 2009), and electrical stimulation of abdomen and bowel (Korsten et al., 2007).

It is important for the correct equipment to be available for an effective bowel program. The recommendations of the experienced rehabilitation team should be followed. Please see the table on Bathroom Equipment, Assistive Devices, and Outcomes by Level of Injury by the Consortium for Spinal Cord Medicine for details (Consortium for Spinal Cord Medicine, 1998).

Nursing Diagnoses To Consider:
- *Bowel Incontinence:* Change in normal bowel habits characterized by involuntary passage of stool
- *Ineffective Self-Health Management:* Pattern of regulating and integrating into daily living a therapeutic regimen for treatment of illness and its sequelae that is unsatisfactory for meeting specific health goals
- *Risk for Compromised Human Dignity:* At risk for perceived loss of respect and honor
- *Caregiver Role Strain/Risk for Caregiver Role Strain:* Difficulty in performing family caregiver role/caregiver is vulnerable for felt difficulty in performing the family caregiver role

Selected Life Care Planning Considerations:
- Incontinence supplies, pads, briefs, skin protection, exam gloves, finger cots
- Stool softeners, laxative suppositories, enemas, rectal stimulator
- Commode chair
- Bathroom modifications
- GI consult for stimulator technology

Spasticity

Spasticity is disordered sensorimotor control, resulting from an upper motor neuron lesion, presenting as intermittent or sustained involuntary activation of muscle. (Pandyan, 2005) Studies indicate that involuntary supraspinal descending inputs, and inhibited spinal reflexes, and changes in muscle properties contribute to clinical spasticity and rigidity, which are frequently linked (SCIRE, Spasticity, 2010). Although spasticity does not typically worsen over time, uncontrolled spasticity has effects on emotional adaptation, dependency, secondary health problems, and environmental integration (Krause, 2007). After SCI, 41% of individuals with SCI give spasticity as a major medical obstacle to community and workplace reintegration (SCIRE, 2010).

Unmanaged spasticity impairs comfort, function, posture, and safety. Spasticity is not all bad; some individuals can take advantage of it to assist with activities of daily living, transfers and other activities. Nevertheless, changes in spasticity in a stable patient should *always* be considered as a potential indicator of a complication in another organ system, e.g., UTI, bladder stone, pressure ulcer, or appendicitis.

Baclofen (Lioresal, Kemstro) is widely used as the first line of pharmacological treatment for spasticity. Tizanidine (Zanaflex), clonidine (Catapres), diazepam (Valium), and dantrolene (Dantrium) may also be useful in treating SCI spasticity. There is inconsistent evidence for the use of Delta(9)-tetrahydrocannabinol (THC, Dronabinol) in reducing spastic pain in SCI individuals (Hagenbach et al., 2006; SCIRE 2010), though it has been extensively studied in multiple sclerosis.

Botulinum neurotoxin (Botox) appears to improve focal muscle spasticity in people with SCI. Phenol block may improve pain, range of motion and function related to shoulder spasticity in individuals with tetraplegia (SCIRE, 2010).

Programmable pumps can be implanted to decrease spasticity, most commonly for intrathecal baclofen, although other drugs or combinations of drugs can be used. Bolus or long-term intrathecal baclofen may improve functional outcomes with low complication rates and is a cost-effective intervention. Intrathecal baclofen improves musculoskeletal pain post SCI and may help dysethetic pain related to spasticity (SCIRE, 2010).

Nonpharmaceutical interventions that can be helpful adjuncts in decreasing spasticity and may produce short-term reductions in spasticity include (SCIRE, 2010):

- hippotherapy
- neural facilitation techniques
- range of motion
- rhythmic passive movements
- prolonged standing
- active exercise interventions
- FES-assisted cycling
- walking

Nursing Diagnoses To Consider:
- *Self-Neglect:* A constellation of culturally framed behaviors involving one or more self-care activities in which there is a failure to maintain a socially accepted standard of health and well-being (Givens, Lauder, and Ludwick, 2006)
- *Self-Care Deficit* (bathing, dressing, feeding, toileting): Impaired ability to perform or complete specified activities for self
- *Chronic Pain:* Unpleasant sensory or emotional experience arising from actual or potential tissue damage or described in terms of such damage (International Association for the Study of Pain); sudden or slow onset of any intensity from mild to severe with an anticipated or predictable end and a duration of greater than 6 months

Selected Life Care Planning Considerations:
- Increased risk of falls, pressure ulcers, pain
- Medications: antispasmodics, oral, parenteral, or via implantable; neuromuscular blockade; pain management
- Implantables: trials, inpatient/outpatient diagnostics, implantation, reservoir refills, battery changes
- Aquatherapy
- Music therapy, hippotherapy
- Functional electronic stimulation
- Neurology or physiatry routine follow up
- DME changes related to altered body positioning: bracing, wheelchair fit, and other DME for safety and comfort
- Surgical release of tendons; postoperative splints, physical therapy, occupational therapy

Intrathecal baclofen is a mainstay of severe spasticity management. The following information is representative and for information only. Please check with the physician and/or suppliers for specifics on any individual case.

Projections:
Botox Injections:
    Surgeon-CPT 42699
    Surgeon-CPT 76536 (ultrasound) Medication-100 IU
    Radiology-CPT 76536

If oral or local injection medications are not sufficient, the treating team may recommend an implantable pump. This will require planning for implantation, monitoring, reprogramming, and replacement as indicated.

Table 5. Implantable baclofen pump replacement schedule

Item or service	Frequency
Baclofen pump replacement, 24 hour inpatient stay CPT 62350 (catheter placement) CPT 62362 (pump placement)	Every seven years
Baclofen pump refill, outpatient or office CPT 95991, 62368, as well as E and M codes.	Every three to four months

Item or service	Frequency
Baclofen pump replacement, 24 hour inpatient stay CPT 62350 (catheter placement) CPT 62362 (pump placement)	Every seven years
Electronic analysis with programming	Every 1-4 months
Electronic analysis without programming	1-2 times per year as needed

Barker, E and Saulino M. Life care planning for the client with severe spasticity: Intrathecal baclofen therapy. Journal of Life Care Planning, Vol. 3, No. 1, 3-14, 2004; Medtronic Corporation, 2010)

The medication used in the pump is billed via J codes (J0475) by the MD or hospital pharmacy. Medication amounts are prescribed by units. The maintenance dose of baclofen is usually 2000mcg/ml concentration, dispensed in 20ml and 40ml kits (Personal communication, K. Emmett, Medtronic Corporation, 2010). The following summarizes procedure and coding often found with implantable pumps. *Current codes and costs should be obtained from the manufacturer, Medtronic, at 763-505-5000 or 800-328-0810 toll-free.*

Intrathecal Programmable Medication Pump:
Pre-Placement Trial/Screening Kit and *Initial Permanent Placement*
> CPT 62311 or 62319 (lumbar puncture)/Surgeon fee
> Screening Kit CPT 8563S

Physical Therapy Session (90 minutes) -CPT 97039
Recovery Room/Observation (RN): 6-12 hours by Registered Nurse
> Facility-CPT 62350 (catheter placement) Facility-CPT 62362 (pump placement)
> Anesthesia/Medication/etc.-CPT 99070
> Anesthesiologist-CPT 00630 (1.5 to 2.0 hours) Pump (ED783) and Pump Kit (A4220)
> Surgeon-CPT 62362 (pump placement) Surgeon-CPT 62350 (catheter placement) Facility-CPT 62367 (programming)
> Surgeon-CPT 77003 (fluoroscopy) Medication: Baclofen J0475

Facility Costs-LOS: 5.0 days
Intrathecal Programmable Medication Pump: *Permanent Replacement*
> Preoperative work up (CBC, Chem Panel, PT, PTT, Type and Cross, Chest X-ray, EKG, Pediatrician/IM Eval)
> Facility-CPT 62362 (placement of new pump)
> Anesthesia/Medication/etc.-CPT 99070
> Anesthesiologist-CPT 00630 (1.5 to 2.0 hours) Pump (ED783) and Pump Kit (A4220)
> Surgeon-CPT 62362 (placement of new pump)
> Surgeon-CPT 62367 (reprogramming)
> Surgeon-CPT 77003 (fluoroscopy) Medication: Baclofen J0475
> Report

Facility Costs-LOS: 5.0 days
Intrathecal Programmable Medication Pump:
Reprogramming/Refill
> Professional-CPT 62368 (reprogramming)
> Professional-CPT 65991
> Facility-CPT 62368

Facility-CPT 65991
Medication: Baclofen J0745

Pain in Spinal Cord Injury

Despite impressive gains in bladder, skin, cardiovascular and respiratory care in SCI, the treatment of chronic pain has not been as successful. Pain is a frequent complication of traumatic spinal cord injury. Severe pain was noted in 10-15% of persons with quadriplegia; 25% of those with thoracic paraplegia and 42-51% of those with lesions of the cauda equine (Ragnarsson, 1997). Reported estimates of the incidence of pain following SCI range anywhere from 11% to 94% with more recent studies reporting an incidence from 48-94% (SCIRE, Pain Management, 2010).

Pain syndromes in SCI can have devastating effects on the capacity to achieve health-related outcomes. Pain is often reported as the most important factor for decreased quality of life. Nepomuceno (1979) noted that 23% of individuals with cervical or high thoracic SCI and 37% of those with low thoracic or lumbosacral injury would trade the loss of sexual and/or bowel and bladder function *and* hypothetical possibility for cure to obtain pain relief. Awareness of the type of pain syndrome the patient is experiencing, the mechanisms involved, and therapies that have demonstrated a positive effect on outcomes can help nurses to advocate for better pain management in this challenging condition (Starkweather, 2007).

Pain Origins

Pain can originate from skin (cutaneous), muscle/ tendons (somatic), internal organs (visceral), nerves (neuropathic), or be referred from a different area of the body. Correctly identifying pain's origin and type of the pain is critical since different types require different treatment. Pain in SCI can be caused by (Siddall, 2000):

- spinal instability
- muscle spasm
- overuse or pressure syndromes
- nerve root entrapment
- pain from cauda equina injury
- segmental deafferentation
- pain at the level of injury
- syringomyelia
- visceral pain

Referral to a pain specialist with SCI experience is recommended. Treatment efficacy can be compromised by an incomplete understanding of pain in individuals with spinal cord injuries and lack of a standardized framework upon which to classify these injuries (Burchiel and Hsu, 2001).

In 1997, the International Association for the Study of Pain developed a classification system that is gaining widespread acceptance (Agency for Healthcare Research and Quality, 2003). The first axis of this classification includes the four major categories or divisions of pain. Of these, musculoskeletal and neuropathic pain syndromes are most common in SCI (Starkweather, 2007).

Musculoskeletal pain after SCI is generally located in the region of preserved sensation close to the site of the spinal injury, although it may radiate (Starkweather, 2007). As the SCI ages, the effects of overuse of functional muscles/structures increases. It is important that the person with a SCI understands the relationship between overwork and musculoskeletal pain. Therapy and exercise programs to maintain and preserve function are very important. In consideration of expected changes with aging, the life care planner should identify equipment that decreases the workload on the shoulders and other functioning units.

Visceral pain is identified by location (abdomen) and by pain features (dull, poorly localized, bloating and cramping in nature), and may be intermittent. Diagnosis when sensory input from visceral structures is not intact is difficult. If investigations fail to find evidence of visceral pathology and treatments directed at visceral pathology do not relieve pain, then consideration must be given to classifying the pain as neuropathic rather than visceral (Siddall et al., 2000).

Neuropathic pain is described as burning, shooting, lancinating, "pins and needles," or strange sensations, e.g., formiculation (like crawling insects). Allodynia, painful response to normally nonpainful stimuli, occurs frequently in SCI (IASP, 2011). It can be seen in three regional presentations (Siddall and Middleton, 2006):

- *Above-level* neuropathic pain is not specific to SCI, and may result from overuse at any time.
- *At-level* neuropathic pain may be due to damage to the nerve roots or the spinal cord. Syringomyelia must always be considered in the person who has delayed onset of at level pain, especially where there is a rising level of sensory loss. MRI establishes the diagnosis.
- *Below-level* neuropathic pain develops sometime after the initial injury. It presents with spontaneous and/ or evoked pain, often diffusely, but is not related to position or movement. It is characterized by sensations of burning, aching, stabbing, stinging, freezing, or electric shocks, often with hyperalgesia. It is constant, but may fluctuate with mood, being occupied, infection, sudden noise, jarring, or other factors. Incomplete injuries are more likely to have an allodynic component due to sparing of tract conveying touch sensations (Siddal and Middleton, 2006)

Wind-up pain is caused by constant stimulation of the second order neurons in the dorsal horn by impulses from referral nerves. The resulting neuroplasticity effect results in a receptor that is extremely fast and appears to be responsible for not only amplifying pain, but also causing opioid tolerance. (D'Arcy Y, 2011)

A basic data set (interview checklist) for clinical evaluation of pain after SCI was recently developed by an international expert panel and endorsed by several major pain organizations and SCI societies. It is available free for the American Spinal Injury Association (ASIA) and the International Spinal Cord Society at http://www.iscos.org.uk/files/PageFile_20_International%20SCI%20Pain%20Basic%20Data%20Set%20incl.%20Training%20cases.pdf or http://tinyurl.com/7rqrwaj

Decubitus ulcers, UTI or stone, AD, increased spasticity, anxiety, depression, psychosocial factors, and other conditions may worsen SCI pain (SCIRE, Pain Management, 2010).

Treatment

Identifying the best treatment plan is difficult and best deferred to clinicians experienced in treating SCI pain. Ideal treatment will include a combination of medication, education, and nonpharmaceutical strategies. SCI patients with more severe pain, in more locations, those with allodynia or hyperalgesia, and those in whom the pain was more likely to interfere with activities were more likely to use pain medications (Widerstrom-Noga and Turk, 2003; SCIRE, 2010).

For persons with musculoskeletal pain, acetaminophen or an NSAID may be effective (Starkweather, 2007). NSAIDS are often ineffective in complete SCI neuropathic pain relief and have potential risks, e.g., gastric ulceration, with prolonged use (SCIRE, 2010). The use of NSAIDs or opioids should be considered on a case-by-case basis (Siddall and Middleton, 2006).

Tricyclic antidepressants appear to be effective in reducing neuropathic pain. SSRIs are not as effective. Amitriptyline is effective in reducing pain in depressed SCI individuals. Trazodone (Desyrel) does not reduce post-SCI pain (SCIRE, 2010). Research has shown that gabapentin (Neurontin) and pregabalin (Lyrica) improve neuropathic pain after SCI, and lamotrigine (Lamictal) may be effective in patients with an incomplete SCI (SCIRE, 2010). Lidocaine through a subarachnoid lumbar catheter and intravenous ketamine (Ketanest, Ketalar) improve post-SCI pain short term (SCIRE, 2010). Evidence points to the fact that tramadol (Ultram) is effective against neuropathic pain, intravenous morphine reduces mechanical allodynia; alfentanil (Alfenta) reduces chronic pain post SCI and is more effective in reducing wind-up-like pain than ketamine (SCIRE, 2010).

Topical capsaicin was used in one study to treat radicular post-SCI pain for one to two weeks. Patients showed improvement in pain and two of the eight patients were still improved for over 2 years (Sandford and Benes, 2000). Ziconotide (Prialt) in combination with low dose morphine was effective in managing chronic pain and improving quality of life without significant side effects in a case study of a patient with refractory pain (Madaris, 2008). This drug has been investigated successfully for use chronic pain (Rauck et al., 2006; Webster, Fisher et al., 2009).

Surgical interventions to alleviate post SCI pain have had some success, as noted:.
- spinal cord stimulation
- DREZ (dorsal root entry zone) myelotomy. Persons with segmental pain are more likely to benefit from this procedure.
- dorsal longitudinal T-myelotomy procedures

There is little evidence that spinal cordotomy is effective. Sympathectomy is not recommended for pain following SCI (SCIRE, 2010). Massage, heat, acupuncture, cognitive behavioral therapy, hypnosis, healing touch, general physical fitness, and overall good preventive health practices can also help to relieve pain after SCI (SCIRE, 2010).

Nursing Diagnoses To Consider:
- *Chronic Pain:* Unpleasant sensory or emotional experience arising from actual or potential tissue damage or described in terms of such damage (International Association for the Study of Pain); sudden or slow onset of any intensity from mild to severe with an anticipated or predictable end and a duration of greater than six months

Selected Life Care Planning Considerations:
- Pain management team consultation and follow up
- Medications: topical, oral/tube, implantable
- Surgical interventions (as above): hospitalization, outpatient care, trials, implants; anticipated repeat therapies
- Recreational therapy
- Psychological support

Cardiovascular

Communication between the brainstem and the autonomic nervous system (ANS) is important for the control of cardiovascular function and is often compromised after SCI (McKinley, 2011). Morbidity and mortality from cardiovascular disease (CVD) in long-term SCI now exceed those caused by renal and pulmonary conditions, the primary causes of mortality in previous decades (Myers, 2007). Although cardiovascular function improves after acute injury, risk of complications associated with cardiovascular and thermoregulation dysfunction continues. Lifelong reassessment is necessary (Nelson, 2001).

Persons with SCI have a greater incidence of obesity, lipid disorders, metabolic syndrome, and diabetes (Myers, 2007). Physiologic changes associated with SCI alone confer a higher risk of CVD. Thus, screening, recognition, and treatment of CVD is an essential component of managing individuals with SCI, and judicious treatment of risk factors can play an important role in minimizing the incidence of CVD in these individuals (Myers, 2007). Regular cardiovascular assessments should be scheduled as the individual ages (Nelson, 2010).

Cardiovascular Issues in SCI (Jacelon, 2010; Myers, 2007)

Inability to regulate temperature by vasoactive means (dilation, constriction)

Hypotension at rest related to lack of muscle tone in lower extremities, abdomen

Orthostatic hypotension This is more common with high thoracic and cervical injuries.

Pharmaceutical interventions (e.g., ephedrine) are used prophylactically or when symptoms occur, only when other methods such as abdominal binders, compression hose, and reclining wheelchairs fail.

Autonomic dysreflexia (see above)

Heart rate variability (HRV) is a measure of beat-to beat variations of the R-R interval on the electrocardiogram. This is measured for a few minutes to 24 hrs. An abnormal (reduced) HRV strongly predicts risk for cardiac events. HRV in SCI is abnormal compared to that of able-bodied individuals (Myers, 2007).

Cardiac arrhythmias can include severe bradycardia, A-V block, and cardiac arrest. Treatment is often atropine, but in rare instances, pacemaker implantation may be required. Arrhythmia management in SCI should be similar to ambulatory individuals, i.e., by the presence or absence of CVD (Myers, 2007).

Blunted cardiovascular response to activity results in reduced capacity to adapt appropriately to exercise, resulting in early fatigue, general avoidance of exertion, and deconditioning, which further contribute to CVD risk (Myers, 2007).

Deep vein thrombosis (DVT) and *pulmonary embolism* (PE) are common complications of acute SCI and major causes of morbidity and mortality. Morbidities from DVT include postphlebitic syndrome, prolonged edema, and pressure ulcers; PE, the most serious, can cause arrhythmias, hypoxia, and death (McKinney, 2011) and may occur despite adequate thromboprophylaxis (McKinney, 2011).

Routine prophylaxis in acute injury is essential (Geerts, 2008). DVT incidence has been shown to range from 7 to 100% even in the presence of anticoagulation therapy, depending on age and severity of injury; 2.7% develop fatal pulmonary embolism. Prophylactic treatment is usually recommended for three months post injury.

DVT incidence is significantly lower when adjusted-dose heparin or low molecular-eight heparin (LMWH) for anticoagulant prophylaxis is administered within 72 hours after spinal cord injury, after active bleeding, evidence of head injury, or coagulopathy are ruled out (Consortium for Spinal Cord Medicine, 1997, 2008). In a retrospective study, 38.6% of patients admitted to a rehabilitation hospital were receiving DVT prophylaxis (Powell, 1999).

The usual symptoms of DVT are sometimes hidden by the fact that the patient is insensate. Presence of lower extremity edema does not always indicate DVT; suspected DVT should be evaluated by objective methods. Ultrasonography is preferred as is noninvasive and sensitive (98-100%) (McKinney, 2011).

Vena cava filter placement is indicated in patients who have not achieved success with anticoagulant prophylaxis or who have a contraindication to anticoagulation (Consortium for Spinal Cord Medicine, 2008). This procedure is not a substitute for thromboprophylaxis, due to the morbidity related to DVT and the propagation of vena cava embolism. Possible complications include vena cava thrombosis, filter migration, and vena cava perforation (McKinney, 2011). For suspected PE, ventilation/perfusion (V/Q) lung scanning is indicated (McKinney, 2011).

Once the diagnosis of DVT is made, the usual treatment regimen includes LMWH initially, and prophylactic warfarin for at least 6 months. The International Normalized Ratio (INR) should be maintained between 2 and 3 (Myers, 2007). Patients with spinal cord injury who have recurrences of thromboembolic disease may also require prolonged therapy (McKinney, 2011).

Prompt and accurate diagnosis and treatment can prevent more serious complications. Therefore, patients, family members, and caregivers should be educated in the recognition and prevention of DVT.

Nursing Diagnoses To Consider:
- *Impaired Gas Exchange:* Excess or deficit in oxygenation and/or carbon dioxide elimination at the alveolar-capillary membrane
- *Impaired Skin Integrity / Risk for Impaired Skin Integrity:* Altered /Risk for altered epidermis and/or dermis
- *Autonomic Dysreflexia / Risk for Autonomic Dysreflexia:* Life-threatening, uninhibited sympathetic response /Risk for life-threatening, uninhibited sympathetic response to a noxious stimulus after a spinal cord injury at T7 or above (has been demonstrated in patients with injuries at T7 and T8).

Selected Life Care Planning Considerations:
- Medications: cardiovascular, anticoagulation; diabetic
- Primary care
  - o routine labs for health monitoring: metabolic panel, CBC
  - o manage anticoagulation; periodic lab studies
  - o monitor for cardiac conditions: laboratory studies, EKG

- Specialty consultation if needed
  - o diagnostic imaging studies
  - o invasive procedures: stents, thrombectomy, umbrella placement
- Inpatient admission

Sexuality / Reproduction

Sexuality is an integral part of being human. While changes to sexual function usually refer to changes in arousal (erection in men and vaginal lubrication in women), ejaculation in men, and orgasm in men and women, in SCI sexuality also includes the psychological and physiological effects of loss of motor and sensory function, bladder and bowel control and alterations to body image, and sexual self esteem (SCIRE, 2010). A study of 684 persons with SCI revealed that for the majority of individuals with paraplegia, regaining sexual function was rated the highest priority. For those with tetraplegia, sexual function was rated as the second highest priority after restoration of hand and arm function (Anderson, 2004).

After injury, sexuality should be introduced and addressed as the patient appears ready. Sexuality should be discussed in a straightforward and nonjudgmental manner, taking into consideration the individual's interest and readiness to learn. Exploring the role of sexuality and ways to express it is encouraged (Consortium for Spinal Cord Medicine, Sexuality, 2010).

Although most persons receive at least some sexuality information during inpatient rehabilitation, most are not ready to address it during the acute phase. When they are ready, they do know how to obtain the information that they need.

The assessment evaluation should be completed by a practitioner who is comfortable discussing the topic (Consortium for Spinal Cord Medicine, Sexuality, 2010). It should include:

- Physical exam to evaluate the impact of the injury on genital responses
- Frank discussion of prior sexual history, including previous sexual trauma, sexual dysfunction, or sexually transmitted disease
- Medication effects on sexual response and fertility, e.g., alcohol, tobacco, and other drugs
- Effects of unhealthy eating habits and obesity
- Presence of depression or other psychological disorders

An evaluation for a diagnosis of testosterone deficiency should be completed in men presenting with suppressed libido, reduced strength, fatigue, or poor response to oral medications for erection enhancement (Consortium for Spinal Cord Medicine, Sexuality, 2010). Genital response depends on the level and completeness of the injury. Psychogenic erections are found in men with incomplete injuries, while higher levels are associated with a better chance of achieving and sustaining erections and ejaculation. Intercourse is difficult without some medical assistance. Women have limited lubrication. Movement of the pelvic area is limited. Women noted the importance of physical closeness and intimate touch regardless of whether intercourse was still enjoyable (Lebowitz, 2007).

Individuals with SCI may need to be encouraged to expand their sexual repertoire to enhance their sexual pleasure following injury (Consortium for Spinal Cord Medicine-Sexuality, 2010). Education should take into consideration age and previous sexual experience and include methods to enhance sensuality by using all available senses, and sexual assistive devices (sex toys) that are sometimes used to enhance sexual experiences. Treatment of sexual dysfunction should include (Consortium for Spinal Cord Medicine, Sexuality, 2010):

- Resources for sex education, counseling, and sex therapy when indicated

- Education about the potential risks related to services or products available without a prescription
- Education for women with SCI about external devices that are available to enhance genital arousal and orgasmic potential

The PLISSIT Model of Intervention (Annon, 1976) is commonly used. PLISSIT is an acronym for four levels of intervention that were developed by psychologist Dr. Jack Anon: permission, limited information, specific suggestions, and intensive therapy.

- **P**ermission, the most basic and general level of intervention, allows the patient to express concerns in this area. Patients are reassured that their feelings are normal, acceptable, and a sign of recovery.

- **Li**mited information relates to patient concerns regarding the impact of their specific condition on sexual expression abilities and may consist of dispelling myths. This level of intervention is often provided in a group setting, includes patients and their sexual partner (if desired), and offers factual information via pamphlets, handouts, and resource lists.

- **S**pecific **S**uggestions are aimed at solving an individual patient's problem and requires advanced knowledge and skill, but may be within the realm of OT service provision. A detailed sexual history is obtained, specific problem(s) identified, and goals collaboratively established that address improved function in the targeted area. Intervention approaches may include problem solving, education, and compensatory strategies.

- The highest level, **I**ntensive **T**herapy, requires formal training and documented competence in sex therapy, sexuality counseling, or psychotherapy. This level of intervention is beyond the scope of typical rehabilitation intervention and indicates the need for referral to a specialist.

Treatment options for erectile dysfunction (ED) after SCI include (SCIRE,2010; Consortium for Spinal Cord Medicine, Sexuality, 2010):

- Oral medications which indirectly relax penile smooth muscle and enhance an erection attained by sexual stimulation, such as the oral phosphodiesterase 5 inhibitors (PDE5i), e.g., sildenafil (Viagra), vardenafil (Levitra), and tadalafil (Cialis)
- Intracavernosal injectable medications, which directly relax the penile smooth muscle creating an erection (prostaglandin E1 penile injections [Caverject® or compounded] and other injectable combinations of papaverine and phentolamine)
- Topical agents for penile smooth muscle relaxation (prostaglandin, minoxidil, papaverine and nitroglycerine)
- Intraurethral prostaglandin E1 (MUSE®)
- Mechanical methods, such as vacuum devices and penile rings
- Surgical penile implants
- Discussion of the potential risk of penile trauma for men
- Behavioral methods (perineal muscle training). Topical agents that cause dilation are not effective for treatment of erectile dysfunction in men with SCI. (SCIRE, 2010)

Implantation of an intrathecal baclofen pump, while effective in managing spasticity, may cause difficulties with erection and sexual function (SCIRE, 2010).

Practical Considerations

Bladder and bowel accidents may occur. These should be anticipated and a contingency plan developed. It is recommended to complete a bowel program prior to sexual activity. Ways to avoid injuring skin or exacerbating existing pressure ulcers should be discussed. Insensate skin surfaces, particularly around the genitalia and buttocks, should be checked after sexual activity for skin tears or signs of pressure. Positioning for sexual activity is dependent on optimal positioning and bed mobility. Individuals must be taught about the potential for risk from the activity itself, autonomic dysreflexia, and safety when using a wheelchair or shower chair for sexual activity.

Fertility (Consortium for Spinal Cord Medicine, 2010)
A woman may not menstruate for months post injury, but fertility remains intact. Women who become pregnant can deliver a healthy child. Women of childbearing age who are sexually active should discuss the risks associated with the various birth control methods with a physician with experience working with SCI; a medical provider with SCI expertise should be involved throughout a pregnancy. The woman's wheelchair will need repeated adjustments throughout the pregnancy. Physical therapy to evaluate the safety of transfers and ADL activities should be recommended. Woman going into labor should anticipate the potential for autonomic dysreflexia.

Male fertility rates have increased to approximately 60% due to technology. However, retrograde (into the bladder) ejaculation is a problem for the majority of men. Semen can be aspirated directly from the vas and banked if necessary; analysis should be carried out for men interested in biological fatherhood to provide information and make recommendations for achieving pregnancy via *in vitro* fertilization or other means. Adoption is an option for some individuals with SCI.

As in any situation, the relationship itself is the most important factor in sexual satisfaction. Counseling and sexual education that promotes a positive body image should involve both persons. Discuss options for providing assistance for activities of daily living, especially bowel and bladder care, from someone other than the romantic partner.

Nursing Diagnoses To Consider:
- *Sexual Dysfunction:* The state in which an individual experiences a change in sexual function during the sexual response phases of desire, excitation, and/or orgasm, which is viewed is unsatisfying, and rewarding, or inadequate
- *Grieving:* A normal complex process that includes emotional, physical, spiritual, social, and intellectual responses and behaviors by which individuals, families, and communities incorporate an actual, anticipated, or perceived loss into their daily lives.

Selected Life Care Planning Considerations:
- Counseling, individual and couple
- Sexuality workshops for SCI
- Reproductive health examination by specialist experienced in SCI
- Sperm retrieval and banking
- IVF
- Specialized prenatal care

Psychosocial

SCI has sudden, drastic effects: helplessness, fear, pain, fatigue, isolation, change in body image, and altered functional abilities. Family and work roles and responsibilities will never be the same. Often the individual is angry: at self, God, or the person or situation that caused the SCI. At this point the patient needs to gain control of something, somehow. Initially, this anger is often expressed in outbursts at staff and family and control is exerted by refusal to participate in rehabilitation.

Depression adjustment disorder Other individuals withdraw. Depression adjustment disorder, also called situational depression, is a stress-related, short-term, nonpsychotic disturbance. It occurs when a person is unable to cope with, or adjust to, a particular source of stress, such as a major life change, loss, or event, and is characterized by being disproportionately overwhelmed or overly intense in responses to stimuli (Benton, 2010). The emergence of depressive symptoms is not surprising; some early investigators have described it as inevitable (SCIRE, 2010).

Major depression Bombardier et al. (2004) found rates of major depression or probable major depression following SCI vary widely across studies and can range from 7% to 31%, with estimates of major depressive disorder typically reported at 15%-23%. Suicidal ideation is reported in 15.4% persons with SCI. (SCIRE, 2010) In one sample of Australians at an average of 19 years post-injury, Migliorini et al. (2008) found 37% were identified as depressed, 30% suffered anxiety, 25% experienced significant stress, and 8.4% reported post-traumatic stress disorder.

Substance abuse can be a significant problem with SCI. Many injuries are incurred as a result of activities involving alcohol or recreational drugs, especially in young males; many persons with depression post-injury self-medicate. This can result in lapses in self-care, causing hospitalization for injuries, infections, pressure ulcers, or other complications. The difficulties are magnified with changes in aging (Craig Hospital, 2010). For more information, RRTC for Substance Abuse and Disability does research and distributes information on the combination of alcohol and disability. Write to the RRTC c/o Wright State University, School of Medicine, 3640 Colonel Glenn Highway, Dayton, OH 45435.

Given the losses and adjustments after SCI, an individual will likely experience repeated strains on available coping resources. Therefore, individual and family counseling with a mental health professional should be made available when needed throughout the lifetime of any person living with SCI. In addition, *cognitive behavioral interventions* provided in a group setting appear helpful in reducing post-SCI depression and related difficulties (SCIRE, 2010).

The benefits of drug treatment for post-SCI depression are largely extrapolated from studies in non-SCI populations (SCIRE, 2010). More study may be needed in this area.

Regular physical exercise may contribute to a reduction of pain, stress, and depression, potentially having a prophylactic effect to prevent recurrent pain and decline in quality of life. Programs that encourage regular exercise, reduce stress, and improve or maintain health appear to reduce depressive symptoms in persons with SCI. Several nontraditional approaches (e.g., massage, transmagnetic stimulation) appear to improve health practices and reduce reported secondary conditions, including depression (SCIRE, 2010).

Nursing Diagnoses To Consider:
- *Disturbed Personal Identity / Risk for Disturbed Personal Identity:* Inability to maintain /Risk of inability to maintain an integrated and complete perception of self
- *Caregiver Role Strain/Risk for Caregiver Role Strain:* Difficulty in performing family caregiver role/caregiver is vulnerable for felt difficulty in performing the family caregiver role)
- *Impaired Parenting/Risk for Impaired Parenting:* Inability/ Risk of inability of the primary caretaker to create, maintain, or regain an environment that promotes the optimal growth and development of the child
- *Dysfunctional Family Processes:* Psychosocial, spiritual, and physiological functions of the family unit are chronically disorganized, which leads to conflict, denial of problems, resistance to change, ineffective problem-solving, and a series of self perpetuating crises
- *Ineffective Coping:* Inability to form a valid appraisal of the stressors, inadequate choices of practice responses, and/or inability to use available resources
- *Grieving:* A normal complex process that includes emotional, physical, spiritual, social, and intellectual

responses and behaviors by which individuals, families, and communities incorporate an actual, anticipated, or perceived loss into their daily lives

- *Powerlessness:* Perception that one's own action will not significantly affect an outcome; perceived lack of control over current situation or immediate happening
- *Hopelessness:* Subjective state in which an individual see limited or no alternatives or personal choices available and is unable to mobilize energy on his own behalf
- *Risk for Compromised Human Dignity:* At risk for perceived loss of respect and honor

Selected Life Care Planning Considerations:
- Individual and family counseling
- Specific therapies: EMD, CBI
- Support groups: BIA, AA, Veterans' groups, Al-Anon
- Recreational therapy
- Gym or health club membership

Aging with a Spinal Cord Injury

As individuals with SCI are living longer and healthier lives with more advanced medical management post-acute SCI, more clinicians are starting to look at other secondary complications such as increased incidence of coronary artery disease, diabetes mellitus, osteoporosis, and pain (Shem, 2006). The general effects of aging complicate the already debilitating effects of the spinal cord injury. These changes are determined by individual factors known to influence the aging process, such as genetics, lifestyle and sociological role (Nelson, 2001). Susan Charlifue, PhD at Craig Hospital in Denver is well-known for her research regarding this topic.

Overall, general life satisfaction is improved over the years. Stress is related to adaptation and coping but not to the level of the injury (Jacelon, 2011).

Skin As a person ages, the skin becomes thinner, with decreased subcutaneous fat (Nelson, 2001) and therefore becomes more prone to pressure ulcers. Persons who have had one pressure ulcer are at more risk to develop another. Also, the risk is higher for unemployed persons and the number of pressure ulcers increase with time (Jacelon, 2011). It would be expected that the aging person will have decreased seating tolerance, and increased need for pressure relief (Nelson, 2001). As skin issues become more probable, it is important to consider changes in DME, sitting, and sleeping surfaces. Increased level of care may be needed when the individual is less able to manage preventive or treatment measures as effectively as before.

Orthopedic Musculoskeletal changes effect strength, endurance and flexibility (Nelson, 2001). This leads to limitations in ability to complete ADLs, transfers, and wheelchair mobility, and will require changes in DME. Persons with SCI have 63% of normal bone density and pathological fractures are more common (Nelson, 2001). Vulnerable joints such as shoulders, elbows and wrists must be protected. Shoulder, elbow, and wrist overuse syndromes are common in manual wheelchair users (Dyson-Hudson et al., 2004; Brose et al., 2008; Yang et al., 2009). Recommendations should consider use of more assistive DME to protect and rest the upper extremities (Consortium for Spinal Cord Medicine, 2005).

Many persons using a manual wheelchair will require surgical treatment of rotator cuff wear-and-tear injury within 10-15 years, and a higher level of care until they have regained the ability to use their arms for all self-care activities. Although a basic principle of rehabilitation is to avoid measures that increase dependence, a power wheelchair may help avoid this complication and may be required postoperatively. In persons with partial use of the hands and arms, tendon transfer surgery may prolong useful function (Shem, 2006).

Cardiovascular The sedentary lifestyle of most persons with SCI, along with a tendency toward obesity and decreased lean body mass, early onset of fatigue with exercise, impaired peripheral circulation, elevated LDL, and low HDL lead to a significantly higher rate of cardiovascular disease than in the able-bodied population, 200% greater on average (Nelson, 2001; Shem 2006; Jacelon, 2011). Lifetime vigilance regarding cardiovascular symptoms is imperative.

Metabolic / Endocrine Endocrine abnormalities commonly seen in SCI include reduced catecholamine metabolism, reduced hepatic blood flow, reduced plasma proteins, glucose intolerance, and insulin resistance. It is estimated that the incidence if diabetes in SCI is 20%, which increases with weight gain. Age-related decreased testosterone levels cause decreased libido, secondary depression, increased risk of osteoporosis, and poor wound healing (Shem, 2006).

Respiratory The respiratory system becomes weaker with age in all persons. However, age-related changes occur earlier with SCI; this is especially true of tetraplegics. Progressive scoliosis and kyphosis related to trunk muscle wasting can interfere with the respiratory process. Persons with SCI at C4 and above and any individuals with vital capacities of less than 1L are generally ventilator-dependent, with significant associated morbidity. One-year survival rate is 90%, at two years 56%, and at five years 33%. 55% of individuals with ventilator have pulmonary complications each year with an average hospital stay of 22 days per year. Individuals who are ventilator dependent need 24 hours per day care, tracheotomy care, suctioning, and respiratory care (Shem, 2006).

Severe spasticity can interfere with the expansion of the diaphragm (Nelson, 2001). Diseases of the respiratory system such as pneumonia, and other respiratory infections are the leading cause of death in persons with SCI after the first year (Nelson, 2001).

Renal Renal function declines with age. There is an increased likelihood of bladder infections, bladder cancer, and other urinary complications as the person with SCI ages. Many of the commonly-used medications cause complications in liver and kidney function related to the metabolism and excretion of these medications and their metabolites.

Gastrointestinal Persons with SCI have a high rate of gallstones and hemorrhoids. Gastric and bowel motility decrease with aging, causing increased problems (Nelson, 2001). Patients may experience chronic gastric dilation and fecal impaction; they may also be at a higher risk for gastroesophageal reflux (GERD, a risk factor for esophageal cancer), hiatal hernia, diverticulosis, and hemorrhoids. There is a higher incidence of gallbladder stones in individuals with SCI. Diagnosis of intra-abdominal pathology can be challenging due to decreased sensation (Shem, 2006).

Psychosocial Psychosocial changes with aging are also significant. Recent reports estimate the prevalence of depression in individuals with SCI to be 16 to 30%, although individual coping styles can be significant influences (Shem, 2006). Spouses and/or parents may no longer be able to provide care due to death or their own disability. Social support decreases as friends have less independence. This can lead to social isolation and depression (Nelson, 2001). Fatigue, depression and decreased life satisfaction should not be left unaddressed (Jacelon, 2011).

Nursing Diagnoses To Consider:
- *Ineffective Self-Health Management:* Pattern of regulating and integrating into daily living a therapeutic regimen for treatment of illness and its sequelae that is unsatisfactory for meeting specific health goals
- *Risk for Impaired Liver Function:* Risk for decrease in liver function that may compromise health
- *Risk for Unstable Blood Glucose:* Risk for variation in blood glucose/sugar levels from the normal range
- *Risk for Electrolyte Imbalance:* Risk for change in serum electrolytes that may compromise health

- *Dysfunctional Gastrointestinal Motility / Risk for Dysfunctional Gastrointestinal Motility*: Increased, decreased, ineffective, or lack of peristaltic activity / Risk for Increased, decreased, ineffective, or lack of peristaltic activity within the gastrointestinal system
- *Impaired Gas Exchange:* Excess or deficit in oxygenation and/or carbon dioxide elimination at the alveolar-capillary membrane
- *Impaired Physical / Bed / Wheelchair / Transfer Mobility:* Limitation of independent movement (specify)
- *Self-Care Deficit:* A constellation of culturally framed behaviors involving one or more self-care activities in which there is a failure to maintain a socially accepted standard of health and well-being (Givens, Lauder, and Ludwick, 2006)
- *Self-Neglect (bathing, dressing, feeding, toileting):* Impaired ability to perform or complete specified activities for self

Selected Life Care Planning Considerations:
- Increased frequency of primary care screening for age-related changes
- Increasing levels of care for temporary or permanent increased disability, e.g., related to orthopedic surgery

References:

American Psychiatric Association. Diagnostic and Statistical Manual of Mental Disorders (DSM IV-TR), 4th edition. Arlington VA 2012

American Therapeutic Recreation Association Home Page. American Therapeutic Recreation Association, July 2009. Retrieved April 14, 2011, from http://atra-online. com

Anderson KD. Targeting recovery: priorities of the spinal cord-injured population. J Neurotrauma. (2004) Oct;21(10):1371-83.

Annon JS. The PLISSIT model: a proposed conceptual scheme for the behavioral treatment of sexual problems. J Sex Educ Ther. 1976;2:1-15.

Barker E and Saulino M. "First-ever guidelines for spinal cord Injuries" RN (2002) Vol 65, No 10.pp 32-37.

Bernstein J. Evidence-based medicine. J Am Acad Orthop Surg. 2004 Mar-Apr;12(2):80-8.

Biering-Sørensen F, Bagi P, Høiby N.(2001) Urinary tract infections in patients with spinal cord lesions: treatment and prevention. Drugs. 2001;61(9):1275-87. Review.

Brose SW et al. Shoulder ultrasound abnormalities, physical examination findings, and pain in manual wheelchair users with spinal cord injury. Archives of Physical Medicine and Rehabilitation 2008, 89(11):2086-93

Burchiel KJ, Hsu FP. Pain and spasticity after spinal cord injury: mechanisms and treatment. Spine 2001;26(24 Suppl):S146-S160.

Consortium of Spinal Cord Medicine, Outcomes Following Traumatic SCI: Clinical Practice Guidelines for Health-Care Professionals, Washington DC, Paralyzed Veterans of America, 1999.

Correa GI, Rotter KP. Clinical evaluation and management of neurogenic bowel after spinal cord injury. Spinal Cord. (2000) May;38(5):301-8.

Chen Y, Deutsch A, DeVivo M, et al. Current Research Outcomes From the Spinal Cord Injury Model Systems, Archives of Physical Medicine and Rehabilitation, Volume 92, Issue 3, March 2011, Pages 329-331, ISSN 0003-9993, 10.1016/j.apmr.2010.12.011.

Christensen P, Bazzocchi G, Coggrave M, et al. A randomized, controlled trial of transanal irrigation versus conservative bowel management in spinal cord-injured patients. Gastroenterology. 2006 Sep;131(3):738-47.

Christensen P, Kvitzau B, Krogh K, et al. Neurogenic colorectal dysfunction-use of new antegrade and retrograde colonic wash-out methods. Spinal Cord. 2000 Apr;38(4):255-61.

Craig Hospital. Alcohol Abuse, retrieved 2/2/12 http://www.
craighospital.org/SCI/METS/alcoholAbuse.asp

D'Arcy Y. Compact clinical guide to acute pain management: an
evidence-based approach, Springer, New York NY, 2011

Davidson PR and Parker KCH. Eye Movement Desensitization
and Reprocessing (EMDR): A Meta-Analysis. Journal of
Counseling and Clinical Psychology, 69 (2), 305-316.
2001

DiMarco AF, Onders RP, Ignagni A, et al. Phrenic nerve pacing
via intramuscular diaphragm electrodes in tetraplegic
subjects. Chest 2005a; 127: 671-678.

DeVivo MJ, Chen Y. Trends in New Injuries, Prevalent Cases,
and Aging With Spinal Cord Injury, Archives of Physical
Medicine and Rehabilitation, Volume 92, Issue 3, March
2011, Pages 332-338, ISSN 0003-9993, 10.1016/j.
apmr.2010.08.031.

Dyson-Hudson TA et al. Shoulder pain in chronic spinal
cord injury, Part I: Epidemiology, etiology, and
pathomechanics. The Journal of Spinal Cord Medicine
2004, 27(1):4-17

Easter Seals and Century 21 System's Easy Access Housing for
Easier Living Program, www.easterseals.com, accessed
March 30, 2012

Emedicine, http://www.emedicinehealth.com/cystoscopy/
article_em.htm accessed January 3, 2012

Evans RJ. Intravesical therapy for overactive bladder. Current
Urology Reports 2005; 6:429-433.

Finnerup NB, Biering-Sorensen F, Johannesen IL, et al.
Intravenous lidocaine relieves spinal cord injury
pain: a randomized controlled trial. Anesthesiology
2005;102(5):1023-1030.

French J. Neurotechnology and life care planning, JNLCP June
2012, vol. XII no. 2, page 589 600

Frye J. Recreational therapy and life care planning. JNLCP June
2011, vol. XI no. 2, page 383-388

Garcia Leoni ME, Esclarin De RA. Management of urinary tract
infection in patients with spinal cord injuries. Clin
Microbiol Infect 2003;9(8):780-785.

Geerts WH, Bergqvist D, Pineo GF, et al. Prevention of venous thromboembolism: American College of Chest Physicians Evidence-Based Clinical Practice Guidelines (8th Edition). Chest. Jun 2008;133(6 Suppl):381S-453S.

Goktepe AS, Yilmaz B, Alaca R, et al. Bone density loss after spinal cord injury: elite paraplegic basketball players vs. paraplegic sedentary persons. Am J Phys Med Rehabil. 2004 Apr;83(4):279-83.

Herdman TH (2012) (Ed.) NANDA-International Nursing Diagnoses: Definitions and Classification, 2012-2014. Oxford: Wiley-Blackwell

Hagenbach U et al. The treatment of spasticity with Delta(9)-tetrahydrocannabinol in persons with spinal cord injury. Spinal Cord. 2007 Aug; 45(8) 551-62Oxford: Wiley-Blackwell

International Association for Study of Pain—allodynia-updated 7-14-11 - retrieved 1/14/12 from http://www. iasp-pain.org/AM/Template.cfm?Section=Pain_Defi ... isplay.cfmandContentID=1728

Jacelon CS (Ed). (2011) The Specialty Practice of Rehabilitation Nursing. A Core Curriculum (Sixth Edition). Rehabilitation Nursing Foundation. Skokie.

Jones T, Ugalde V, Franks P, et al. Venous thromboembolism after spinal cord injury: incidence, time course, and associated risk factors in 16,240 adults and children. Arch Phys Med Rehabil. Dec 2005;86(12):2240-7.

Joseph A. (1998) Nursing Clinical Practice Guideline Neurogenic Bladder Management. SCI Nursing. Pp 21-56.

Kalisvaart JF et al. Bladder cancer in spinal cord injury patients. Spinal Cord 2010, Mar; 48(3) 257-261

Kirshblum SC, Burns SP, Biering-Sorensen F, et al. (2011) International standards for neurological classification of spinal cord injury (Revised 2011). Journal of Spinal Cord Medicine, Volume 34, Number 6, November 2011, pp. 535-546(12)

Krause JS, Vines CL, Farley TL, et al. An exploratory study of pressure ulcers after spinal cord injury: relationship to protective behaviors and risk factors. Arch Phys Med Rehabil. 2001 Jan;82(1):107-13.

Krause JS. Self-reported problems after spinal cord injury: Implications for rehabilitation practice. Topics in Spinal Cord Injury Rehabilitation 2007;12(3):35-44.

Korsten MA, Singal AK, Monga A, et al. Anorectal stimulation causes increased colonic motor activity in subjects with spinal cord injury. J Spinal Cord Med. 2007;30(1):31-5.

Leibowitz RQ, Stanton AL. Sexuality after spinal cord injury: A conceptual model based on women's narratives. Rehabilitation Psychology, Vol 52(1), Feb 2007, 44-55.

Lynch S, Vickery S. Steps to reducing hospital-acquired pressure ulcers. Nursing:2010 November 2010-Volume 40-Issue 11-p 61-62

Madaris L. Ziconotide: A Non-Opioid Alternative for Chronic Neuropathic Pain, A Case Report. SCI Nursing. 2008. Vol 24 #2.

Maïmoun L. Fattal, C. Micallef, et al. Bone loss in spinal cord-injured patients: from physiopathology to therapy. Spinal Cord (2006) 44, 203-210.

Makhsous M, Priebe M, Bankard J, et al. Measuring tissue perfusion during pressure relief maneuvers: insights into preventing pressure ulcers. J Spinal Cord Med 2007a;30:497-507.

Makhsous M, Lin F, et al. Promote Pressure Ulcer Healing in Individuals with Spinal Cord Injury Using an Individualized Cyclic Pressure-Relief Protocol. Advances in skin and wound Care. 2009

McHale DJ and Carlson KK. (ed) (2003) AACN Procedure Manual for Critical Care (4ᵗʰ edition) WB Saunders Co., Philadelphia. pp 625-638.

McKinley W. Cardiovascular Concerns in Spinal Cord Injury. Medscape Reference. Online. Updated 10/28/11 retrieved on 1-19-12 from http://emedicine.medscape.com/article/321771-overview

McKinney D. Prevention of Thromboembolism in Spinal Cord Injury. Medscape Reference.online Updated 8/11/11

retrieved on 1-17-12 from http://emedicine.medscape.
com/article/322897-overview

Merenda L. "The Pediatric Patient with SCI - Not a Small Adult!"
SCI Nursing. 2001.Vol 18, No 1. pp 43-44.

Moore DA, Edwards K. Using a Portable Bladder Scanner to
Reduce the Incidence of Nosocomial Urinary Tract
Infections. MedSurg Nursing. 1997;6:39-53

Morales V. "Bladder Management of the Pediatric Spinal Cord
Injury Patient", SCI Nursing. Vol. 18, No 2. pp 102 - 104.

Myers J, Lee M, Kiratli J. Cardiovascular disease in spinal cord
injury: an overview of prevalence, risk, evaluation,
and management. Am J Phys Med Rehabil. 2007
Feb;86(2):142-52.

National Center for PTSD, U.S. Department of Veterans Affairs.
Understanding PTSD treatment. February 2011. www.
ptsd.va.gov, retrieved 3/26/2012

Nelson A. (ed) (2001) Nursing Practice Related to Spinal Cord
Injury and Disorders: A Core Curriculum. EPVA. New
York City

Nelson AL. Motacki K. Menzel N.(ED) The Illustrated Guide
to Safe Patient Handling and Movement. Springer
Publishing Co. NY, NY(2009)

Nepomunceno C, Fine PR, Richards JS, Gowens H, Stover SL,
Rantanuabol U, Houston R.Â Pain in patients with spinal
cord injury.Â Arch Phys Med Rehabil 1979;60:595-608.

Myers J, Lee M, Kiratli J. Cardiovascular disease in spinal cord
injury: an overview of prevalence, risk, evaluation,
and management. Am J Phys Med Rehabil. 2007
Feb;86(2):142-52.

Pandyan AD, Gregoric M, Barnes MP, Wood D, Van Wijck
F, Burridge J, Hermens H, Johnson GR. Spasticity:
clinical perceptions, neurological realities and
meaningful measurement. Disabil Rehabil. 2005 Jan
7-21;27(1-2):2-6.

Powell M, Kirshblum S, O'Connor KC. Duplex ultrasound
screening for deep vein thrombosis in spinal cord
injured patients at rehabilitation admission. Arch Phys
Med Rehabil. Sep 1999;80(9):1044-6.

Puet TA, Jackson H, Amy S. Use of pulsed irrigation evacuation in the management of the neuropathic bowel. Spinal Cord. 1997 Oct;35(10):694-9.

Ragnarsson KTÂ Management of pain in persons with spinal cord injury.Â Spinal Cord Med 1997;20:186-199.

Rauck RL, Wallace MS, Leong MS, et al. Ziconotide 301 Study Group. A randomized, double-blind, placebo-controlled study of intrathecal ziconitide in adults with severe chronic pain. J Pain Symptom Manage. 2006 May;31(5):393-406.

Regan MA. Teasell RW. Wolfe DL, et al. for the SCIRE Research Team. "A Systematic Review of Therapeutic Interventions for Pressure Ulcers After Spinal Cord Injury" Archives of Physical Medicine and Rehabilitation. Volume 90, Issue 2, February 2009, Pages 213-231(2009)

Regan MA, Teasell RW, Keast D, Aubut JL, et al. (2010). Pressure Ulcers Following Spinal Cord Injury. In Eng JJ, Teasell RW, Miller WC, et al., editors. Spinal Cord Injury Rehabilitation Evidence. Version 3.0

Richards JS, Waites K, Chen YY, et al. The epidemiology of secondary conditions following spinal cord injury. Top Spinal Cord Inj Rehabil 2004;10:15-29.

Romero-Ganuza J, Gambarrutta C, Merlo-Gonzalez VE, et al. Complications of tracheostomy after anterior cervical spine fixation surgery, American Journal of Otolaryngology, Volume 32, Issue 5, September-October 2011, Pages 408-411, ISSN 0196-0709, 10.1016/j.amjoto.2010.07.020. (http://www.sciencedirect.com/science/article/pii/S0196070910001419)

RRTC Wright State University, School of Medicine, 3640 Colonel Glenn Highway, Dayton, OH 45435

Sandford PR, Benes PS. Use of capsaicin in the treatment of radicular pain in spinal cord injury. J SPINAL CORD MED 2000;23(4):238-243.

Shafik A, El-Sibai O, Shafik IA. Physiologic basis of digital-rectal stimulation for bowel evacuation in patients with spinal cord injury: identification of an anorectal excitatory reflex. J Spinal Cord Med. 2000;23(4):270-5.

Sheel AW, Reid WD, Townson AF, Ayas N Respiratory Management. In: Eng JJ, Teasell RW, Miller WC, et al., editors. Spinal Cord Injury Rehabilitation Evidence. Volume 3.0. Vancouver: p. 1-46. (2010).

Shem K, Aging with spinal cord injury. JNLCP January 2006 vol. 6, no. 1, p. 3-8

Siddall PJ. Middleton JW. A proposed algorithm for the management of pain following spinal cord injury. Spinal Cord (2006) 44, 67-77

Siddall, PJ, Yezierski, RP, Loeser JD Pain Following Spinal Cord Injury: Clinical Features, Prevalence, and Taxonomy from IASP Newsletter 2000-3

Singh R, Singh R, Rohilla RK, et al. Surgery for pressure ulcers improves general health and quality of life in patients with spinal cord injury. J Spinal Cord Med. 2010;33(4):396-400.

Smith, BM. Evans, CT. Kurichi, JT, et al. Acute Respiratory Tract Infection Visits of Veterans With Spinal Cord Injuries and Disorders: Rates, Trends, and Risk Factors. J Spinal Cord Med. 2007; 30(4): 355-361

Sniger, W. Garshick, E. Alendronate increases bone density in chronic spinal cord injury: A case report. Archives of Physical Medicine and Rehabilitation. Volume 83, Issue 1, Pages 139-140, January 2002

Starkweather A. Chronic Pain After SCI: An Overview of Treatment Options. SCI Nursing. October 2007.

Taricco M, Adone R, Pagliacci C, Telaro E. Pharmacological interventions for spasticity following spinal cord injury. Cochrane Database of Systematic Reviews 2000, Issue 2.

Taylor G. Pressure and Shear - Definitions, Relationships and Measurements www.pressuremapping.com/File/ ShearTerms/pdf Accessed 4/02/2012

Teasell RW, Mehta S, Aubut J, et al. (2010). Pain Following Spinal Cord Injury. In Eng JJ, Teasell RW, Miller WC, et al., editors. Spinal Cord Injury Rehabilitation Evidence. Version 3.0. http://www.scireproject.com/

rehabilitation-evidence/pain-management (accessed 1-13-12)

Tescher AN, Rindflesch AB, Youdas JW, et al. Range-of-Motion Restriction and Craniofacial Tissue-Interface Pressure From Four Cervical Collars Journal of Trauma-Injury Infection and Critical Care: November 2007-Volume 63-Issue 5-pp 1120-1126

Vallès M, Rodríguez A, Borau A, Mearin F. Effect of sacral anterior root stimulator on bowel dysfunction in patients with spinal cord injury. Dis Colon Rectum. 2009 May;52(5):986-92.

Vernillion C. Life care planning and case management for the elderly: introduction to geriatric medicine and geriatric specialists. JNLCP June 2010 vol. X no. 2, p. 236-241

Vogel, L and DeVivo, M (1997) Pediatric spinal cord injury issues: Etiology, demographics, and pathophysiology. Topics in Spinal Cord Injury Rehabilitation, 3 (2) 1-8.

Wardell DW. Rintala DH. Duan Z. Tan G. A Pilot Study of Healing Touch and Progressive Relaxation for Chronic Neuropathic Pain in Persons With Spinal Cord Injury. Journal of Holistic Nursing, Vol. 24, No. 4, 231-240 (2006)

Webster LR, Fisher R, Charapata S, Wallace MS. Long-term intrathecal ziconotide for chronic pain: an open-label study. J Pain Symptom Manage. 2009 Mar;37(3):363-72. Epub 2008 Aug 19.

Weiss, D. Osteoporosis and Spinal Cord Injury. Updated 8-16-11. Medscape Reference. Accessed 1-19-12 from http://emedicine.medscape.com/article/322204-overview

Wolfe DL, Ethans K, Hill D, Hsieh JTC, et al. Bladder Health and Function Following Spinal Cord Injury. In Eng JJ, Teasell RW, Miller WC, et al., editors. Spinal Cord Injury Rehabilitation Evidence. Version 3.0. (2010). Vancouver: p 1-19.

Yang J et al. Carpal tunnel syndrome in manual wheelchair users with spinal cord injury: a cross-sectional multicenter study. American Journal of Physical

Medicine and Rehabilitation / Association of Academic Physiatrists 2009, 88(12):1007-16

Yezierski RP Spinal cord injury: a model of central neuropathic pain; Neurosignals, 2005;14(4):182-193

Wadsworth BM, Haines TP, Cornwell PL, Paratz JD. Abdominal binder use in people with spinal cord injuries: a systematic review and meta-analysis. Spinal Cord 2009; 47(4): 274-285.

Widerstrom-Noga EG, Felipe-Cuervo E, Yezierski RP.Â Relationships among clinical characteristics of chronic pain after spinal cord injury.Â Archive Phys Med Rehab 2001;82:1191-1197.

Widerstrom-Noga EG, Turk DC. Types and effectiveness of treatments used by people with chronic pain associated with spinal cord injuries: influence of pain and psychosocial characteristics. Spinal Cord 2003;41(11):600-609.

CHAPTER 2

Traumatic Brain Injury

Terri Brandley, BSN, RN, CCM
Linda Husted, MPH, RN, CNLCP, LNCC, CCM, CDMS, CRC
Shelly Kinney, MSN, RN, CCM, CNLCP
Jacquelyn Morris, BSN, RN, CRRN, CNLCP
Kathy Pouch, MSN, RN-BC, CCM, CNLCP, CNCC
Karen Yates, RN, LNC, NLCP
Jean Beaubien, BSN, RN, CRRN, CDMS, CCM, CNLCP, contributor

"As even mild injury can lead to disabling consequences, the long-term consequences of TBI need to be better understood, especially as the survival rate has increased dramatically in the last few decades" (Colantonio, 2004).

The Centers for Disease Control and Prevention (CDC) defines traumatic brain injury (TBI) as a blow to the head or penetrating head injury that disrupts the function of the brain. This is the typical explanation of a brain injury when one thinks about TBI. The Brain Injury Association of America (BIAA) defines TBI as "an alteration in brain function, or other evidence of brain pathology, caused by an external force" (BIAUSA 2011).

BIAA further differentiates TBI from an *acquired brain injury* (ABI) (BIAA, 2011). An ABI is an injury or insult to the brain that affects the flow of oxygen to the brain, at the cellular level throughout the brain, and not just at the site of trauma. It is an injury to the brain, which is not hereditary, congenital, degenerative, or induced by birth trauma. It is an injury to the brain that has occurred *after* birth. There are several types of ABI:

- Anoxic brain injury (the brain gets little or no oxygen)
- Anemic anoxia (low oxygen-carrying capacity in the blood going to the brain)

- Toxic anoxia (toxins or metabolites block oxygen metabolism in the brain)
- Hypoxic injury (the brain receives inadequate oxygen) This is most often caused by a critical reduction in blood flow or blood pressure

Incidence

Approximately 1.7 million people sustain brain injuries in the US each year (CDC, 2011). Although the nature and severity of their injuries vary, a large number of people live with the long-term effects. Two percent of the population, an estimated 5.3 million Americans, are living with some disability due to traumatic or acquired brain injury (CDC, 2011). This makes brain injury-related disability a major public health concern.

- Males are more likely than females to sustain TBI. The ages at highest risk for TBI are less than 4 years, 15 to 19 years, and age 65 and older (CDC, 2011).
- The leading causes of TBI are: falls (35.2%), especially among 0 to 4 year olds and the elderly; motor vehicle/ traffic crashes (17.3%); struck by/against (16.5%); and assaults (10%) (CDC, 2011). Among active duty military personnel in war zones, blasts are a leading cause of TBI (CDC 2011).
- Approximately 75% of TBIs are concussions or other forms of mild TBI (CDC 2011).
- An estimated 300,000 sports-related brain injuries of mild to moderate severity occur in the United States each year (Sosin, et al. 1996).
- Firearm use is the leading cause of death related to TBI with firearms accounting for 40% of TBI-related deaths (CDC 2011).

This points to a growing need for preventive measures as well as a tremendous need for post-injury resources for individuals and families. The CDC identifies survivors of TBI as having a long-term or lifelong need for help to perform activities of daily living. The most frequently identified unmet needs were improving memory and problem solving, managing stress and emotional upsets, controlling temper, and improving job skills.

TBI can cause a wide range of functional changes affecting thinking, sensation, language, and emotions. It can also cause epilepsy and increase the risk for conditions such as Alzheimer's disease, Parkinson's disease, and other brain disorders that become more common with aging (CDC 2011).

Prevention

Falls are the cause of the greatest number of TBIs, especially among those over 65. Fall prevention measures are attracting greater attention as the population ages:

- Exercise
- Medication review with modification
- Education about risk factors can reduce falls among community dwelling older adults (Tinetti 1994)
- Combining attention to individual patients' needs
- Reducing environmental hazards (e.g., putting in grab bars and removing tripping hazards)
- Increasing the safety and fit of wheelchairs
- Limiting psychoactive drug use can reduce falls among nursing home residents (Ray 1997; CDC 2011).

To decrease the number of motor vehicle accidents, lower speed limit, stricter law enforcement, and public safety awareness are key. The CDC and the BIAA suggest the following:

- Wear a seat belt every time you drive or ride in a motor vehicle.
- Always buckle your child into a child safety seat, booster seat, or seat belt (according to the child's height, weight, and age) in the car.
- Never drive while under the influence of alcohol or drugs.

Schools are a great place to incorporate prevention efforts. The National SAFE KIDS Campaign website and the National Program for Playground Safety website have teacher plans and student handouts about motor vehicle, sports and recreation, and playground safety. CDC has developed a toolkit for high school coaches to raise awareness about sports-related concussions. This toolkit provides information on preventing and managing sports-related concussions (CDC 2005). The CDC has developed a kit for primary care physicians called *Heads Up: Brain Injury in Your Practice.* The kit is available free of charge, and contains practical, easy-to-use clinical information and provides patient education materials in English and Spanish (CDC 2011).

Causes of Brain Injury
Causes of brain injury include the following:

- Airway obstruction
  o Near-drowning, anaphylaxis, foreign body, strangulation
- Electrical shock or lightning strike
- Trauma to the head, chest, or neck
  o Gunshot wound, motor vehicle crashes, sports injury
- TBI with or without skull fracture
- Vascular disruption
  o Blood loss from open wounds, artery impingement from forceful impact, shock
  o Myocardial infarction with shock, stroke
  o Arteriovenous malformation (AVM), aneurysm, intracranial surgery
- Infectious disease
  o Meningitis, certain venereal diseases, AIDS, insect-borne and parasitical diseases
- Intracranial tumors
- Metabolic disorders
  o Hypo/hyperglycemia, hepatic encephalopathy, uremic encephalopathy
- Seizure disorders

- Toxic exposure
  - o   Illicit drugs, alcohol, lead, carbon monoxide, toxic chemicals, chemotherapy

Measurement Tools

Three tools used to evaluate or classify an individual following a brain injury are the *Glasgow Coma Scale*, the *Glasgow Outcomes Classification*, and the *Rancho Los Amigos* scale.

The Glasgow Coma Scale (Table 1) was derived by Graham Teasdale and Bryan J. Jennett, professors of neurosurgery at the University of Glasgow's Institute of Neurological Sciences, as a means to assess consciousness. First published in 1974, it scores the level of consciousness and coma severity by assessing the opening of eyes, motor response, and verbal response to stimuli. Coma is defined as: (1) not opening eyes, (2) not obeying commands, and (3) not uttering understandable words (Neuroskills 2006).

The total score is calculated by adding scores for eye opening, best motor response, and best verbal response (E+M+V=3 to 15).
- Scores of less than or equal to 8 indicate coma
- Scores greater than or equal to 9 indicate the patient is not in coma
- Fifty percent of patients with a Glasgow Coma Score less than or equal to 8 die within 6 hours
- Scores of 9 to 11 indicate moderate severity
- Scores greater than or equal to 12 indicate minor injury

The Glasgow Outcomes classification (Table 2) also originates from the Institute of Neurological Sciences. It describes anticipated functional outcomes associated with injury classifications.

Table 1. Glasgow Coma Scale. Teasdale and Jennet, 1974. Reprint permission from Russ Rowlett and the University of North Carolina at Chapel Hill.

Eye-opening response, E	Spontaneous, open with blinking, baseline	4
	Opens to command, speech, or shout	3
	Opens to pain not applied to face	2
	None	
Verbal response, V	Oriented	5
	Confused, but answers questions	4
	Inappropriate response, words discernible	3
	Incomprehensible speech	3
	None	1
Motor response, M	Obeys commands for movement	6
	Purposeful movement to painful stimulus	5
	Withdraws to pain	4
	Abnormal (spastic) flexion, decorticate posturing	3
	Extensor (rigid) response, decerebrate posturing	2
	None	1

Adjusted verbal response for children under age 5:		
Score	**2-5 years**	**0-23 months**
5	Appropriate words or phrases	Smiles or coos appropriately
4	Inappropriate words	Cries and consolable
3	Persistent cries and/ or screams	Persistent inappropriate crying and/or screaming
2	Grunts	Grunts, or is agitated and restless
1	No response	No response

Table 2. Glasgow Outcome Scale (Jennett and Bond, 1975)

Death	Severe injury or death without recovery of consciousness
Persistent vegetative state	Severe damage with prolonged state of unresponsiveness and a lack of higher mental functions
Severe disability	Severe injury with permanent need for help with daily living
Moderate disability	No need for assistance in everyday life, employment is possible but may require adaptive equipment
Low disability	Light damage with minor neurological and psychological deficits

The Rancho Los Amigos scale (Los Amigos Research and Educational Institute, 1990) (Table 3) evaluates level of cognitive function ranging from "not responsive" to "purposeful and appropriate responses."

Table 3. Rancho Los Amigos Cognitive Scale, Revised (Los Amigos Research and Educational Institute, 1990)

Levels of Cognitive Functioning

Level I - No Response: Total Assistance

Complete absence of observable change in behavior when presented visual, auditory, tactile, proprioceptive, vestibular or painful stimuli.

Level II - Generalized Response: Total Assistance

- Demonstrates generalized reflex response to painful stimuli.
- Responds to repeated auditory stimuli with increased or decreased activity.

- Responds to external stimuli with physiological changes generalized, gross body movement and/or not purposeful vocalization.
- Responses noted above may be same regardless of type and location of stimulation.
- Responses may be significantly delayed.

Level III - Localized Response: Total Assistance

- Demonstrates withdrawal or vocalization to painful stimuli.
- Turns toward or away from auditory stimuli.
- Blinks when strong light crosses visual field.
- Follows moving object passed within visual field.
- Responds to discomfort by pulling tubes or restraints.
- Responds inconsistently to simple commands.
- Responses directly related to type of stimulus.
- May respond to some persons (especially family and friends) but not to others.

Level IV - Confused/Agitated: Maximal Assistance

- Alert and in heightened state of activity.
- Purposeful attempts to remove restraints or tubes or crawl out of bed.
- May perform motor activities such as sitting, reaching and walking but without any apparent purpose or upon another's request.
- Very brief and usually non-purposeful moments of sustained alternatives and divided attention.
- Absent short-term memory.
- May cry out or scream out of proportion to stimulus even after its removal.
- May exhibit aggressive or flight behavior.

- Mood may swing from euphoric to hostile with no apparent relationship to environmental events.
- Unable to cooperate with treatment efforts.
- Verbalizations are frequently incoherent and/or inappropriate to activity or environment.

Level V - Confused, Inappropriate Non-Agitated: Maximal Assistance

- Alert, not agitated but may wander randomly or with a vague intention of going home.
- May become agitated in response to external stimulation, and/or lack of environmental structure.
- Not oriented to person, place or time.
- Frequent brief periods, non-purposeful sustained attention.
- Severely impaired recent memory, with confusion of past and present in reaction to ongoing activity.
- Absent goal directed, problem solving, self-monitoring behavior.
- Often demonstrates inappropriate use of objects without external direction.
- May be able to perform previously learned tasks when structured and cues provided.
- Unable to learn new information.
- Able to respond appropriately to simple commands fairly consistently with external structures and cues.
- Responses to simple commands without external structure are random and non-purposeful in relation to command.
- Able to converse on a social, automatic level for brief periods of time when provided external structure and cues.

- Verbalizations about present events become inappropriate and confabulatory when external structure and cues are not provided.

Level VI - Confused, Appropriate: Moderate Assistance

- Inconsistently oriented to person, time and place.
- Able to attend to highly familiar tasks in non-distracting environment for 30 minutes with moderate redirection.
- Remote memory has more depth and detail than recent memory.
- Vague recognition of some staff.
- Able to use assistive memory aide with maximum assistance.
- Emerging awareness of appropriate response to self, family and basic needs.
- Moderate assist to problem solve barriers to task completion.
- Supervised for old learning (e.g. self care).
- Shows carry over for relearned familiar tasks (e.g. self care).
- Maximum assistance for new learning with little or nor carry over.
- Unaware of impairments, disabilities and safety risks.
- Consistently follows simple directions.
- Verbal expressions are appropriate in highly familiar and structured situations.

Level VII - Automatic, Appropriate: Minimal Assistance for Daily Living Skills

- Consistently oriented to person and place, within highly familiar environments. Moderate assistance for orientation to time.

- Able to attend to highly familiar tasks in a non-distraction environment for at least 30 minutes with minimal assist to complete tasks.
- Minimal supervision for new learning.
- Demonstrates carry over of new learning.
- Initiates and carries out steps to complete familiar personal and household routine but has shallow recall of what he/she has been doing.
- Able to monitor accuracy and completeness of each step in routine personal and household ADLs and modify plan with minimal assistance.
- Superficial awareness of his/her condition but unaware of specific impairments and disabilities and the limits they place on his/her ability to safely, accurately and completely carry out his/her household, community, work and leisure ADLs.
- Minimal supervision for safety in routine home and community activities.
- Unrealistic planning for the future.
- Unable to think about consequences of a decision or action.
- Overestimates abilities.
- Unaware of others' needs and feelings.
- Oppositional/uncooperative.
- Unable to recognize inappropriate social interaction behavior.

Level VIII - Purposeful, Appropriate: Stand-By Assistance

- Consistently oriented to person, place and time.
- Independently attends to and completes familiar tasks for 1 hour in distracting environments.
- Able to recall and integrate past and recent events.

- Uses assistive memory devices to recall daily schedule, "to do" lists and record critical information for later use with stand-by assistance.
- Initiates and carries out steps to complete familiar personal, household, community, work and leisure routines with stand-by assistance and can modify the plan when needed with minimal assistance.
- Requires no assistance once new tasks/activities are learned.
- Aware of and acknowledges impairments and disabilities when they interfere with task completion but requires stand-by assistance to take appropriate corrective action.
- Thinks about consequences of a decision or action with minimal assistance.
- Overestimates or underestimates abilities.
- Acknowledges others' needs and feelings and responds appropriately with minimal assistance.
- Depressed.
- Irritable.
- Low frustration tolerance/easily angered.
- Argumentative.
- Self-centered.
- Uncharacteristically dependent/independent.
- Able to recognize and acknowledge inappropriate social interaction behavior while it is occurring and takes corrective action with minimal assistance.

Level IX - Purposeful, Appropriate: Stand-By Assistance on Request

- Independently shifts back and forth between tasks and completes them accurately for at least two consecutive hours.

- Uses assistive memory devices to recall daily schedule, "to do" lists and record critical information for later use with assistance when requested.

- Initiates and carries out steps to complete familiar personal, household, work and leisure tasks independently and unfamiliar personal, household, work and leisure tasks with assistance when requested.

- Aware of and acknowledges impairments and disabilities when they interfere with task completion and takes appropriate corrective action but requires stand-by assist to anticipate a problem before it occurs and take action to avoid it.

- Able to think about consequences of decisions or actions with assistance when requested.

- Accurately estimates abilities but requires stand-by assistance to adjust to task demands.

- Acknowledges others' needs and feelings and responds appropriately with stand-by assistance.

- Depression may continue.

- May be easily irritable.

- May have low frustration tolerance.

- Able to self monitor appropriateness of social interaction with stand-by assistance.

Level X - Purposeful, Appropriate: Modified Independent

- Able to handle multiple tasks simultaneously in all environments but may require periodic breaks.

- Able to independently procure, create and maintain own assistive memory devices.

- Independently initiates and carries out steps to complete familiar and unfamiliar personal, household, community, work and leisure tasks but may require more than usual amount of time and/or compensatory strategies to complete them.

- Anticipates impact of impairments and disabilities on ability to complete daily living tasks and takes action to avoid problems before they occur but may require more than usual amount of time and/or compensatory strategies.

- Able to independently think about consequences of decisions or actions but may require more than usual amount of time and/or compensatory strategies to select the appropriate decision or action.

- Accurately estimates abilities and independently adjusts to task demands.

- Able to recognize the needs and feelings of others and automatically respond in appropriate manner.

- Periodic periods of depression may occur.

- Irritability and low frustration tolerance when sick, fatigued and/or under emotional stress.

- Social interaction behavior is consistently appropriate.

Original Rancho Los Amigos Cognitive Scale co-authored by Chris Hagen, Ph.D., Danese Malkmus, M.A., Patricia Durham, M.A., Rancho Los Amigos Hospital, 1972. Revised 11/15/74 by Danese Malkmus, M.A., and Kathryn Stenderup, O.T.R.

Brain Injury Classifications
Mild

Mild TBI accounts for 80% of all TBI. It is usually caused by a contusion-type injury and may or may not result in loss of consciousness up to thirty minutes (NCIPC, 2003; Gennarelli, 1986). A person with mild TBI has a 50% or better chance of sustaining no permanent injury (Maniker, 2003).

A person with a *complicated mild TBI* will have a positive computed tomography (CT) finding (Kennedy et al., 2006) and the following:

- Glasgow Coma Scale score range is 13 to 15
- Loss of consciousness less than 20 minutes
- Post-traumatic amnesia less than one day
- Alteration in mental status
- Usually returns to the community at or near premorbid state
- Glasgow Outcome classification considers mild TBI normal, classifies as no disability (Patterson, 1993; BIAA, 2005).

Cognitive deficits include poor short-term memory, poor concentration, irritability, and depression. These symptoms may affect the person's previous work status and may cause personality changes (Salazar, 2002). Physical symptoms include headaches, visual disturbances, dizziness, tinnitus, olfactory deficits, fatigue, and nausea. These symptoms may occur intermittently throughout the person's lifetime, and varies from individual to individual (Patterson, 1993).

Moderate

A moderate TBI presents with more extensive injury pattern that can be caused by contusion and acceleration/deceleration injuries. Symptoms can linger several months or be permanent; however, with proper treatment there may be a good recovery with learned compensatory techniques (BIAA, 2005; DOD, 1999).

- Glasgow Coma Scale score between 9 and 12
- Loss of consciousness between 20 minutes and 24 hours
- Post-traumatic amnesia from 1 to 7 days
- Should have inpatient rehabilitation for intensive treatment
- An altered return-to-work setting is most likely
- Ongoing extensive post-concussion symptoms remain
- Usually returns to the community at independent-to-moderate independent in daily life
- Glasgow Outcome classification is usually moderate disability (Patterson, 1993; BIAA, 2005)

Severe

Severe TBI is characterized by extensive diffuse axonal damage within the cortex and upper and lower brainstem, causing focal damage from hemorrhage, hematoma and complications such as cerebral edema and neurological or pulmonary deficits.

- Glasgow Coma Scale score between 3 and 8
- Loss of consciousness greater than 24 hours
- Post-traumatic amnesia 1 day to less than 7 days
- Requires inpatient and possibly post-acute facilities admissions for treatment
- Potential ongoing deficits result
- Usually returns to the community or supervised living as conscious but will need moderate-to-severe maximum assistance in daily life
- Glasgow Outcome classification is usually severe disability (Patterson, 1993; BIAA, 2005)

Closed Head Injury

A closed head injury is defined as brain injury caused by an external forceful impact without fracture or displacement of the skull. However, severe brain injury may occur due to internal brain swelling.

Types of closed head injury are:

- *Concussion* is the most common brain injury and can occur in both open and closed injury. It can involve a brief loss of consciousness (< 20 minutes) or no loss of consciousness, with a feeling of being dazed. CT scan may or may not demonstrate injury. Effects, such as headache, fatigue, and disturbed concentration, may take months to years to resolve, or be permanent.
- *Contusion* is bruising or bleeding of the brain caused by direct impact. Large blood collections associated with contusions may need to be surgically removed.

- *Coup-contre coup (from the French, strike-counterstrike)* describes brain contusion at the site of the impact and on the opposite side of the skull. These contusions are due to the force with which the brain is slammed from one side to the other, as in a violent blow, fall, or whiplash.
- *Diffuse axonal injury* is caused by shaking, as with *shaken baby syndrome*, or by rotational forces, as with a car accident. There is extensive tearing and shearing of brain tissues, with temporary or permanent damage, coma, or death. Shaken baby syndrome results in lifelong disability if the child survives (National Center on Shaken Baby Syndrome (2011).

Open Head Injury

Open head injury occurs with depressed, compound, or basilar skull fractures from direct impact, or penetrating injury as from the impact of a bullet, knife, or other sharp object. Open injury may involve hair, skin, bone, or other foreign bodies forced into the brain. Low-impact penetrating objects can ricochet inside the skull, while high impact objects can cause shearing and rupture of brain tissues. Ninety-one percent of bullet wounds result in death and are the largest cause of TBI deaths (BIAA, 2011).

Fracture of the petrous bone causes *Battle's sign* (bruising at the ear and jaw) with cerebral spinal fluid leaking out of the ear, and often results in hearing loss due to damage to the eighth nerve.

Anterior fossa fractures cause *raccoon eyes* (bruising about the eyes) and cerebrospinal fluid (CSF) to leak into the sinuses. Loss of smell or vision deficits may occur due to damage to the cranial nerves. Cribiform plate fracture, fracture at the bridge of the nose, also causes CSF leak into the nose.

Diastatic skull fractures are fractures in infants' and children's skulls before the cranial sutures are closed.

Second impact injury, also termed "recurrent traumatic brain injury," is a second brain injury sustained by a person before the symptoms of a first traumatic brain injury have resolved. These injuries may occur in contact sports and have resulted in death due to cerebral edema. The American Academy of Neurology (AAN) has set guidelines to manage and prevent these types of injuries (American Academy of Neurology, 2013).

Complications
Post-Concussion Syndrome (PCS)

Post-concussion syndrome (PCS), or mild TBI, has been called the silent epidemic, affecting an estimated 800,000 persons each year. Recent studies have shown biochemical and physiological changes occur from a decrease of cerebral blood flow to neurons, with deficient oxygen supply leading to metabolic disturbances, neuronal instability due to lack of blood glucose, and neuron death from immediate release of excitatory neurotransmitters (BIAA, 2006).

Post-concussive syndrome presents with somatic complaints, cognitive impairments, and emotional and behavioral changes. Recovery generally occurs after three months from injury. However, approximately 15% of patients note symptoms more than 12 months after injury.

Neuropsychological assessment is used to evaluate post-concussive symptoms. Testing may include measurements of attention, language, memory, emotional functioning and other neurobehavioral parameters. Medications, cognitive rehabilitation, psychotherapy, stress management, and vocational counseling are used to manage symptoms of post-concussive syndrome (Legome and Alt, 2010).

Characteristic symptoms include the following (BIAA, 2006):

- Sensory
  - o Inner ear edema, dizziness, vertigo, hearing changes
  - o Visual disturbance, sensitivity to light
  - o Post-traumatic headaches
  - o Altered taste and smell
  - o Noise intolerance
- Physical
  - o Amplification of symptoms
  - o Balance and spatial disorientation
  - o Fatigue (physical, psychological, and mental) (RMRBIS, 2003).
  - o Musculoskeletal complaints
  - o Sleep disturbances
- Cognitive/Mental
  - o Increased irritability
  - o Depression and anxiety
  - o Reading and auditory comprehension deficits
  - o Decreased attention and concentration
- Other manifestations
  - o Avoids social or recreational activities
  - o Becomes a loner/isolation in family and social situations
  - o Functional deficits at home and work
  - o Suicidal ideation and attempts
  - o Behavior leading to legal issues
  - o High-risk behaviors

Post-Traumatic Amnesia (PTA).

PTA is a common symptom of TBI. PTA duration was found to be a reliable index of severity and has been used for this since 1961 (Russell, 1961). PTA is variable, resolving quickly or lingering for months, varying individual to individual, hour to hour, and day to day. Longer duration of PTA indicates more extensive brain damage (May, 1992). PTA symptoms may be random, with episodes of clarity and episodes of confusion. (May, 1992). Some PTA characteristics are as follows (Russell, 1961):

- Misidentification of family, friends, and providers
- Short-term memory loss for daily events
- Disorientation
- Impaired attention
- Delusions

Nursing Diagnoses To Consider

- *Fatigue:* An overwhelming sustained sense of exhaustion and decreased capacity for physical and mental work at the usual level.
- *Risk for Acute Confusion:* At risk for reversible disturbances of consciousness, attention, cognition, and perception that develop over a short period of time.
- *Impaired Memory:* Inability to remember or recall bits of information or behavioral skills.
- *Risk for Impaired Attachment:* At risk for disruption of the interactive process between parent/significant other and child that fosters the development of a protective and nurturing reciprocal relationship.
- *Impaired Social Interaction:* Insufficient or excessive quantity or ineffective quality of social exchange.
- *Sexual Dysfunction:* The state in which an individual experiences a change in sexual function during the sexual response phases of desire, excitation, and/or orgasm, which is viewed as unsatisfying, unrewarding, or inadequate.
- *Anxiety:* Vague uneasy feeling of discomfort or dread accompanied by an autonomic response (the source often nonspecific or unknown to the individual); a feeling of apprehension caused by anticipation of danger. It is an alerting signal that warns of impending danger and enables the individual to take measures to deal with threat.
- *Ineffective Coping:* Inability to form a valid appraisal of the stressors, inadequate choices of practiced responses, and/or inability to use available resources.

Sensory Problems

An individual who has suffered a TBI may experience decreased ability to feel parts or areas of the body. Decreased or absent ability to sense pressure or pain, changes in body or environmental temperature, or the use of hot or cold therapy all can substantially increase the risk of skin breakdown. Decreased cognitive awareness preventing self-repositioning puts patients with TBI at a very high risk of developing pressure ulcers or other types of skin injury.

Head, Ears, Eyes, Nose, and Throat.

Focal neurological deficits affect a specific body location or function, such as speech, vision, or unilateral neglect (Medline Plus, 2006). Additional examples of focal deficits might include:

- Anosmia: Loss of the sense of smell caused by traumatic injury to the first cranial nerve occurs in 2% to 38% of patients with TBI (Brain Injury, 1998; Shephard, 2006).
- Diplopia: Injuries to the fourth cranial nerve, the trochlear nerve, are quite common and can cause a positional diplopia, in which those affected experience diplopia when they look down and toward the eye in which the trochlear nerve is injured (Brain Injury, 1998; Shephard, 2006).
- Visual problems: Among the most common complications (Padulo, 2006). Individuals post TBI can exhibit a variety of visual disturbances. An individual can also have a constellation of symptoms called post trauma vision syndrome (PTVS). This syndrome is a cognitive dysfunction of the ambient visual process (inability to organize spatial information with other sensory-motor systems) with symptoms such as exotropia, exophoria, accommodative insufficiency, convergence insufficiency, and oculomotor dysfunction. (Padulo, 2006).
- Hearing deficits can occur and need to be assessed to define the type of hearing loss: conductive hearing, loss

of sensorineural hearing at a certain frequency range, or hearing changes, such as tinnitus. Tinnitus is ringing in the ears and may be related to visual as well as auditory brain activity. For example, gaze-evoked tinnitus (GET) is an unusual condition in which tinnitus loudness and pitch increase during lateral gaze. This can be caused by an imbalance between the auditory and visual parts of the brain (Center of Neuro, 2006).

- Hearing deficits can be caused by cochlear nerve injury, especially in patients with temporal bone fractures (Shephard S, 2006; Traumatic Brain, 2006).

Nursing Diagnoses To Consider:
- *Disturbed Sensory Perception* (Specify visual, auditory, kinesthetic, gustatory, tactile, olfactory): Change in the amount or patterning of incoming stimuli accompanied by diminished, distorted, or impaired response to such.
- *Impaired Verbal Communication:* Decreased, delayed, or absent inability to receive, transmit, and/or use a system of symbols.

Cardiovascular.
Prolonged immobility with dependent edema, fractures of extremities and other factors can contribute to the development of deep vein thrombosis (DVT) and pulmonary embolus (PE). DVT is a common but serious medical condition that occurs in approximately two million Americans each year (Geerts, 2004).

Anticoagulation treatment for a one-time acute DVT with warfarin (Coumadin) or other medications usually lasts for 3 to 6 months. Anticoagulated patients must be monitored regularly to keep the international normalized ratio (INR) level elevated (2-3) to decrease clot formation, and follow a stable diet that is low in vitamin K and products that interfere with the anticoagulant effect of warfarin.

Mortality due to cardiovascular and respiratory causes were leading causes of death among brain injury survivors in several studies, particularly associated with reduced mobility. The risks were increased in the first one to five years post injury, and decreased after the first five years (Shavelle, 2001).

Respiratory
Pneumonia and purulent bronchitis
One of the major risk factors in home care for an immobilized brain injury or stroke patient is aspiration pneumonia due to dysphagia, due to neurological deficit or associated throat or cervical injury (Shavelle, 2001). This is often overlooked, and gives pause to home caregivers when routinely feeding a patient. Being immobilized or having a weak cough makes it more difficult to mobilize and expel secretions.

Underlying lung disease or smoking contribute to the risk of pneumonia and bronchitis. The NLCP should consider include preventive measures to prevent recurrence of future lung problems with routine pulmonary therapy, incentive spirometry, lung and oral exercises, high-frequency chest wall oscillation devices, and specialist involvement, such as a pulmonologist. Periodic chest x-rays and other diagnostic tests may be indicated.

Tracheal stenosis and sleep apnea
Long-time ventilator patients and those who are ventilator-dependent are more prone to tracheal stenosis. Tracheal stenosis can lead to difficulty breathing, poor endurance, fatigue, and sleep apnea. Brain injury patients may have an increased risk for problems with sleep and nerves in the immediate post-injury phase and many years post-injury (Colantonio, 2004).

Sleep apnea is also caused by vocal cord stenosis from prolonged nasotracheal or orotracheal intubation or autonomic nerve damage to the respiratory center.

Based on individual assessment, the NLCP should consider providing for speech therapy to strengthen oral and accessory chest muscles; otolaryngology and/or pulmonary specialist referral; sleep studies; pulmonary studies to assess oxygenation levels, and MRI or CT of the cervical spine and chest.

Nursing Diagnoses To Consider:
- *Impaired Spontaneous Ventilation:* Decreased energy reserves resulting in an inability to maintain independent breathing that is adequate to support life.
- *Ineffective Breathing Pattern:* Inspiration and/or expiration that does not provide adequate ventilation.

Genitourinary
Urethral strictures
Genitourinary complications with TBI vary from mild to severe, depending on the nature and extent of the head injury itself, the nerves involved and associated injuries such as spinal cord injury or co-morbid conditions such as diabetes. Strictures of the urethra can occur due to nerve or muscle damage. An enlarged prostate can cause similar symptoms. Future care with an urologist should be included in the plan as well as future urodynamic and other diagnostic urologic studies. Aging considerations, medications and the possible involvement of a nephrologist should be considered, as kidney damage can occur from backflow from the bladder, frequent infections, and other urologic conditions.

Urinary tract infection.
Genitourinary problems after brain injury can occur in as many as 45% of persons with brain injury, with bladder infection occurring in over a third. Neurogenic bladder is caused by the interruption of the signals between the brain and spinal cord, allowing voluntary control of the sphincter muscles utilized in bladder elimination. Urologic specialist consultation and urological diagnostic testing, including

urodynamic studies, are integral in diagnosing and managing the condition.

Some medications can cause problems with urinary incontinence, such as dantrolene sodium (Dantrium). Bladder training with catheter use, electrical stimulation, and even surgery can be helpful with various genitourinary conditions. Adequate hydration is important for optimum urologic functioning. Future care concerns might include cueing the individual to drink adequate amounts of fluids, particularly in humid climates, routine diagnostic screening tests with urinalysis and urine culture, and urodynamic studies to monitor for early signs of urinary tract infection with a patient who is less vigilant about self-care.

Sexual Dysfunction

Medications, fatigue, and the brain injury itself can interfere with sexual functioning. Sexual counseling after brain injury may include an urologist, sex therapist, counselor, and/or fertility specialist. Changes in roles and relationships also contribute to problems. Depending on the etiology, counseling, medication, therapy, erectile pumps, and injections may be beneficial.

Nursing Diagnoses To Consider:

- *Impaired Urinary Elimination:* Dysfunction in urine elimination.
- *Sexual Dysfunction:* The state in which an individual experience a change in sexual function during the sexual response phases of desire, excitation, and/or orgasm, which is viewed as unsatisfying, unrewarding, or inadequate.

Gastrointestinal
Stress ulcers

Initial medical management of the patient with acute TBI includes stress ulcer prophylaxis due to the traumatic event (Phillips, 2005). In 2006, researchers found the pathogenesis of the gastric destruction caused by severe TBI was related to release of endothelin-1, inducible nitric oxide synthase, and macrophage inflammatory protein-1, and that prophylaxis with IV omeprazole reduced the severity of the stomach ulcers (Hsieh, 2006).

Dysphagia
Dysphagia, swallowing inability or difficulty, is common after a TBI with ventilator management. Early detection is the key to preventing aspiration pneumonia. There was evidence of dysphagia in 68% of pediatric patients with severe TBI, 15% with moderate TBI, and 1% in mild TBI (Morgan, 2003).

Bowel incontinence
According to Leary (2006) 50% of 238 ABI patients had an impaired bladder or bowel sub scores, when admitted to a Regional Neurological Rehabilitation Unit. At discharge, 36% had residual impairment and 3.5% had ongoing bowel and bladder malfunction. It was Leary's (2006) conclusion that, "Incontinence was common in patients with brain injury on a neurological rehabilitation unit. Significant improvement was seen upon discharge."

Elevated liver function
Elevated liver function (ELF) can be related to the trauma itself or anticonvulsant therapy; premorbid findings of alcohol or drug abuse or overuse should not be overlooked (Smith, 2003).

Periodic liver function studies should be included if dantrolene sodium (Dantrium) is used to manage muscle tightness, spasms, or pain (Meythaler, 2003).

Nursing Diagnoses To Consider:
Ineffective Airway Clearance: Inability to clear secretions or obstructions from the respiratory tract to maintain a clear airway.

Bowel Incontinence: Changes in normal bowel habits characterized by involuntary passage of stool.

Musculoskeletal

Musculoskeletal problems associated with TBI can occur immediately following injury or may become apparent after the first year as the brain recovers. The original mechanism of injury may have also caused traumatic musculoskeletal injuries with acute and long-term sequelae.

Heterotrophic ossification

Heterotrophic ossification (HO) is ectopic bone formation in soft tissue surrounding joints, most commonly the hip, elbow and shoulder (Pape et al., 2011). Accelerated rate of fracture healing has also been reported with the formation of exuberant callus at fracture site. In TBI, the incidence of neurogenic heterotrophic ossification (NHO) ranges from 11% to 76%, with a 10% to 20% incidence of clinically significant NHO (Melamed, 2002). NHO generally causes joint pain and decreased range of motion, low-grade fever, warmth and swelling around the joint, and in extreme cases, complete joint fusion. The specific cause of HO is not clear, but it is thought to be a combination of the circulating calcium following traumatic injury, soft tissue edema, hypoxia, and the inappropriate differentiation of fibroblasts into bone-forming cells (Bruno, 2004).

Elevated serum alkaline phosphatase levels and increased sedimentation rate can be an early sign of HO and warrant further radiology workup by radiograph, ultrasound, and three phase bone scan. Bone scans can pick up HO in the earliest stages prior to complete calcification of the affected areas.

Maintaining range of motion plays a key role in the prevention and treatment of HO in TBI. Nonsteroidal anti-inflammatory drugs (NSAIDs) and etidronate (Didronel) can help with pain management, and the risk and benefits of these drugs in established HO should be assessed. HO may result in functional impairment. If so, surgical excision is delayed 12 to 18 months to allow the heterotrophic bone to mature (Pangilinan, 2006). HO often recurs even after surgical excision. It is important for the life care planner to ask the treating rehabilitation physician to opine as to the anticipated incidence of recurrence and the plan for future treatment.

Contractures

Joint contractures can result if spasticity is not controlled or if joints are frozen because of heterotrophic ossification. Surgery may be necessary to release or lengthen tight tendons or remove areas of abnormal bone growth. The nurse life care planner should ask the physician's opinion on medications, physical therapy, Botox therapy, and splinting to address developing and potential contractures.

Falls

Many survivors of TBI at are increased risk of falls due to musculoskeletal problems, impaired judgment and other cognitive difficulties, sensory deficits, medication side effects, vestibular problems, dizziness, impulsivity, and the effects of concurrent traumatic injuries. Interventions may include caregiver education, mobility aides, cognitive aids, careful medication monitoring and in extreme cases, manipulation of the physical environment. All interventions must be geared towards maintaining safety while promoting a maximum level of independence.

Nursing Diagnoses To Consider:
* *Chronic Pain:* Unpleasant sensory or emotional experience arising from actual or potential tissue damage or described in terms of such damage (International Association for the Study of Pain); sudden or slow onset of any intensity from mild to severe with an anticipated or predictable end and a duration of greater than 6 months

- *Risk for Falls:* At risk of increased susceptibility to falling that may cause physical harm.

Movement Disorders
Spastic hypertonia (spasticity)
Damage to the brain stem, cerebellum or mid-brain affects the reflex centers by interrupting the flow of messages along various nerve pathways. This can cause changes in muscle tone, movement, sensation, and reflexes. The areas of the body affected are determined by the location of the brain injury. It can be a significant problem for individuals with TBI, with a profound impact on function and skin integrity.

In the acute phase of recovery, decelerate or decorticate posturing may be noted. As the individual recovers, nerve signals controlling motor functions may change and continue to develop and change dramatically over the first year following injury. Insuring the highest quality of life is the goal of spasticity management. There can be both advantages and disadvantages of spasticity:

- Advantages of spasticity
  o Substitutes for strength, allowing standing, walking, transfers
  o Maintains muscle tone and mass
  o Increases metabolic requirements to promote blood circulation and improve breathing
  o Warns when there is a problem in areas where the body has no feeling
  o May improve circulation and prevent DVT and edema
  o May reduce the risk of osteoporosis

- Disadvantages of spasticity; morbidity
  o Orthopedic deformity, e.g., hip dislocation, contractures, scoliosis
  o Impaired ADLs
  o Impaired mobility

o Skin breakdown secondary to positioning difficulties and shearing pressure

o Pain or abnormal sensory feedback

o Increased caloric needs due to energy expenditure

o Sleep disturbance

o Depression secondary to lack of functional independence

o Limited range of motion

o Inability to sit comfortably, maintain balance, or change positions

o Adds to the cost of medications and attendant care (Meythaler, 2003)

Decisions to treat spasticity should be based on the affect on the individual's quality of life and functional potential. Limitations in function, pain, prevention of contractures, and positioning are all areas to be considered. Correct positioning and range of motion exercises and stretching are the first line treatment. This can be aided with splinting, casting, and specialized seating guided by a seating evaluation if a wheelchair is necessary. The life care plan should include a seating assessment each time a new wheelchair is required.

Medications may be necessary if physical means of spasm control are not effect. Common medications used for muscle spasms are dantrolenesodium (Dantrium), baclofen, tizanidine, clonidine, and benzodiazepines. The sedative and cognitive effects may limit their use. It is important to assess the effects these medications may have on other organs.

In extreme cases, intrathecal baclofen may be warranted. This is provided through a pump surgically implanted beneath the skin of the abdomen with a thin tube infusing the medication into the intrathecal area of the spine. The pump requires refilling every 2 to 4 months by a specially trained provider. Most frequent complications are pump failure and infection. Sources are treated accordingly and may require surgical intervention to repair or remove the pump and/or line. The pump normally has a life of 5 to 7 years. Decreased cognitive side effects are noted when the medication is infused directly instead of circulating throughout the whole body. (*See Chapter 1, Spinal Cord Injury, for more information on implanted pumps*)

Botulinum (Botox) can be highly effective, but it requires repeat injections 3 to 4 times per year to maintain the effect. "Local treatments for spasticity include chemical neurolysis with phenol or alcohol injections or botulinum toxin A and B (Botox) injections. They differ mainly in their onset and mechanism of action" (Burnett, 2003). Referral for surgery to release and/or lengthen tight tendons may be necessary if poorly controlled spasticity has led to joint contracture. A team assessment is important to assess needs, set goals of treatment, and maximize the level of functioning by reducing spasticity.

Tremors
Tremors and dystonia decrease with time after injury, but still affect as many as 12% of survivors 2 years after the initial trauma. Assessment and treatment for tremor is similar to spasticity. Effect on quality of life and risk benefit analysis is important when considering treatment for tremor.

Parkinsonism
Individuals who have experienced a TBI may be at higher risk for Parkinson's-like tremors and conditions as they age. For more information, see "TBI and Aging."

Myoclonus
Myoclonus is sudden, involuntary jerking of a muscle or muscle group. Sudden muscle contractions are called *positive myoclonus*; sudden muscle relaxation, *negative myoclonus*. Uncontrollable myoclonus may occur singly or repetitively; with or without a pattern; and infrequently or many times per minute.

Treatment of myoclonus focuses on medications that may help reduce symptoms. Many, such as barbiturates, phenytoin (Dilantin), and primidone (Mysoline), are also used to treat epilepsy. Clonazepam (Klonepin) may be used; however, tolerance can develop. Barbiturates slow down the central nervous system and cause tranquilizing or antiseizure effects. Phenytoin and primidone are effective antiepileptic medications, although phenytoin can cause liver failure. Sodium valproate (Depakene, Depakote) is an alternative therapy for myoclonus and can be used either alone or in combination with clonazepam (National Institute of Neurological Disorders and Stroke, 2012). The NLCP should consider providing for regular laboratory studies for side effects.

Hemiballismus

Hemiballismus is a movement disorder characterized by unilateral wild, large amplitude flinging movements of the arm and leg, normally causing falls and preventing postural maintenance. Treatment is similar to the other movement disorders.

Other Neurological Complications
Seizures

There is a 5% chance of developing seizures any time after brain injury associated with CHI. With open head injuries, this increases to 30% to 50%. Posttraumatic seizures are a major complication, indicating a worse prognosis and causing additional cognitive and behavioral changes. Seizures can exacerbate TBI cognitive changes and impairments in social interaction. Anticonvulsant therapy can also cause cognitive changes. All these factors complicate rehabilitation.

Fifty percent of those individuals who develop posttraumatic seizures will no longer have seizures 5 to 10 years post injury, 50% will have good seizure control with anticonvulsants, and only 25% will continues to experience seizures. Younger patients and those with more severe injuries are more likely to develop early-onset post-traumatic seizures. Subcortical atrophy or impaired local cerebral blood flow are most predictive of late-onset seizures occurring 8 to 12 months post injury.

Seizures can be generalized or partial. The major diagnostic tool is the electroencephalogram (EEG). A sleep EEGs is four times more likely to show an abnormality than a waking EEG. Single photon emission computed tomography (SPECT) has been a useful tool in demonstrating seizure focus. A rise in prolactin levels has been shown to also be of some usefulness in diagnosis. Seizures are associated with increases in psychopathology, from personality disorders to frank episodic or chronic psychosis, but it is not clear if the presence of seizures increase the risk for psychopathology (Silver, 2005).

Pain

Chronic pain is common. Headache is the primary complaint in post-concussive syndrome. Up to 90% of individuals experience posttraumatic headache immediately; up to 44% have headache six months post injury. Other pain problems, such as back pain, complex regional pain syndrome, and fibromyalgia can also occur.

Autonomic dysfunction syndrome

Autonomic dysfunction syndrome (ADS) can occur in TBI, hydrocephalus, brain tumors, subarachnoid hemorrhage, and intracerebral hemorrhage. Temperature elevations in spastic limbs, subnormal temperature in flaccid limbs, hyperhidrosis, hypohidrosis, electrocardiogram alterations, arrhythmias, hypertension, tachycardia, fever, neurogenic lung disease, increased intracranial pressure (ICP), and the dystonias that occur after traumatic brain injuries may also be due to dysregulation of the autonomic system. Certain cortical and subcortical areas influence the activity of the hypothalamus. Cortical and subcortical damage result in dysregulation of the overall autonomic balance; this causes deficits in the control of temperature and blood pressure (Kishner, 2006).

Hydrocephalus

Posttraumatic hydrocephalus can occur two weeks to years after an injury. The term *communicating* denotes patency of flow between ventricles and from the fourth ventricle to the spinal subarachnoid space. *Non-communicating (obstructive) hydrocephalus* occurs when the flow through or from the ventricular system is obstructed. *Communicating hydrocephalus* occurs when products of inflammation obstruct the arachnoid villi after hemorrhage. Severe skull fractures and meningitis may also predispose patients to hydrocephalus in this way (Pangilinan, 2006).

Fatigue and sleep disorders

Sleep disturbances are commonly reported 36% to 70% in individuals post injury. These often continue for more than three months; approximately 20% of individuals still experience fatigue after one year. Difficulties initiating and maintaining sleep as well as excessive daytime somnolence may occur. After secondary causes are ruled out, sleep studies can be performed. Objective tests, such as polysomnography and multiple sleep latency tests can be used. Actinography may also be used (Silver, 2005).

Cognitive disorders

Cognitive deficit severity depends on a number of critical factors, such as severity of diffuse axonal injury as indicated by length of post traumatic amnesia; extent of generalized atrophy; and location, depth, and volume of focal cerebral lesions. Age, comorbidities, and the other significant cranial or systemic condition, e.g., hypoxia or hypotension, also contribute. Four major domains are commonly impaired after closed TBI:

- *Attention*: Range of attention may vary from impaired awareness and wandering attention, such as with posttraumatic amnesia, to inability to concentrate and distractibility in the early recovery phase to impairments later revealed only under rigorous testing.

Attention underpins all aspects of cognition and even mild impairments can affect other processes, such as new learning.

- *Memory:* Verbal and nonverbal memory dysfunction can occur across a range of severity. Tasks that require effortful, controlled, and generally conscious processing usually show the greatest degree of disruption. Short-term memory, such as recall of lists or misplacing objects, such as keys, is the most common deficit.

- *Executive function:* These higher-level tasks include establishing goals and planning; initiating and sequencing; and inhibiting responses; conceptual reasoning and self-regulation. Reduced verbal fluency, at least early in the course of recovery, is a frequent finding in mild TBI. Deficits in higher order functions may be apparent only under certain circumstances as in response to situations in which the correct response is not readily suggested by the task itself.

- *Language and communication:* Communication functions cannot be viewed in isolation. Associated relationships between basic linguistic faculties and divided attention, working memory, and frontal control functions are all important.

Aphasia

Anomic aphasia is the most frequent type of aphasia syndromes, a fluent aphasia with marked inability to identify objects and proper names, frequent paraphasias and circumlocution, and preserved comprehension. Wernicke's or *receptive aphasia*, involves difficult understanding spoken or written language. *Expressive aphasia* involves difficulty in conveying thoughts through speech or writing. *Global aphasia* results from severe and extensive damage to the language areas of the brain (Ninds, 2006; Silver, 2005). The NLCP may consider providing for adaptive communications devices as appropriate after comprehensive evaluation.

Speech disorders

Dysarthria is relatively common after severe TBI (Ninds, 2006; Silver, 2005). *Prosodic dysfunction* is defined as disturbances in intonation or the inability to impart tonal color to one's language. This dysfunction can influence both the ability to convey affect in speech and to perceive affect in speech (Silver, 2005).

Nursing Diagnoses To Consider:

- *Sleep Deprivation:* Prolonged periods of time without sleep (sustained, natural, periodic suspension of relative consciousness)
- *Fatigue:* An overwhelming sense of exhaustion and decreased capacity for physical and mental work at the usual level.
- *Impaired Verbal Communication:* Decreased, delayed, or absent ability to receive, process, transmit, and/or use a system of symbols.
- *Impaired Environmental Interpretation:* Consistent lack of orientation to person, place, time, or circumstances over more than 3 to 6 months, necessitating a protective environment.

Conditions of Altered Consciousness
Minimally responsive vs. persistent vegetative state

Minimally responsive state is characterized by primitive reflexes, an inconsistent ability to follow simple commands, and retain an awareness of environmental stimulation.

Vegetative state is characterized by spontaneous eye-opening; however, there are no purposeful movements or communicative abilities.

Persistent vegetative state (PVS) is a vegetative state lasting for more than a month. Criteria include:

- Arousal present, but the ability to interact with the environment is not
- Eye opening spontaneous or in response to stimulation
- General responses to pain, such as increased heart rate, increased respiration, posturing, or sweating
- Sleep-wake cycle, respiratory functions, and digestive functions return

Coma

Coma is loss of consciousness with no response to stimulation, no awareness of the environment, inability to follow commands or verbalize, and without purposeful or defensive movement. Glasgow Coma Scale score range is 1 to 2, Rancho Los Amigos Scale is I to II with only localized response (ARN Core, 2007). An inpatient rehabilitation admission for coma stimulation program may be done. Return of neuropsychological function would be rare, and Glasgow Outcome classification is usually long-term persistent unresponsiveness (ARN Core 2007; BIAA, 2005; Patterson, 1993; Venes, 2005).

Locked-in syndrome

This rare neurological condition occurs in pontine injury. The person has no control over any part of the body (quadriplegia) except blinking the eyes; this residual ability can be used to operate environmental controls. The person is both conscious and able to think (ARN Core, 2007; BIAA, 2011).

Psychological effects of TBI
Temporolimbic syndrome

Kolb and Wishaw (1990) identified eight principal symptoms of temporal lobe damage: 1) disturbance of auditory sensation and perception, 2) disturbance of selective attention of auditory and visual input, 3) disorders of visual perception, 4) impaired organization and categorization of verbal material, 5) disturbance of language comprehension, 6) impaired long-term memory, 7) altered personality and affective behavior, and 8) altered sexual behavior. The limbic system controls emotions, hormonal secretions, mood, motivation, and pain and pleasure responses. It operates by influencing the endocrine system and the autonomic nervous system and manages the fight or flight chemicals. Neuropsychiatric disorders from the temporolimbic lobes may include; amnesia, delusions and hallucinations, emotional and mood, anxiety and disassociative, and neurovegetative conditions. Frontotemporal contusions following head injury can produce behavioral and emotional effects of personality changes, depression, and delusion in left sided lesions, and posttraumatic mania from right-sided involvement (Kolb and Wishaw, 2009).

Affective mood disorders.

Affective disorders primarily affect mood, and interfere with ADLs. They are a frequent complication of TBI and can delay recovery process and outcomes. Symptoms may include insomnia, non-restorative sleep, appetite disturbance, and anhedonia. Approximately 25-40% of TBI survivors will experience a major depressive disorder (Handel, Ovitt, Spiro, Rao, 2007). Individuals with prior psychiatric history and impaired social support are at higher risk for developing mood disorders.

Personality Disorders

The most common personality disorders (avoidant, paranoid, and schizoid) have been diagnosed in approximately 23% of persons with TBI at 30-year follow-up (Ruocco and Swirsky-Sacchetti, 2007). Patients with personality disorders often exhibit problems in social relationships perceiving and responding to others and stressful situations. Personality disorders are categorized into three clusters. *Cluster A* may present as a delusional disorder or schizophrenia. *Cluster B* appears as an antisocial personality disorder. *Cluster C* is described as an avoidant personality disorder associated with anxiety disorders. Psychotherapy is the foundation for treatment of personality disorders to improve perceptions and responses to stressors, because of poor or limited coping skills. Medications may be necessary to allow the patient to productively participate in psychotherapy and may include; anti-depressants, anti-convulsants, and antipsychotics (Beinenfeld, 2010).

Psychosis

A small percentage of individuals may experience psychosis after mild or severe TBI. The most common symptoms are paranoia or persecutory delusions. Prevalence of psychosis following TBI is increased by damage to the frontal and temporal structures, impairment of the dopamine system, and increased stress from cognitive, emotional, and behavior deficits (Fujii and Ahmed, 2001). Treatment may include neuroleptics, anticonvulsants, and lithium. Caution and frequent monitoring is recommended in treatment with antipsychotic medications due to the increased sensitivity of the injured brain.

Aggression

Aggression can be defined as both verbal and physical against self, others, and objects. It often occurs after brain injury in the acute stages, and can have a variety of underlying causes. Treatment varies with behavior strategies and pharmacological intervention, which may include antipsychotics, and antidepressants (Sudgen, Kile, Farrimond, Hilty, Bourgeouis, 2006).

Frontal Lobe Syndrome

This is often characterized by the contrast of the report of a patient who is unable to do anything but who scores normal or mildly impaired on mental status testing. Symptoms may include aphasia, severe impairment of attention, gait impairment, impaired normal response inhibition, diminished cognitive flexibility, praxis, poor judgment and insight, memory deficits, inappropriate emotional reactions, and incontinence. Diagnosis is determined through laboratory studies; imaging studies such as CT or MRI; and neuropsychological testing. Treatment is provided by neuropsychology and/or behavioral neurologist in conjunction with physical, occupational, and speech therapists. Medications are rarely effective in frontal lobe syndrome (Espay and Jacobs, 2010).

Affective Mood Disorders

Affective disorders primarily affect mood, and interfere with the activities of daily living. They are a frequent complication of traumatic brain injury and can delay recovery process and outcomes. Symptoms may include depressed mood, decreased self-esteem, mood-congruent delusions, insomnia, appetite disturbance, and anhedonia. Approximately 25%-40% of patients with TBI will experience a major depressive disorder. Diagnosis is made following a complete neuropsychological exam including mental status examination and neuroimaging. Treatments for mood disorders with pharmacological options include antidepressants and mood stabilizers (Handel, Ovitt, Spiro, Rao, 2007).

Neuropharmacological management

Patients with brain injury are sensitive to medications and require close monitoring during pharmacological treatment. Medications should be started at a low dose and gradually increased as the patient responds. Psychostimulants, dopaminergic agents, antidepressants, opioid antagonists, beta-blockers, and anticonvulsants are commonly used medications to treat the neuropsychiatric sequelaee of TBI (Rao and Lyketsos, 2000).

Methylphenidate (Concerta, Ritalin) and dextroamphetamine (Dextrostat) are psychostimulants used in the treatment of inattention, distractibility, disorganization, hyperactivity, impulsivity, hypoarousal, apathy, and hypersomnia. Treatment may result in improvement of mood and cognition in TBI. Side effects include paranoia, dysphoria, agitation, and irritability (Rao and Lyketsos, 2000).

Dopaminergic agents supplement the decreased dopamine activity following TBI. Amantadine enhances the release of dopamine and is used for the treatment of mutism, impulsivity, aggression, information processing, apathy, and inattention. Side effects include confusion, hallucinations, edema, and hypotension. Dopamine agonists Levodopa and bromocriptine (Parlodel) can be effective in treating mood, cognition, and behavior. Side effects include nausea, psychosis, and sedation (Rao and Lyketsos, 2000).

Selective serotonin reuptake inhibitors; citalopram (Celexa), escitalopram (Lexapro), fluoxetine (Prozac), and sertraline (Zoloft) are useful in the treatment of depression, mood, lability, and impulsivity. Side effects may include nausea, dry mouth, headache, diarrhea, nervousness, erectile dysfunction, weight gain, drowsiness, and insomnia (Mayo Clinic, 2010).

Carbamazepine (Tegretol) and valproic acid (Depakene) are examples of anticonvulsants used to treat seizure disorder, mood lability, mania, impulsivity, aggression, and rage. Phenytoin and barbiturates are not recommended in TBI due to their ability to decease cognitive function and motor performance (Rao and Lyketsos, 2000). A neuropsychiatrist working in close collaboration with patient and family to resolve persistent neuropsychiatric sequelaee may also prescribe other agents to treat self-injurious behavior such as opioid antagonists (naltrexone), selective serotonin antagonist buspirone), or beta-blockers (propranolol) (Rao and Lyketsos, 2000).

Nursing Diagnoses To Consider:
- *Risk for Other-Directed Violence:* At risk for behaviors in which an individual demonstrates that he or she can be physically, emotionally, and/or sexually harmful to others.
- *Risk for Self-Directed Violence:* At risk for behaviors in which an individual demonstrates that he or she can be physically, emotionally, and/or sexually harmful to self.

- *Impaired Verbal Communication:* Decreased, delayed, or absent ability to receive, process, transmit, and/or use a system of symbols.

Endocrine effects

Basilar skull fracture, hypothalamic edema, prolonged unresponsiveness, hyponatremia, and/or hypotension are associated with a higher occurrence of endocrinopathy. Significant endocrine failure may be caused by direct injury to the hypothalamic-pituitary axis (HPA), neuroendocrinological effects from catecholamines and cytokines, or from systemic infection or inflammation causing primary gland failure. Autopsy evidence of HPA hemorrhage or ischemia is common. Delayed diagnosis of hypopituitarism is often mistaken for symptoms of residual head injury.

In the Powner study (2006), some kind of chronic hormone deficiency occurred in 30% to 40% of selected patients; 10% to 15% had more than one deficiency. These included deficient levels of growth hormone in 15% to 20%, gonadal hormones in 15%, and hypothyroidism in 10% to 30%. All clinical symptoms responded favorably to replacement therapy.

Practitioners may miss subtle signs of endocrinopathy or attribute symptoms to the brain injury itself, delaying diagnosis and treatment (Powner, 2006). Endocrine problems can interfere with the progress of rehabilitation and are detrimental to rehabilitation outcome if not recognized and treated properly (Klein, 2005).

Hypopituitarism

Autopsy and other studies have shown that TBI may be associated with impairments of pituitary and hypothalamus function, which may contribute to long-term physical, cognitive, and psychological disability. In two major studies, the occurrence and risk factors of pituitary dysfunction, including GHD in patients with TBI over 5 years showed 54% to 57%

had pituitary dysfunction of some type (Bondanelli, 2004; Tanriverdi, 2006).

Hypopituitarism is a treatable cause of morbidity after TBI. In order to improve outcome and quality of life of TBI patients, an adequate replacement therapy as indicated is of paramount importance (Bondanelli, 2005). Endocrine workup includes serum hormonal assays for cortisol, testosterone, tri-iodothyronine (T3), thyroxine (T4), thryotropin, follicle-stimulating hormone (FSH), leuteinizing hormone (LH), and estrogen (females). Growth hormone testing is another screening factor.

The most common alterations in hypopituitarism appear to be gonadotropin and somatotropin deficiency, followed by corticotropin and thyrotropin deficiency. Hyper-or hypoprolactinemia may also be present. Diabetes insipidus (DI) may be common in the early, acute phase post-TBI, but it is rarely permanent. Treatment involves multiple hormonal replacement therapies and monitoring of serum levels. Clinical response of the patient will gauge effectiveness of the treatment, and should include improved vital signs, increased endurance and participation in rehabilitation, and improved overall appearance. Hormonal replacement therapy is usually required long term. Involvement of the endocrinologist and brain injury specialist are essential in addressing long term and initial rehabilitation treatment needs.

Growth hormone deficiency
Patients with a history of TBI frequently develop pituitary dysfunction, especially growth hormone deficiency (GHD). Therefore, evaluation of pituitary hormone secretion, including growth hormone, should be included in the long-term follow-up of all TBI patients to guide hormone replacement therapy.

According to the Tanriverdi study (2006), GHD is the most common pituitary deficit 12 months after TBI, and 50.9%

of the patients had at least one anterior pituitary hormone deficiency. Pituitary function may improve or worsen in a considerable number of patients over 12 months (Tanriverdi, 2006).

Insulin-like growth factor-I (IGF-I) is the screening assay for growth hormone deficiency. Testing will need to be done to confirm the diagnosis. Treatment involves multiple hormonal replacement therapies and monitoring of serum levels, as well as the improvements in the patient's clinical status, including vital signs and endurance. Growth hormone replacement therapy outcomes include increased muscle mass, increased exercise tolerance and improved quality of life. Hormonal replacement therapy usually is required long term and should be considered in future care planning needs, as well as the involvement of an endocrinologist.

Syndrome of inappropriate antidiuretic hormone
The most common endocrine complication in the post-acute period is the syndrome of inappropriate antidiuretic hormone (SIADH); incidence post TBI is reportedly as high as 33%. SIADH can also be induced medications commonly used in TBI, such as carbamazepine (Tegretol), major tranquilizers, and antidepressants.

SIADH prevents water excretion by the kidneys, leading to dilutional hyponatremia. Hyponatremia causes cerebral edema resulting in lassitude, seizures, confusion, and coma; increasing cerebral edema increases intracranial pressure, decreasing cerebral blood flow.

Other causes of hyponatremia include iatrogenic or psychogenic water overload, large gastrointestinal fluid losses, and renal sodium wasting. Hypothyroidism can also masquerade as SIADH, with similar symptoms. Unresolved SIADH leads to serious consequences, including coma and death.

Diabetes insipidus

DI is rare, with an estimated one case per 100,000 hospital admissions. Posttraumatic DI occurs in 2% to 16% of all cases (Klein, 2005). The most common causes of posttraumatic DI include severe TBI with basilar skull fractures, craniofacial trauma, thoracic injury, cranial nerve injury, and post-cardiopulmonary arrest. It is centrally caused by hypopituitarism. The usual onset is 5 to 10 days following trauma. Delayed onset of DI is associated with a poor prognosis and permanent DI. Acute DI following mild to moderate TBI indicates a posterior pituitary lesion with only a temporary antidiuretic hormone (ADH) deficiency. Untreated DI may cause poor neurological outcome, including death.

Cerebral salt wasting

Cerebral salt wasting (CSW) is caused by impaired renal function, resulting in the inability of the kidneys to conserve sodium. The syndrome is thought to be neurologically caused. Salt wasting with volume depletion is the hallmark of this syndrome. Patients become dehydrated, lose weight, have orthostatic hypotension, and demonstrate a negative fluid balance. It is common after central nervous system injury, yet often remains unrecognized. Treatment of CSW consists of hydration with IV normal saline and salt replacement (Zafonte, 2004). Rehydration is essential to reducing the risks of cerebral ischemia or cerebrovascular accident due to dehydration and associated vasospasm.

Brain Injury Treatment Options

A statistical study was published by the CDC in 2002 reviewing TBI data for 12 states finding 66% of TBI patients were discharged from the acute care hospital without further health care, 17% were discharged to outpatient therapy, home health care, or residential/rehabilitation facilities and 3% were transferred to acute rehabilitation hospitals (1% left against medical advice, 6% died, and 6% had no coding) (CDC, 2003, 2006).

Post-Acute Rehabilitation Facilities

It is unclear how many of the 17% of TBI survivors noted above are transferred to post-acute rehabilitation (PARF) (CDC, 2002). However, in order to meet admission criteria, the survivor must demonstrate definite cognitive or behavioral deficits and may have ongoing physical or medical needs. The focus of these facilities is neurorehabilitation to maximize physical, medical, cognitive, and emotional condition with the ultimate goal of community re-entry.

Another option is a neurobehavioral program for ultra-high risk TBI survivors with unwanted or dangerous behaviors that prevent community living (Mentor-ABI, 2005). The facility should be evaluated for the some of the following aspects for the severe behavior problems as follows:

- Trained staff, with neuropsychologists, neuropsychiatrists, and doctorate-level behavior analysts
- Clinical staff (occupational therapy, physical therapy, speech-language pathology, teachers, vocational rehabilitation) experienced with severe TBI
- Close supervision and secure environment
- A natural, home-like setting
- Age and functional-level appropriate activities, including recreational
- Discharge planning is appropriate to the individual's culture, life-setting and the discharge setting (Page, 2001)

Residential Care

Residential care availability can vary from state to state. This may mean placement in a long-term facility without any program or placement in a facility with a structured TBI program. These placements may be funded privately or Medicaid. An outcome-based study found that TBI survivors who were transferred to residential care or long-term care were typically older, funded by Medicaid, and had the poorest reported outcomes (Mellick, 2003).

Group Homes

Group homes are usually apartment-style living with other TBI survivors, with oversight and supervision of TBI-trained staff. This facility ensures medication adherence, provides structure for everyday living skills, appointments (e.g., physical therapy, physician), perhaps work programs, and support from TBI survivor peers and families. Group homes may be near someone's home or located in another state (Mentor-ABI, 2005).

Home Care (With and Without Support)

Since 66% of people with a TBI are released to home without services, one would presume there was no need for services. However, many times these people have difficulty returning to school, work or families due to effects of post-concussion syndrome (Fralish, 1996) and discover that they need help. A physician paper recommends more evaluations and treatment planning for the 66% (most likely mild TBI) group, as nearly half have continued post-concussion syndrome with some cognitive deficits at 6 months and further interventions were needed (Cushman, 2008).

Home Health Care, Outpatient Therapies, and Day Programs

Cognitive therapy from a speech-language pathologist or occupation therapist can be provided in a home or outpatient setting depending on the TBI survivor's physical ability. A survivor may also transition to a day program after hospital discharge to receive these services (Mentor ABI, 2005). The focus is on the individual's deficits in attention and concentration, learning and memory, judgment and perception, problem solving, communication, and swallowing (NICDC, 2002 NINDS, 2006).

Independent Living

Most people who suffer a TBI at any level have some type of cognitive deficit. Achieving the best recovery outcome depends on post-injury therapies and support systems or, in the case of mild TBI, the ability to self-learn new adaptive behaviors and learning techniques.

Many young TBI survivors wish to return to an independent lifestyle, living alone without parents. Other survivors may find themselves alone when they lose their families to divorce or other situations. Federal and state governments and non-profit organizations have developed support systems to make it possible for TBI survivors to remain in the community in independent living situations. Two aspects will be discussed below.

Traumatic Brain Injury Waivers In 1991 the first traumatic brain injury waiver was initiated in the United States—a Federal and state program providing

- Community skills training
- Assistance with medical and wellness appointments
- Caregiver support
- Drug and alcohol prevention and treatment
- Legal assistance
- Housing
- Education
- Transportation
- Information and resources

All therapy disciplines, especially intensive cognitive therapy, are provided; there is also a transitional living specialist who provides coaching.

These community-based programs (CBP) are very successful, as noted in a 2000 study comparing them to the standard inpatient neurobehavioral rehabilitation program (IRP). Outcomes were based on the Community Integration

Questionnaire (CIQ) and Quality of Community Integration Questionnaire (QCIQ). The CBP demonstrated twice as high in the confidence interval and had a perceived self-efficacy on community cognitive functioning (Cicerone, 2004).

Independent Living Centers In many states, the physical assistance portion of the traumatic brain injury waiver are provided through independent living centers. They are private, non-profit, consumer-controlled community-based organizations that provide services, resources, and advocacy to TBI survivors and their families. They also focus on assisting TBI survivors achieve their highest maximum potential while living in the community. Services include self-directed employment and caregiver training. Independent living centers receive state, national, and federal funding (Ilusa, 2002).

Outcome Measurement Resources

The *Center for Outcome Measurement in Brain Injury (COMBI)* is an online resource on brain injury outcomes. The COMBI is a collaborative project of 16 brain injury centers, most of which are members of the Traumatic Brain Injury Model Systems. COMBI has more than 25 scales or instruments measuring outcomes, some of which are described below. The COMBI is coordinated by the Rehabilitation Research Center at Santa Clara Valley Medical Center CA.

Functional Independence Measure (FIM)

FIM is an 18-item instrument used by clinicians to measure disability and is considered the most widely accepted functional assessment measure in use in the rehabilitation community. It covers self-care, sphincter control, transfers, locomotion, communication, and social cognition (Wright, 2000).

Functional Assessment Measure (FAM)

FAM is a 12-item adjunct to the FIM with more brain injury/stroke related items. Scoring is done by clinicians who assess abilities from total assistance to complete independence on a variety of skills. The scores for the same categories as the FIM are evaluated periodically from admission to discharge to follow-up. The 12 items on the FAM do not stand alone, but are intended to be added to the 18 items of the FIM. The total 30-item scale combination is referred to as the FIM +FAM (Wright, 2000).

Disability Rating Scale (DRS)

The DRS is an 8-item instrument used by clinicians to measure disability in older juveniles and adults with moderate to severe TBI in inpatient rehabilitation. One advantage of the DRS is its ability to track an individual from coma to community, because various items in this scale address all three World Health Organization categories: impairment, disability and handicap (WHO, 1980). Items measured in the DRS are eye opening, communication ability, motor response, feeding, toileting, grooming, level of functioning, and employability.

The maximum DRS score is 29, for extreme vegetative state. No disability would be scored as a zero. This rating scale is intended to measure general functional changes over the course of recovery. The DRS has been proven reliable and valid. DRS is relatively insensitive for mild TBI because it is unable to reflect subtler but sometimes significant changes (Wright, 2000).

High level Mobility Assessment Tool (HiMAT)

The High-level Mobility Assessment Tool (HiMAT) quantifies mobility required for participation in physically demanding employment roles, leisure activities, social roles, and sporting activities. This was developed to quantify high-level mobility outcomes suitable for any individual with a TBI who has a goal that requires a level of mobility beyond independent level walking. The HiMAT consists of 13 items for a maximum score of 54 (Williams, 2006).

Other Resources

One important resource for information on outcomes after TBI is the *National Institute on Disability and Rehabilitation Research (NIDRR)*. NIDRR's mission is to generate new knowledge and promote its effective use to improve the abilities of people with disabilities to perform activities of their choice in the community, and expand society's capacity to provide full opportunities and accommodations for its disabled citizens (NIDRR 2008).

In 1999, the *Agency for Health Care Policy and Research (AHCPR)* through its Evidence-based Practice Center conducted a meta-analysis of research articles to examine the effectiveness of rehabilitation methods at various phases of recovery following traumatic brain injury in adults. 3,098 research articles were included in the analysis. Key questions were posed including (Chestnut et al., 1999):

- How should the concepts of recovery, functional status, and disability be defined?
- How should the type and severity of injury itself be measured?
- Which therapies are effective?
- What are the best ways to match patients with treatment approaches to facilitate effectiveness?

The *International Brain Injury Association (IBIA)* is another resource for evaluating evidence for the clinical effectiveness of cognitive rehabilitation in stroke and traumatic brain injury. In the U.S., systematic reviews of cognitive rehabilitation have been conducted through the *American Congress of Rehabilitation Medicine (ACRM)* and the *Academy of Neurogenic Communication Disorders and Sciences*. Efforts to evaluate the effectiveness of treatments for cognitive rehabilitation in Europe have been conducted through the Cochrane Collaboration.

In 1999 a task force on Cognitive Rehabilitation was developed under the auspices of the European Federation of Neurologic Societies (EFNS). Guidelines were proposed in 2003 and more recently, an update has been published. One conclusion was that electronic memory aids, such as computers, paging systems, or portable voice recorders have been shown to be effective in several Class III studies and recommended as "probably effective" for improving performance of everyday activities for people with TBI or stroke (IBIA 2006).

For the past 20 years, the *Brain Trauma Foundation (BTF)* has been dedicated to improving outcomes for individuals with a TBI nationwide. Given that all brain damage does not occur at the moment of impact, but evolves over the next hours and days due to brain swelling, BTF has developed evidence-based guidelines to address secondary damage. Guidelines available for physicians, trauma centers, and other healthcare professionals, are (BTF 2011):

- Guidelines for Pre-Hospital Management
- Guidelines for Surgical Management of Traumatic Brain Injury
- Management and Prognosis of Severe Traumatic Brain Injury
- Guidelines for Acute Medical Management of Severe Traumatic Brain Injury in Infants, Children, and Adolescents
- Guidelines for Field Management of Combat-Related Head Trauma

Five indicators have been found to have prognostic significance. These are age, Glasgow Coma Scale score, pupil reactivity, brainstem reflexes, and the presence of post-traumatic hypotension. The presence of midline shift is also of prognostic significance. Another important prognostic indicator is the presence of subarachnoid hemorrhage on CT scan, particularly in the region of the suprasellar or ambient cisterns (BTF 2011).

As of 2006, Craig Hospital in Englewood, Colorado, has been designated the *Traumatic Brain Injury Model Systems National Data and Statistical Center (TBINDSC)*. It is a central resource for researchers and data collectors in the Traumatic Brain Injury Model Systems (TBIMS) program. Each of the 16 TBI model systems in the United States conducts individual studies. The TBINDSC provides technical assistance, training, and methodological consultation to 16 TBIMS centers as they collect and analyze longitudinal data from people with TBI in their communities and conduct research on evidence-based TBI rehabilitation interventions. To access the latest information on outcome studies and effective rehabilitation interventions, go to the individual websites of the 16 TBI model systems (TBINDSC 2011).

Assessing Cognitive and Behavioral Patterns

The following interviewing questions will focus on cognitive and behavioral deficits. These questions are generally asked of the patient first, and then information is gathered from significant family members to account for the possibility of patient's cognitive deficits, especially confabulation.

Interview questions focus on behavior and emotional deficits. It is critically important to ascertain the severity of behavior. Assess for tangential sentence structure, confabulation or perseveration during the interview.

- Have you ever been so frustrated with yourself that you have tried hitting, biting, or other ways of hurting yourself?
- Have you been physically hurtful to others?
- Have people told you that you have behaved unacceptably in social situations (e.g., spitting, yelling verbal harassments, bullying, or doing physical inappropriate acts)?

- Have you wandered away from home unexpectedly? (If yes, was this due to a frustrating circumstance, high level of noise, or confusion.)
- Do you find yourself avoiding people or situations that you normally would attend?

Assess judgment or self-protection ability by questions related to door-to-door or telephone salesman and receiving the correct change back from store clerks.

- Do you find yourself easily distracted, cannot follow the conversation, or do not understand the important message someone is saying?
- Do you have trouble organizing your normal daily routine tasks? (To assess short-term memory, ask "what did you have for dinner last night?" Verify this information with another person.)
- Has someone said or done something that offends you and they say they didn't mean it that way?
- If a fire started in the kitchen, what would you do first?

Conclusion

Brain injury is the leading cause of death and disability worldwide (IBIA, 2012). This chapter provides nurse life care planners with a solid foundation in the types of injury, incidence, causes and possible interventions to prevent brain injuries. Measurement tools used to evaluate level of consciousness, outcome severity and level s of cognitive and physical function are included.

While each individual with brain injury is unique, a comprehensive list of medical complications provides the nurse life care planner with an organized means to review, system by system, current injuries and deficits as well as consider possible future complications. Various treatment options are described with a range of functional outcomes discussed. The nurse life care planner determines which information in this chapter is relevant and applicable.

References

Agency on Health Care Policy and Research. (1999). Rehabilitation for TBI. Retrieved from http://archive.ahrq.gov/clinic/epcsums/tbisumm.htm

Agha A, Rogers B, et al. (2004). Anterior pituitary dysfunction in survivors of traumatic brain injury. Journal of Clinical Endocrinology and Metabolism, 10(89), 4929-4936.

Agha A, Thornton, E et al. (2004)Posterior pituitary dysfunction after traumatic brain injury. The Journal of Clinical Endocrinology and Metabolism, 12(89), 5987-5992.

American Academy of Neurology. (2013) Brain injury guidelines. Retrieved from http://www.aan.com/Guidelines/Home/ByTopic?topicId=13

American Urological Association. (2011, January). Neurogenic bladder. Retrieved from http://www.urologyhealth.org/urology/index.cfm?article=9

Ayello EA. (2003). Preventing pressure ulcers and skin tears. In Mezey MD, Fulmer TT, et al., (Eds.), Geriatric nursing protocols for best practice (2nd ed., pp. 165-184) New York, NY: Springer Publishing Company.

Bahoul M, Chaari AN, et al. (2006). Neurogenic pulmonary edema due to traumatic brain injury: Evidence of cardiac dysfunction. American Journal of Critical Care, 15(5), 462-470.

Bienenfeld D and Ahmed I. (2010, June 14). Personality disorders. Retrieved from http://emedicine.medscape.com/article/294307-overview

Blackwell T. (1994). Life care planning for traumatic brain injury. Athens, GA: Elliott and Fitzpatrick.

Blackwell T, Krause, et al. (2001). Spinal cord injury desk reference: Guidelines for life care planning and case management. New York, NY: Demos Medical.

Bondanelli M, Ambrosio MR et al. (2005). Hypopituitarism after traumatic brain injury. European Journal of Endocrinology, 152(5), 679-691.

Bondanelli M., De Marinis L et al. (2004). Occurrence of pituitary dysfunction following traumatic brain injury. Journal of Neurotrauma, 21(5), 685-696.

Brain Injury Association of America. (n.d.). About brain injury. Retrieved from http://www.biausa.org/about-brain-injury.htm

Ibid. Brain injury facts. Retrieved from http://www.biausa.org/LiteratureRetrieve.aspx?ID=104991

Ibid. (2001). The road to rehabilitation series. Retrieved from http://www.biausa.org

Ibid. (2006). Types of brain injuries. Retrieved from http://biausa.fyrian.com/about-brain-injury.htm#types

Brain Injury Resource Center. (1998). TBI glossary. Retrieved from http://www.headinjury.com/tbiglossary.htm

Brooks N. (1984). Closed head injury: psychological, social and family consequences. New York, NY: Oxford University Press.

Centers for Disease Control and Prevention. (2006). Incidence rates of hospitalization related to traumatic brain injury-12 states. MMWR Morbidity and Mortality Weekly Reports, 55(8), 201-204.

Ibid. (2006) CDC injury fact book. Atlanta GA. Retrieved from http://www.cdc.gov/Injury/publications/FactBook/InjuryBook2006.pdf

Ibid. (2012, February 29). Falls, older adults. Retrieved from http://www.cdc.gov/ncipc/pub-res/toolkit/SummaryofFalls.htm

Chesnut RM, Carney N, et al. (1998). Evidence report on rehabilitation of persons with traumatic brain injury. Rockville, MD: Agency for Health Care Policy and Research

Cicerone KD, Mott T, et al. (2004). Community integration and satisfaction with functioning after intensive cognitive rehabilitation for traumatic brain injury. Archives of Physical Medicine and Rehabilitation, 85(6), 943-950.

Cicerone KD. (2006). Evidence-based guidelines for cognitive rehabilitation: A European perspective. Retrieved from http://www.internationalbrain.org/articles/

evidencebased-guidelines-for-cognitive-rehabilitation-a-european-perspective/

Colantino A, Ratcliff G, et al. (2004). Aging with traumatic brain injury: Long term health complications. International Journal of Rehabilitation Research, 27(3), 209-214.

Commission for Accreditation of Rehabilitation Facilities. (n.d.). Accreditation. Retrieved from http://www.carf.org/Accreditation/

Crippen, D. W. (2012, June 21). Head trauma. Retrieved from http://emedicine.medscape.com/article/433855-overview

Cushman JG, Agarwal N, et al. (2001). Practice management guidelines for the management of mild traumatic brain injury: The EAST practice management guidelines work group. Journal of Trauma, 51(5), 1016-1026.

Dugdale DC. (2011, July 31). Focal neurological deficits. Retrieved from http://www.nlm.nih.gov/medlineplus/ency/article/003191.htm

Edwards P. (2000). The specialty practices of rehabilitation nursing: a core curriculum (3rd ed.) (Skokie, IL: Rehabilitation Nursing Foundation.

Espay AJ. (2010, April 27). Frontal lobe syndromes. Retrieved from http://emedicine.medscape.com/article/1135866- overview

Fleminger S. (2003). Managing agitation and aggression after head injury. British Medical Journal, 327(7405), 4-5.

Foxx-Orenstein A, Kolakowsky-Hayner S, et al. (2003). Incidence, risk factors, and outcomes of fecal incontinence after acute brain injury: Findings from the Traumatic Brain Injury Model Systems national database. Archives of Physical Medicine and Rehabilitation, 84(2), 231-237.

Fralish K. (1996). Characteristics of persons with head injury. Brain Injury, 10(10), 763-778.

Fujii D. (2002). Neuropsychiatry of psychosis secondary to traumatic brain injury. Psychiatric Times, XIX (9), 1.

Geerts WH, Pineo GF, et al. (2004). Prevention of venous thromboembolism: The Seventh ACCP Conference on

Antithrombotic and Thrombolytic Therapy. Chest, 126, 2297-2298.

Gennarelli TA. (1986). The mechanism and pathophysiology of a cerebral concussion. Journal of Head Trauma, 1, 23-29.

Goldstein G, Ruthven L. (1983). Rehabilitation of the brain-damaged adult. New York, NY: Springer.

Guerrero JL, Thurman D J et al. (2000). Emergency department visits associated with traumatic brain injury: United States 1995-1996. Brain Injury, 14(2), 181-186.

Harrison-Felix C., Whiteneck G et al. Mortality following rehabilitation in the Traumatic Brain Injury Model Systems of Care. NeuroRehabilitation, 19, 45-54.

Herdman TH (2012) (ed.) NANDA International. Nursing diagnoses: Definitions and Classification, 2012-2014. Oxford, United Kingdom: Wiley-Blackwell.

Herrmann BL, Rehder, et al. (2006). Hypopituitarism following severe traumatic brain injury. Experimental and Clinical Endocrinology and Diabetes, 114(6), 316-321.

Horlander KT, Mannino DM, et al. (2003). Pulmonary embolism mortality in the United States, 1979-1998: An analysis using multiple-cause mortality data. Archives of Internal Medicine, 163, 1711-1717.

Hsieh JS, Howng SL, et al. (2006). Endothelin-1, inducible nitric oxide synthase and macrophage inflammatory protein-1alpha in the pathogenesis of stress ulcer in neurotraumatic patients. Journal of Trauma, 4(61), 873-878.

Independent Living Centers of the United States of America. (2008, September 11). Independent living centers. Retrieved from http://www.ilusa.com/links/ilcenters. htm

International Brain Injury Association. (n.d.). Brain injury facts. Retrieved from http://www.internationalbrain. org/?q=Brain-Injury-Facts

Leary, Cheesman, et al. (2006) Incontinence after brain injury: prevalence, outcome and multidisciplinary management on a neurological rehabilitation units. Clinical Rehabilitation 2006 Dec; 20(12): 1049-9

Jackson RM. (1993). Respiratory failure after cerebral injury. In R. Demling (Ed.) Acute respiratory failure (p. 440). Far Hills, NJ: New Horizons Press Books.

Jorge R, Robinson RG. (2003). Mood disorders following traumatic brain injury. Internal Review of Psychiatry, 15(4), 317-327.

Kalsotra, A., Zhao, J., Anakk, S., Dash, P. K., and Strobel, H. W. (2007). Brain trauma leads to enhanced lung inflammation and injury: Evidence for role of P4504Fs in resolution. Journal of Cerebral Blood Flow and Metabolism, 27, 963-974.

Kaschak Newman, D., and Jakovac-Smith, D. (1991). Geriatric care plans. Springhouse, PA: Springhouse Publisher Co.

Kearon, C. (2003). Natural history of venous thromboembolism. Circulation, 107, 22-30.

Kennedy, R.E., Livingston, L., Marwitz, J.H., Gueck, S., Kreutzer, J.S., and Saunders, A.M. (2006). Complicated mild traumatic brain injury on the inpatient rehabilitation unit: A multicenter analysis. Journal of Head Trauma Rehabilitation, 21(3), 260-271.

Kishner S, Strum S. (2011, July 7). Post head injury autonomic complications. Retrieved from http://emedicine. medscape.com/article/325994-overview

Klein M. (2012, January 18). Post head injury endocrine complications. Retrieved from http://emedicine. medscape.com/article/326123-overview

Knudson M and Ikossi DG. (2004). Venous thromboembolism after trauma. Current Opinion in Critical Care, 10, 539-48.

Los Amigos Research and Educational Institute (1990) Rancho Los Amigos cognitive scale, revised. Levels of cognitive functioning.

Lubit RH. (2011, June 14). Postconcussive syndrome. Retrieved from http://emedicine.medscape.com/ article/292326- overview

Lehrer M. (2005). Pressure ulcer. Retrieved from http:// emedicine.medscape.com/article/319284-overview

May D, Potter R, et al. (1992, January/February). Predicting post traumatic amnesia patients' performance on specific cognitive tasks. The Journal of Cognitive Rehabilitation, 34-40.

Manker A, Greenwald B. (2003). Giving a head up on mild traumatic brain injury. Retrieved from http://www.theuniversityhospital.com/healthlink/archives/articles/ brain_injurys.html

Marwitz JH, Cifu DX et al. (2001). A multi-center analysis of rehospitalizations five years after brain injury. The Journal of Head Trauma Rehabilitation, 16(4), 307-317.

Mauk KL. (Ed.). (2007). The specialty practice of rehabilitation nursing: a core curriculum (5th ed.). Glenview, IL: Association of Rehabilitation Nurses.

Mentor ABI. (2005). Post-Acute Neuro-Rehabilitation Centers. Retrieved from http://thementornetwork.com/standard/page.aspx?guide705be6e-1254-48a8-89ac-0b0ea699bb28

Mellick D, Gerhart KA et al. (2003). Understanding outcomes based on the post-acute hospitalization pathways followed by persons with traumatic brain injury. Brain Injury, 17(1), 55-71.

Meythaler JM. (2003). Traumatic brain injury inform-spastic hypertonias following traumatic brain injury. Retrieved from http://main.uab.edu/tbi/show.asp?durki=56147

Moberg-Wolf EA. (2011, November 17). Physical medicine and rehabilitation for spasticity. Retrieved from http://emedicine.medscape.com/article/318994-overview

Montejo JC. (1999). Enteral nutrition-related GI complications in critically ill patients: a multi-center study. The Nutritional and Metabolic Working Group of the Spanish Society of Intensive Care Medicine and Coronary Units. Critical Care Medicine, 27(8), 1447-1493.

Morgan A, Ward E, et al. (2003). Incidence, characteristics, and predictive factors for dysphagia after pediatric traumatic brain injury. Journal of Head Trauma Rehabilitation, 18(3), 239-251.

National Center for Injury Prevention and Control. (2003). Report to Congress on mild traumatic brain injury in the United States: Steps to prevent serious health problem. Atlanta, GA: Center for Disease Control and Prevention.

National Data and Statistical Center. (n.d.). The Traumatic Brain Injury Model System Outcomes. Retrieved from http://www.tbindsc.org

National Institute on Disability and Rehabilitation Research. (2004). Brain Injury Outcomes. Retrieved from http://www2.ed.gov/legislation/FedRegister/proprule/2002-1/030502c.html

National Institute of Health Consensus Development Program. (1998). Rehabilitations of persons with traumatic brain injury. Retrieved from http://consensus.nih.gov/1998/1998traumaticbraininjury109html.htm

NIDCD. (2002). Traumatic Brain Injury (Version 98-4315). Retrieved from http://www.nidcd.nih.gov

National Institute of Neurological Disorders and Stroke. (2012, June 14). What disabilities can result from TBI? Retrieved from http://www.ninds.nih.gov/disorders/tbi/ detail_tbi.htm#193673218

National Institute of Neurological Disorders and Stroke. (2012, July 9)., NINDS aphasia information page. Retrieved from http://www.ninds.nih.gov/disorders/aphasia/aphasia.htm

National Institute of Neurological Disorders and Stroke. (2012, July 20). Myclonus fact sheet. Retrieved from http://www.ninds.nih.gov/disorders/myoclonus/detail_myoclonus.htm

National Institute of Neurological Disorders and Stroke. (2012). What is dysarthia. Retrieved from http://www.ninds.nih.gov/doctors/NIH_Stroke_Scale_Booklet.pdf

Olszewski J. (2006). Causes, diagnosis and treatment of neurological dysphagia, an interdisciplinary clinical problem. Otolaryngologia polska, 60(4), 491-500.

Padulo WV, Argyris S. (n.d.). Vision and brain injury: Post trauma vision syndrome. Retrieved from http://www.neuroskills.com/tbi/vision1.shtml

Pape, Marsh, et al. (2004). Current concepts in the development of heterotopic ossification. Journal of Bone and Joint Surgery 86B: 6 p 783-787

Page TJ. (2001). Navigating the curves: Navigating behavior changes and brain injury. In The Road to Rehabilitation (pp. 1-16). Washington, DC: Brain Injury Association of America.

Pangilinan PH, Kelly BM et al. (2012, May 29). Classification and complications of traumatic brain injury. Retrieved from http://emedicine.medscape.com/article/326643- overview

Pangilinan PH, Kelly BM et al. (2011, November 17). Posttraumatic hydrocephalus. Retrieved from http://emedicine.medscape.com/article/326411-overview

Patterson T. (1993). Traumatic brain injury. In Emick-Herring B (Ed.), The specialty practice of rehabilitation nursing: A core curriculum (3rd ed., pp. 52-58). Skokie, IL: Rehabilitation Nursing Foundation.

Pentland B. (2003). Acquired brain injury: Early rehabilitation and long term outcome. In BSDH (Ed.), British Society of Disability and Oral Health (pp. 1-46). London: BSDH. http://www.bsdh.org.uk/reports/Brian_Pentland.ppt

Phillips B J, Fujii, TK. (2005). Traumatic brain injury: A review. The Internet Journal of Surgery, 6(1). doi:10.5580/307 Retrieved from http://www.ispub.com/journal/the-internet-journal-of-surgery/volume-6-number-1/traumatic-brain-injury-a-review.html

Powner DJ, Boccalandro C, et al. (2006). Endocrine failure after traumatic brain injury in adults. Neurocritical Care, 5(1), 61-70.

Reichmann R. (1987). Aging with a disability. New York, NY: Demos Medical Publishing. Rocky Mountain Regional Brain Injury System. (2003). Fatigue and TBI. Thinking Ahead, 5(1), 1-7.

Russell R, Smith A. (1961). Post-traumatic amnesia in closed head injury. Archives of Neurology, 5, 16-29.

Salazar AM. (2002). Traumatic brain injury: Mild traumatic brain injury. Journal of Neurology, 249, 1-3.

Sbordone RJ. (2000). Neuropsychology for health care
     professionals and attorneys (2nd ed.). Boca Raton, FL:
     CRC Press.
Schurr MJ. (1999). Formal swallowing evaluation and therapy
     after traumatic brain injury improves dysphagia
     outcomes. Journal of Trauma, 46(5), 817-821.
Scottish Intercollegiate Guidelines Network (2004).
     Management of patients with stroke: identification and
     management of dysphagia: A national clinical guideline.
     Edinburgh, Scotland: Author. Retrieved from http://
     www.sign.ac.uk/pdf/sign78.pdf
Sehnert KW, Croft AC. (1996). Basal metabolic temperature
     and laboratory assessment in post-traumatic
     hypothyroidism. Journal of Physiological Therapy, 1,
     6-12.
Shavelle RM, Strauss D, et al. (2001). Long term causes of
     death after traumatic brain injury. American Journal of
     Physical Medicine and Rehabilitation, 80, 510-516.
Shavelle R, Strauss DJ. et al.(2006). Life expectancy. In N. Zasler,
     D.Katz, R. Zafonte (Ed.), Brain injury medical: Practice
     and principles (pp. 247-261). New York, NY: Demos
     Medical Publishing.
Silver J, McAllister TW et al. (2011). Textbook of traumatic
     brain injury. Arlington, VA: American Psychiatric
     Publishing
Strauss D, Shavelle RM, DeVivo MJ. et al. (2004). Life expectancy
     after traumatic brain injury. NeuroRehabilitation, 19,
     257-258.
Smith-Hammond CA, Goldstein LB. (2006). Cough and
     aspiration of food and liquids due to oral-pharyngeal
     dysphagia: ACCP evidence-based clinical practice
     guidelines. Chest, 129(1 Suppl), 154S-168S.
Tanriverdi F, Senyurek H, et al. (2006). High risk of
     hypopituitarism after traumatic brain injury: A
     prospective investigation of anterior pituitary function
     in acute phase and 12 months after trauma. Journal
     of Clinical Endocrinology and Metabolism, 91(6),
     2105-2111.

Teasdale G, Jennett B (1974). "Assessment of coma and impaired consciousness: A practical scale". The Lancet 2 (7872): 81-4.

Trimble MR, Mendez MF, et al. (1997). Neuropsychiatric symptoms from the temporolimbic lobes. Journal of Neuropsychiatry Clinical Neuroscience, 9, 429-438.

Varney NR, Roberts RJ. (1999). The evaluation and treatment of mild traumatic brain injury. Mahwah, NJ: Lawrence Erlbaum Associates.

Venes D. (Ed.). (2005). Taber's cyclopedic medical dictionary (20th ed.). Philadelphia, PA: F.A.Davis Company

Walsh K. (1987). Neuropsychology: A clinical approach. New York, NY: Churchilland Livingstone.

Weed R, Berens DE. (Eds.) (1999). Life care planning and case management handbook.New York, NY: CRC Press.

Williams G. (2006). The High Level Mobility Assessment Tool. Retrieved from http://www.tbims.org/combi/himat

Winternitz WW, Dzur JA. (1976). Pituitary failure secondary to head trauma. Case report. Journal of Neurosurgery, 44(4), 504-505.

World Health Organization. (1948). Disability Rating. Retrieved from http://www.tbims.org/ combi/drs/index.html

Wright, J. (2000). Introduction to the Disability Rating Scale. Retrieved from http://www.tbims.org/combi/drs

Wright, J. (2000). Introduction to the Functional Assessment Measure. Retrieved from http://www.tbims.org/combi/ FAM

Wright J. (2000). Introduction to the FIM(TM). Retrieved from http://www.tbims.org/ combi/ FIM

Zafonte RD, Mann NR. (1997). Cerebral salt wasting syndrome in brain injury patients: A potential cause of hyponatremia. Archives of Physical Medicine and Rehabilitation, 78(5), 540-542.

CHAPTER 3

Chronic Pain

Nicki Bradley, BS, RN-BC, CCM, CNLCP, MSCC
Sandra Callaghan, MSN, RN, BS, NP-C, CLCP, CNLCP, MSCC
Barbara Greenfield, BSN, RN, CCM, CNLCP
Barbara Malloy, BSN, RN, CCM, CLCP, MSCC, LNCC
Catherine Winslow, BSN, RN, CCM, CDMS, CNLCP
Peggie Nielson, BSN, RN, CNLCP, MSCC, contributor

Introduction

Chronic pain is a common problem in nursing, long-term disability, and rehabilitation. It is often a focus for life care planning, either as a stand-alone condition or as related to other conditions. This chapter will give the foundation for management of chronic pain and serve as a guide for the life care planner.

The Institute Clinical Systems Improvement (ICSI) has adopted the IASP's definition in its 2009 Assessment and Management of Chronic Pain. The ICSI defines chronic pain as "persistent; either continuous or recurrent, and of sufficient duration and intensity to adversely affect a patient's well-being, level of function, and quality of life." The period mentioned here notes that at 6 weeks "or longer than the anticipated healing time," patients should be evaluated for the presence of chronic pain. It also defines chronic pain as a constellation of behaviors related to persistent pain that represents significant life role disruption that occurs at the end of the spectrum of chronic pain.

The Institute for Clinical Systems Improvement (ICSI) has differentiated distinct biological mechanisms that contribute to chronic pain. Each patient may have multiple and/or overlapping contributors. An important definition of pain is nociception, which ISCI notes as the process of detection and signaling the presence of a noxious stimulus. It is a "noxious stimulus or a stimulus that would become noxious if prolonged. Activity induced in a nociceptive pathway by a noxious stimulus is not pain.

Many people have mixed and or overlapping types of pain. Most pain researchers agree on the following information on the biological and psychological sources of pain:

Biological sources of pain

- Neuropathic "pain arising as direct consequence of a lesion or disease affecting the somatosensory system" (Geber, 2009)
- Peripheral (CRPS, HIV, sensory neuropathy, metabolic, phantom limb pain).
- Central (Parkinson's disease, MS, myelopathic, post stroke pain, fibromyalgia syndrome)

Alternatively classified by:
- Mononeuropathy (traumatic or other)
- Polyneuropathy (can include metabolic, nutritional, drug or toxin related, hereditary, and malignant, infection related or other).
- Muscle pain (myofascial pain syndrome, fibromyalgia).
- Inflammatory pain often of acute nature. Chronic types: inflammatory arthropathies, infection, tissue injury.
- Mechanical/compressive pain: acute injuries (fracture, dislocation); low back pain, neck pain, musculoskeletal disorders, visceral pain.
- Low back pain, the most common chronic pain may be a result of neuropathic, muscle, inflammatory and mechanical/compressive problems. This is illustrative of the need for a multifactorial approach to assessment and treatment. Some writers classify fibromyalgia as muscular, others as neuropathic. Many researchers feel it is likely of a mixed etiology.

Psychological sources of pain

In addition to the ICSI mechanisms, other guidelines (such as the Chronic Pain Disorder Medical Treatment Guidelines, 2009) suggest evaluation for psychological contributors or comorbidities (Colorado, 2009). Specific examples that are either associated with or contribute to chronic pain include:

- Depression
- Anxiety
- Personality disorders
- Somatization
- Post-traumatic stress

Comorbid psychopathology can affect the course of chronic pain treatment. In a recent analysis, patients with panic disorder, antisocial personality disorder and dependent personality disorder were more than two times more likely to not complete an interdisciplinary program. Personality disorders in particular appear to hamper the ability to successfully complete treatment. The prevalence of depression and anxiety in patients with chronic pain is similar. The possibility of underlying substance abuse should also be assessed.

Another possible confounding factor is *secondary gain*. Indemnity and ongoing litigation may affect pain resolution. Gatchel (2009) suggests more important social contributors, citing primary losses such as physical health and functioning and secondary losses such as loss of financial stability and relationships, both personal and work-related.

Specific guidelines for suggested and required psychological testing are included in the procedure summaries in this chapter. These are performed by psychologists and should be part of the life care plan.

Complex Regional Pain Syndrome: CRPS

The International Association for the Study of Pain (IASP) has defined this diagnosis as:

> ... a variety of painful conditions following injury which appear regionally, having a distal predominance of abnormal findings, exceeding in both magnitude and duration the expected clinical course of the inciting event and often resulting in significant impairment of motor function, and showing variable progression over time (Stanton-Hicks, 2011).

Diagnostic criteria defined by IASP in 1995 were the following:

- The presence of an initiating noxious event or cause of immobilization that leads to development of the syndrome
- Continuing pain, allodynia, or hyperalgesia which is disproportionate to the inciting event and/or spontaneous pain in the absence of external stimuli
- Evidence *at some time* of edema, changes in skin blood flow, or abnormal sudomotor activity in the pain region
- The diagnosis is excluded by the existence of conditions that would otherwise account for the degree of pain or dysfunction

The Harden Criteria later redefined pain using the following four criteria:

- Continuing pain, which is disproportionate to any inciting event
- Should report at least one symptom in three of these four:
  - o hyperesthesia and/or allodynia
  - o temperature asymmetry

o   skin color changes
o   skin color asymmetry

CRPS Assessment

Criteria two through four should be satisfied to make the diagnosis when looking specifically at CRPS. To improve specificity the IASP suggested the following criteria:

- Continuing pain disproportionate to the inciting event
- A report of one *symptom* from each of the following four categories and one *physical finding* from two of the following four categories:
  o   Sensory: hyperesthesia,
  o   Vasomotor: temperature asymmetry or skin color changes or asymmetry,
  o   Sudomotor/edema: edema or sweating changes or sweating asymmetry, or
  o   Motor/trophic: reports of decreased range of motion or motor dysfunction (weakness/tremor or dystonia) or trophic changes: hair, nail, skin.

A comparison between three sets of diagnostic criteria for CRPS concluded that there was a substantial lack of agreement between different diagnostic sets.

An important part of pain assessment includes identifying barriers to effective pain management that are related to the professionals involved, and other factors in the health care delivery system, such as patients who "fall through the cracks." Assessment of these factors is beyond the scope of this paper, but should be kept in mind.

The nurse life care planner should assess pain when completing the onsite visits. Questions include:

- Pain location(s)
- Pain duration

- Management of pain, both from health care provider prescription and patient's personal management strategies
- What makes the pain worse?
- What makes the pain easier to manage?

Assessment Tools
Pain

Many tools are available for pain assessment. The ICSI published *Chronic Assessment and Management* in 2009, which addresses the management of chronic pain for physiologically mature adolescents (between 16-18 years) and adults. It can be applied to pediatric populations in some circumstances. It is not intended for the treatment of migraine headaches, cancer pain, advanced cancer pain, or in the context of palliative care or end-of-life management.

The ICSI includes an assessment algorithm in this document. It also includes assessment tools developed by others. These include:

- Oswestry Low Back Disability Index (included in the ISCI Adult Low Back Pain Guidelines)
- Brief Pain Inventory (Short Form): pain diagram, 0-10 ratings worst/ least/average/current; % improvement over last 24 hours, general activity, mood, sleep, relationships, walking ability, enjoyment of life; simple numerical grading scale (Charles Cleeland, PhD, Pain Research Group, 1991)
- Patient Health Questionnaire (PHQ): symptoms of depression (Pfizer, 2005), scoring card

Symptoms

Studies demonstrate a significant correlation between pain, depression, fatigue, and other symptoms commonly seen in those with cancer. These co-occurring symptoms are commonly referred to as symptom clusters. The use of multidimensional scales incorporating the most common symptoms would ensure systematic assessment. Several currently available instruments that measure symptom clusters and have demonstrated validity and reliability include:

- Edmonton Symptom Assessment Scale (ESAS)
- MD Anderson Symptom Inventory (MDASI)
- Memorial Symptom Assessment Scale (MSAS)
- Rotterdam Symptom Checklist (RSC)

It is important for the nurse life care planner to have training in the use of these assessments prior to using them in practice.

Psychological

The following 26 tests are described and use for professional evaluations by health care providers and psychologists. Even though most nurse life care planners are not trained to use these tests, they are important to have a common knowledge of how to understand the tests and result applications.

- BHI™ 2 (Battery for Health Improvement - 2nd edition)
- MBHI™ (Millon Behavioral Health Inventory) [Has been superseded by the MBMD. The updated version of the test, the MBMD, should be administered instead.]
- MBMD™ (Millon Behavioral Medical Diagnostic)
- PAB (Pain Assessment Battery)
- MCMI-111™ (Millon Clinical Multiaxial Inventory, 3rd edition)
- MMPI-2™ (Minnesota Inventory-2nd edition ™)
- PAI™ (Personality Assessment Inventory)
- BBHI™ 2 (Brief Battery for Health Improvement - 2nd edition)
- MPI (Multidimensional Pain Inventory)
- P-3™ (Pain Patient Profile)
- Pain Presentation Inventory
- PRIME-MD (Primary Care Evaluation for Mental Disorders)

- PHQ (Patient Health Questionnaire)
- SF 36 ™
- (SIP) Sickness Impact Profile
- BSI® (Brief Symptom Inventory)
- BSI® 18 (Brief Symptom Inventory-18)
- SCL-90-R® (Symptom Checklist -90 Revised)
- BDI ®-II (Beck Depression Inventory-2nd edition)
- CES-D (Center for Epidemiological Studies Depression Scale)
- PDS™ (Post Traumatic Stress Diagnostic Scale)
- Zung Depression Inventory
- MPQ (McGill Pain Questionnaire)
- MPQ-SF (McGill Pain Questionnaire - Short Form)
- Oswestry Disability Questionnaire
- Visual Analogue Pain Scale (VAS

Diagnostic Tools

Pain management health care providers, to understand the pathways and form support for pain management, commonly use the following diagnostic tools. Nurse Life Care Planners should understand how these tests are used, the costs of the testing, and the future need for repeat tests.

Evoked Potential Studies

Evoked potential studies are a group of tests that measure electrical signals along nerve pathways. Stimulation travels along the nerves and through the spinal cord to specific regions in the brain and are picked up by the electrodes and measured, then interpreted. Somatosensory evoked potentials record transmission of nerve impulses from the limbs to the brain, and can be used to diagnose nerve damage or degeneration in the spinal cord or nerve roots. Somatosensory EPs differentiate central versus peripheral nerve disease when combined with results from a nerve conduction velocity test, which measures nerve function in the extremities. The amount of time the stimulation takes to travel along the nerve to the brain is measured. It can detect problems with the spinal cord as well as numbness and weakness of the extremities.

Changes in the electrical tracings may indicate damage to or degeneration of nerve pathways to the brain from the eyes, ears, or limbs. No discernible activity may mean complete loss of nerve function in that pathway. Other changes may provide evidence of the type and location of nerve damage.

Nerve Blocks

Lumbar sympathetic block is useful for diagnosis and treatment of pain of the pelvis and lower extremities. This block consists of an injection of anesthetic into the sympathetic nerves that cover the extremity on the same side of the injection. It. is commonly used for differential diagnosis and is the recommended treatment of pain involving the lower extremity. For diagnostic purposes, one to three blocks may be performed over a one to three week duration.

Regional blocks (lumbar, stellate ganglion, thoracic, lumbar sympathetic) There is limited role for intravenous regional sympathetic blocks for the diagnosis of CRPS.

Electromyography / Nerve conduction Velocity Studies

Electromyography (EMG) is a test for the health of the muscles and the nerves that control those muscles during rest or activity. The motor neurons transmit electrical signals that cause muscles to contract. The EMG translates these signals into values that are interpreted. An EMG uses tiny needle electrodes inserted directly into a muscle to record the electrical activity of that muscle.

Nerve Conduction Velocity (NCV) tests the speed of the electrical signals through a nerve. In NCV studies, only surface electrodes are used to measure the speed and strength of signals traveling between two or more points. These tests can reveal nerve dysfunction, muscle dysfunction or problems with nerve-to-muscle signal transmission (www.mayoclinic.com, 2012).

Monofilament Testing

The nylon monofilament test is a test to diagnose patients at increased risk for injury to the foot due to peripheral sensory neuropathy. The test is abnormal if the patient cannot sense the touch of the monofilament when it is pressed against the foot with just enough pressure to bend the filament. Not recommended by ODG as a sole diagnostic test.

Quantitative Sensory Testing

Quantitative sensory testing (QST) has been used to assist in the diagnosis and management of a variety of conditions such as diabetic neuropathy and other neuropathies, as well as carpal tunnel syndrome and other nerve entrapment and compression disorders or damage. Because QST combines objective physical sensory stimuli with subjective patient response, it is psychophysical in nature and requires that it be used in patients who are alert, able to follow directions, and cooperative.

Due to the subjective component of testing, psychological factors should be taken into consideration during testing and results analysis, thus reducing the degree of objectivity QST can provide. *QST is considered experimental or investigational, as there are no quality published studies to support any conclusions regarding the effects of this testing on health outcomes. Many insurance companies deny funding for this testing.* They cite a 2010 study that shows intrinsic value of the test, mainly for research purposes although it does have some use in differential diagnosis. They also state the test is not useful for medicolegal purposes (Clinical Testing, (2012).

Autonomic Test Battery

Resting skin temperature (RST), resting sweat output (RSO), and quantitative sudomotor axon reflex test (QSART) are a recently developed test battery with some evidence to support its limited use in the diagnosis of CRPS-I There is no current evidence to support the use of cytokine DNA testing for the diagnosis of pain, including chronic pain.

Opioid Testing

The patient should be screened for risk of addiction prior to initiating opioid therapy. It is important to attempt to identify individuals who have the potential to develop aberrant drug use both prior to the prescribing of opioids and while actively undergoing opioid treatment. Most screening occurs after the claimant is already on chronic opioid therapy, and consists of screens for aberrant behavior/misuse.

Healthcare Provider Subspecialties Working with Chronic Pain

- Anesthesiology
- Physical Medicine and Rehabilitation
- Psychiatry
- Neurology

Treatment for Chronic Low Back Pain

Chronic low back pain can be treated via intensive multidisciplinary rehabilitation. A recent Cochrane study (2006) updated the research completed in 1998. Studies selected included a physical dimension treatment and at least one other treatment dimension (psychological, social, or occupational). Back schools were not included unless they included the above criteria. There was strong evidence that intensive multidisciplinary biopsychosocial rehabilitation with functional restoration improved function when compared to inpatient or outpatient nonmultidisciplinary rehabilitation. Intensive (> 100 hours), daily interdisciplinary rehabilitation was moderately superior to noninterdisciplinary rehabilitation or usual care for short-and long-term functional status (standardized mean differences, -0.40 to -0.90 at three to four months, and -0.56 to -1.07 at sixty months). There was moderate evidence of pain reduction. There was contradictory evidence regarding vocational outcome. Less intensive programs did not show improvements in pain, function, or vocational outcomes.

Pain Rehabilitation Programs
Multidisciplinary Pain Management Program

A multidisciplinary pain management (MPM) or comprehensive pain program (CPP) affords an interdisciplinary treatment approach. The program may be in one clinical setting or involve interdisciplinary coordination managed by a nurse case manager or primary care health. These programs focus on pain reduction through functional restoration (Gatchel, 2009).

Multiple diagnoses respond to these programs. However, comprehensive research resulting in guidelines is limited. Low back pain is found to be associated with improved outcomes with CPP and has been widely studied. CPP has been found to have an evidence rating of C (Recommended) for the treatment of chronic low back pain (NGC, ACOEM, 2007). CPP programs often include a physical therapist and occupational therapy, psychologist, physical medicine and rehabilitation specialist or pain management specialist, biofeedback therapist, sleep evaluation, and nurse case manager. Other models include passive modalities such as acupuncture, and massage, or active community reintegration modalities such as therapeutic recreation.

The patient is referred to a pain management specialist or directly to the pain management specialty clinic. A comprehensive pain assessment is critical in assessing the patient's pain.

Treatment ranges from 3 weeks of inpatient care to approximately 6 weeks of outpatient treatment depending on type of program and level of functional improvement. The best programs are individualized. Length of stay is based on realistic functional goals and continued treatment should be based on the success of the individual. Measurement criteria include medication use, improved community access, ability to return to activities of daily living, and ultimately return to work or productive activities (Gallagher, 2002)

Multidisciplinary biopsychosocial rehabilitation with functional restoration produces greater improvements in pain and function for patients with disabling chronic low back pain than less intensive multidisciplinary or nonmultidisciplinary rehabilitation or usual care.

Outpatient

Outpatient rehabilitation and management may be included in the life care plan if the focus is on improvable outcomes. The nurse life care planner evaluates the different programs for criteria that they will meet the individual's needs. Outpatient pain rehabilitation may be medically necessary in the following circumstances:

- The patient has a chronic pain syndrome with evidence of loss of function that persists beyond three months and has evidence of three or more of the following:
    o Excessive dependence on health-care providers, spouse, or family
    o Secondary physical deconditioning due to disuse and/or fear-avoidance of physical activity due to pain
    o Withdrawal from social activities or normal contact with others, including work, recreation, or other social contacts
    o Failure to restore pre-injury function after a period of disability such that the physical capacity is insufficient to pursue work, family, or recreational needs
    o Development of psychosocial sequelae that limit function or recovery after the initial incident, including anxiety, fear-avoidance, depression, sleep disorders, or nonorganic illness behaviors (with a reasonable probability to respond to treatment intervention)

- The diagnosis is not primarily a personality disorder or psychological condition without a physical component.

- There is evidence of continued use of prescription pain medications (particularly those that may result in tolerance, dependence or abuse) without evidence of improvement in pain or function.

- Previous methods of treating chronic pain have been unsuccessful and there is an absence of other options likely to result in significant clinical improvement.

- An adequate and thorough multidisciplinary evaluation has been made. This should include pertinent validated diagnostic testing that addresses the following:
  o A physical exam that rules out pain-related conditions that require treatment prior to initiating the program.
  o All diagnostic procedures necessary to rule out treatable pathology related to the pain site, including imaging studies and invasive injections (used for diagnosis), should be completed prior to considering a patient a candidate for a program. The exception is diagnostic procedures that were repeatedly requested and not authorized by a pay source. Although the primary emphasis is focused on function, underlying pathology that contributes to pain may need to be addressed and treated by a primary care health care provider prior to or coincident to starting treatment
  o Evidence of a screening evaluation should be provided when addiction is present or strongly suspected.
  o Psychological testing, using a validated instrument to identify pertinent areas to be addressed in the program (including but not limited to mood disorder, sleep disorder, relationship dysfunction, distorted beliefs about pain and disability, coping skills and/or locus of control regarding pain and medical care).

o   An evaluation of social and vocational issues that require assessment.

If a goal of treatment is to prevent or avoid controversial or optional surgery, trials of 10 visits of conservative treatments may be implemented to assess whether surgery may be avoided.

If a primary reason for treatment in the program is addressing possible substance use issues, an evaluation with an addiction clinician may be indicated upon entering the program to establish the most appropriate treatment approach (pain program vs. substance dependence program). This should address evaluation of drug abuse or diversion (and prescribing drugs in a non-therapeutic manner). In this particular case, once drug abuse or diversion issues are addressed, a 10-day trial may help to establish a diagnosis, and determine if the patient is not better suited for treatment in a substance dependence program.

Addiction consultation can be incorporated into a pain program. If there is indication reflection substance dependence, there should be evidence the program has the capability to address this pathology prior to approval. Once the evaluation is completed, a treatment plan should be presented with specifics for treatment of identified problems, and outcomes that will be followed. There should be documentation that the patient has motivation to change, and is willing to change the medication regimen (including decreasing or actually weaning substances known for dependence). There should be documentation the patient is aware successful treatment may change compensation and/or other secondary gains. In questionable cases, an opportunity for a brief treatment trial may improve assessment of patient motivation and/or willingness to decrease habituating medications.

Negative predictors of success (as outlined above) should be identified, and if present, the pre-program goals should indicate how they will be addressed. If a program is planned for a patient that has been continuously disabled for greater than 24 months, the outcomes for the necessity of use should be clearly identified, as there is conflicting evidence that chronic pain programs provide improvement beyond this period. These other desirable types of outcomes include decreasing post-treatment care including medications, injections and surgery.

Treatment is not suggested for longer than two weeks without evidence of compliance and significant demonstrated efficacy as documented by subjective and objective gains. (Note: Patients may get worse before they get better. For example, objective gains may be moving joints that are stiff from lack of use, resulting in increased subjective pain.) However, it is also not suggested that a continuous course of treatment be interrupted at two weeks solely to document these gains, if there are preliminary indications that they are being made on a concurrent basis. The life care plan including outpatient pain treatment programs should include a trial period and the additional needs to reach outcomes.

Integrative summary reports that include treatment goals, compliance, progress assessment with objective measures and stage of treatment, should be made available (some require requests) at least on a bi-weekly basis during the course of the treatment program.

At the conclusion and subsequently, neither re-enrollment in repetition of the same or similar rehabilitation program (e.g. work hardening, work conditioning, outpatient medical rehabilitation) is medically warranted for the same condition or injury (with possible exception for a medically-necessary organized detox program). Prior to entry into a program the evaluation should clearly indicate the necessity for the type of program required, and providers should determine upfront which program their patients would benefit more from. A chronic pain program should not be considered a "stepping stone" after less intensive programs, but prior participation in a work conditioning or work hardening program does not preclude an opportunity for entering a chronic pain program if otherwise indicated.

Suggestions for treatment post-program should be well documented and provided to the health care provider referring health care provider. The patient may require time-limited, less intensive post-treatment with the program itself. Defined goals for these interventions and planned duration should be specified.

Post-treatment medication management is particularly important. Patients that have been identified as having substance abuse issues generally require some sort of continued addiction follow-up to avoid relapse.

Inpatient

These programs typically consist of more intensive functional rehabilitation and medical care than their outpatient counterparts. They may be appropriate for patients who:

- lack minimal functional capacity to participate effectively in an outpatient program
- have medical conditions that require more intensive oversight
- are receiving large amounts of medications necessitating medication weaning or detoxification
- have complex medical or psychological diagnosis that benefit from more intensive observation and/or additional consultation

The most effective programs combine intensive daily biopsychosocial rehabilitation with a functional restoration approach. If a primary focus is drug treatment, the initial evaluation should attempt to identify the most appropriate treatment plan (drug treatment/detoxification approach vs. multidisciplinary/interdisciplinary treatment).

Conservative and Complementary Treatment

Each person responds differently to conservative modalities based on personal experience, culture, and beliefs. The nurse life care planner should evaluate conservative treatment modalities the injured person has had following the injury and what seemed to produce the most pain relief. When assessing the different modalities for the injured worker, the treatments should correspond to the overall pain management program for the individual injury.

Massage therapy

This includes techniques such as Swedish, deep tissue and specific trigger point massage. All techniques use some form of manipulating the soft tissue. Hands and fingers are commonly used for this manipulation but some techniques use elbows, forearms, and feet. Massage is used to manage chronic pain by reducing stress and increasing blood flow to reduce tension in the affected area. Spasms and chronic muscle tension caused by daily living, strain and sprain, or certain systemic conditions are possible indications for massage therapy to release soft tissue tension.

The patient and therapist determine frequency of treatment. Sessions may be brief or they may last an hour or longer.

There are few risks if massage is used appropriately by a trained licensed massage professional. Side effects can include temporary discomfort or pain, bruising or swelling.

Contraindications should be discussed with the treating health care provider health care provider. Several conditions such as deep vein thrombosis, weakened bones from various causes, and bleeding disorders would be considered contraindications. Massage should not be undertaken if there are open wounds, tumors or inflammation in the areas to be massaged.

Massage therapy should be discussed with the treating health care provider, and undertaken only with a trained massage professional. Many states now regulate massage therapy by requiring graduation from an approved school or training program with ongoing continued education in that field. The governing body for massage therapy is the National Certification Board for Therapeutic Massage and Bodywork.

Facilities offering massage therapies vary from hospitals and private offices, and to sport and fitness locations. Many massage therapists will travel to the patient's home.

Scientific studies continue with a focus on understanding the outcomes of massage therapy. Some claims suggest that release of certain chemicals such as serotonin or endorphins is achieved. Typically, massage therapy enhances relaxation, reduces stress and improves sleep.

Physical Therapy

Physical therapy (PT) incorporates conservative measures to treat nervous, muscular and skeletal problems. Following an in-depth assessment, the physical therapist initiates a plan including both active and passive interventions. PT is a vital component of the collaborative effort to achieve effective control of pain. There are no invasive interventions involved in physical therapy. Active PT includes stretching, exercises for strengthening and often low-impact aerobic activities. Commonly used passive modalities include heat/cold packs, ultrasound, and TENS units. Other functional sessions may include light exercise, followed by modalities to increase function. The goal is to prevent loss of muscle mass and strength and increase endurance.

The treating medical provider will prescribe PT frequency. Typically, formal active therapy involves two to four sessions a week with one day of rest between session days. As condition improves, the program frequency decreases and transitions to an independent home program. Successful rehabilitation is achieved by understanding the pain problem, by self-pacing during the activity, and by setting realistic goals.

Physical therapy may cause pain and/or injury or aggravate a pre-existing conditions. During the initial phases of a therapy program, the patient may note muscle soreness or temporarily increased pain. Patients should be taught to expect and how to manage this.

Before prescribing PT, the health care provider will assess the patient's medical stability. Any cardiac, pulmonary, neurologic or musculoskeletal limitations will be addressed before undertaking a PT program.

The desired outcome is not necessarily pain reduction, because this not always possible with chronic pain. Improved function, increased activity, and improved coping skills are appropriate goals for people suffering from chronic pain.

Aquatic Therapy (hydrotherapy, water therapy).
Water therapy is whirlpool therapy and strengthening and endurance exercises performed in water. It is prescribed as a non-weight bearing exercise to regain function prior to more strenuous land-based PT, or to maintain function in chronic conditions.

Warm water assists in healing, reduces pain, and helps with muscle relaxation and vasodilation, increasing blood flow to injured areas. This is useful for patients with muscle spasms or pain attributed to fibromyalgia. Buoyancy provides arthritic, obese, or other patients with conditions limiting weight bearing with support for weight, thus enabling them to exercise without adding additional strain on affected joints. Water exercise can mobilize joints, increase range of motion, and help the individual to regain balance and stability. Muscle groups can be exercised and strengthened.

Until the patient is released from supervision, a therapist should be present throughout the sessions to teach, evaluate, and promote safety.

Hydrotherapy increases venous return and central blood volume, leading to an increase in cardiac preload. Some cardiovascular patients cannot tolerate this, and cardiovascular patients should obtain medical clearance for this reason. Contraindications for aquatherapy include some forms of cardiac disease, infection/fever, bowel/bladder incontinence, and some surgeries. Many facilities will not allow patients with open wounds in a shared pool.

At the conclusion of therapy, the patient can transition into a home exercise program, or utilize a local pool facility of choice for ongoing exercise.

Acupuncture

The cultures of Asia have practiced the healing art of acupuncture for centuries. The skin and underlying muscles are penetrated with hair-thin metal needles along meridians to release obstructions or blockages in the flow of energy (qi). Treatments are enhanced with electrical stimulation, heat, and needle manipulations (NCCAM, Introduction 2007). Acupuncture is used most commonly to treat back pain and is used for joint pain, neck pain, and headaches.

The National Center for Complementary and Alternative Medicine (NCCAM), established in October of 1998, is a branch of the National Institute of Health (NIH). This organization conducts scientifically based protocols to determine the practices of alternative and complementary medicine (NCCAM, 2009). The American Pain Society and the American College of Health Care Providers have included acupuncture in their clinical practice guidelines, issued in 2007.

The bio-mechanisms of acupuncture are new additions (since 1995) in the Western medical model. Studies are underway using functional MRIs to determine the response to brain neurochemistry with acupuncture treatment. A placebo effect and effects on opiate receptors have been proposed; however, the research is not definitive (NCCAM, Pain 2009).

Indications

According to the NCCAM research on use of acupuncture for the treatment of fibromyalgia was found to be insufficient. This same paper notes that the research for treatment of migraines and tension headaches have shown evidence of effectiveness; a study in 2009 showed results were equal to conventional treatment. Treatment for chronic back pain, neck pain, menstrual cramps, osteoarthritis and lateral epicondylitis have shown benefits (NCCAM, Pain 2009). According to the NCCAM article on pain, although acupuncture is "a promising alternative" (NCCAM, Pain 2009), further research is needed for many diagnoses such as carpal tunnel, post-operative dental pain, and osteoarthritis of the knee.

Using acupuncture for the treatment of chronic low back pain has been recommended by the American Pain Society and the American College of Health care providers (2007) and should be considered when other conventional treatment has failed (NCCAM, Pain 2009).

Treatment recommendations for acute conditions are one to three sessions. The initial treatment for chronic conditions (those conditions which continue 30 days beyond the usual course of an acute disease or for injury to heal), [Title 8 California Code of Regulations, Section 9792.2, p. 2]) are three to six visits. If symptoms improve, treatment may continue for as many as 10 to 12 visits for up to one to two months. Treatment may continue if functional gains are documented.

Acupuncture is safe when provided by a licensed practitioner. There is a high rate of infection if acupuncture needles are not sterilized and reused. Disposable needles are used by most practitioners to assist reduce the infection rate. The Food and Drug Administration (FDA) regulates distribution and supply of acupuncture needles in the U.S. (NCCAM, Introduction 2010).

Diabetics and others with nerve or circulatory problems should have medical clearance. Frail patients, confused or demented patients, and those with chronic illness may not tolerate acupuncture. Patients with implanted mechanical devices such as pacemakers and medication pumps should not be treated with electrical stimulation during acupuncture treatments. The nurse life care planner should be aware of the following contraindications:

- Allergies to metals
- Uncontrolled movements
- Bleeding disorders or anticoagulation therapy
- Lymphedema from cellulitis
- First trimester of pregnancy
- Provider type/qualifications

Most states have guidelines for certifying or licensing acupuncturists, including health care providers, usually registered nurses or physicians. The abbreviation for a licensed acupuncturist is *L.Ac.* The National Certification Commission for Acupuncture and Oriental Medicine is a national private and voluntary certifying board. Sixteen of 50 states (plus the District of Columbia) recognize the NCCAOM certification. Another 22 states require NCCAOM certification.

Outcomes are based on goals set by the clinician and patient. Functional goals include improved ability to provide self-care, improved sleep, resumption of leisure activities, ability to maintain posture, improved ability to return to work and engage in school, improved organ function (e.g. urinary, gastrointestinal), and general improved mood (Seems, 2006/2007).

Psychotherapy

The nurse life care planner understands that the triad of pain health care provider, therapy, and psychologist is an essential feature of successful pain management programs. When developing rationales for the usage of psychological services related to pain management, the nurse life care planner should identify the different psychological interventions.

Typically, the psychologist (in cooperation with the rest of the team) and patient meet once per week in sessions lasting 50 minutes. Therapy is individualized and the patient may treat in private sessions, group, or family sessions. The length of psychotherapy varies according to the type of situation, severity of the symptoms, how quickly progress is made and how positive the support system appears to be.

Very little risk is documented with psychotherapy. Feeling emotionally uncomfortable at certain points in therapy can result from exploring painful feelings.

Anticipated outcomes with psychotherapy include enhanced relationships, increased self-esteem, and improved ability to manage the daily stress associated with chronic pain.

Trigger Point Injections.

Trigger point injections are used to treat sensitive bands of skeletal muscle fibers called trigger points, especially those in the neck, low back, and extremities. These trigger points are often painful to touch and can spread throughout the muscle as well as cause referred pain in another location. The injection consists of dry needling or injection of a local anesthetic with or without corticosteroid. The goal of trigger point injections is to relax the muscles and inhibit pain nerves, reduce swelling, and facilitate active stretching and PT.

Several different trigger points may be injected during one visit. Repeated injections to the same area are not recommended until the post injection soreness has resolved. If two or three previous attempts have not produced good results, additional injections are not recommended. Immediately following the injections, stretching and movement of the muscle groups is suggested to increase the efficacy of the treatment. It may be immediate or two or three days before the patient notices more function.

Most sources recommend injecting no greater than four sites per session per week. The optimum duration is four sessions although some patients may require the repetition of two to four series of injections over a one or two year period.

Trigger point injections are minimally invasive and usually well tolerated. Corticosteroids are contraindicated in a variety of medical conditions. This will be determined by the administering health care provider.

It is anticipated that a trigger point injection or series of injections will relax the knotted muscle fibers, decrease swelling, and alleviate direct or referred pain. The result would include expected increase in range of motion, pain relief, and increased joint function.

Biofeedback
Biofeedback, neurofeedback, or brainwave biofeedback (hereinafter collectively referred to as biofeedback) is a non-invasive, self-regulatory treatment to normalize and optimize brain functioning. Biofeedback is a young and relatively new practice that is gaining use in pain management program. It functions outside most understanding, but it works on a sound scientific principle. Biofeedback can be used

to treat numerous conditions including depression, anxiety disorders, sleep problems, concentration difficulties, memory problems, fine motor skill deficiencies, attention deficit disorder, alcoholism, headaches, high blood pressure, urinary incontinence and chronic pain. Direct feedback is provided to the patient about the state of a particular brainwave activity. Techniques include:

- Electromyography biofeedback - provides information about the body's muscle tension so relaxation can be practiced
- Temperature (Thermal) biofeedback - temperature tends to drop when one is under stress, a low reading can prompt one to begin relaxation techniques
- Galvanic skin response training - sensors measure the activity of the sweat glands and the amount of perspiration on the skin alerting one to anxiety
- Heart rate variability biofeedback - monitors heart rate allowing one to control blood pressure, lung function and therefore, stress and anxiety
- Electroencephalography - measures brain wave activity allowing one to control the brain waves to achieve desired goals, which may include behavior modification, headaches and pain

Biofeedback is used to help treat many physical and mental conditions including anxiety, stress, pain, and addictions. It is noninvasive, can reduce need for medications for those who do not tolerate medications well or for those who want to reduce medication intake. It can be an option when medication does not work and can be used to allow the patient to take greater control over healthcare needs.

Biofeedback treatments are individually prescribed. Treatments typically begin on a weekly basis, and as sleep improves and pain is reduced, sessions can be spread out to once per month to allow time to gradually reduce medications and introduce new physical activities into daily activity.

Biofeedback can be prescribed to coincide with cognitive behavioral / psychological therapeutic sessions to maximize improvements.

Sessions typically last thirty to sixty minutes and the number of sessions are determined based on the individual's condition and the individual's ability to learn control of the physical responses. Some individuals may require ten sessions, others may require fifty sessions.

Biofeedback is considered safe. No negative side effects have been reported. Biofeedback is not recommended for persons with psychosis or psychopathic personalities. Diabetics and patients with other endocrine disorders should be monitored by their providers as biofeedback may change the insulin metabolism and dosage requirements. The health care provider should evaluate medications both dosages and effectiveness when incorporating biofeedback into treatment plan.

Expected outcomes are reduced depression, anxiety, and pain; improved sleep, physical and mental functioning and quality of life.

Medications

The nurse life care planner utilizes the current medication list in the life care plan and is encouraged to research any medications prescribed in appropriate resources. Many medications have undesirable side effects; it may be appropriate to consider measures in the life care plan to manage these.

Projected medication needs can be listed in the rationale for future needs including local costs. As in rationales, the cost is not included in the total costs listed in the plan.

Over-the-counter medications

Over the counter (OTC) pain medications are those that can be purchased without a prescription. These include oral preparations such as aspirin, acetaminophen, nonsteroidal anti-inflammatory drugs, topical corticosteroids (e.g., Cortaid) and other topical medications (e.g., Ben-Gay, Icy Hot, Capzacin-P).

Prescription medications

Prescription medications are used at every stage of medical treatment for pain, from initial onset of acute pain through rehabilitation, and include a number of medication classifications that provide relief for a variety of pain types.

NSAIDs Nonsteroidal anti-inflammatory medicatons are often initiated before opiates in the treatment of mild to moderate pain but their therapeutic outcomes may not be adequate. Types of NSAIDs include salicylic acid, acetylsalicylic acid (Bayer, Ecotrin), choline magnesium trisalicylate (trilisate), ibuprofen (Advil, Motrin), naproxen, diclofenac (Voltaren), indomethacin (Indocin), meloxicam (Mobic), nabumetone (Relafen), etodalac (Iodine), ketorolac (Toradol), and celecoxib (Celebrex). NSAIDs are available over the counter in low doses, but the higher doses require a prescription. Some may be taken intramuscularly, subcutaneously, intravenously, as a transdermal patch, or topically as a gel.

Narcotics (Opioids) Narcotic medications have a dissociative effect that helps the patient manage pain. They can be natural, synthetic, or semi-synthetic, short acting and long acting. The short acting opioids are often used for acute pain. The long acting narcotics are used for chronic pain and are designed to provide a timed released dose over a longer period. As dosages increase, so do the undesirable side effects.

Examples of narcotic pain medications include codeine, hydrocodone (Vicodin), oxycodone (Percocet, Oxycontin), morphine, hydromorphone (Dilaudid), fentanyl, methadone, and tramadol (Ultram).

Muscle Relaxants Typically, muscle relaxants are prescribed early in the course of a pain syndrome on a short-term basis. Muscle relaxants can cause dizziness, fatigue, nausea and can be addictive. Examples include baclofen, metaxalone (Skelexan), cyclobenzaprine (Flexeril), carisoprodol (Soma) and diazepam (Valium). Metaxalone is powerful and the least addictive. Diazepam is a strong muscle relaxant but very addictive. Carisoprodol and cyclobenzaprine effectively treat painful muscle spasms.

Neuroleptic Agents Neuroleptic (anticonvulsants, anti-epileptic) drugs are often prescribed for neuropathy and/or radiculopathy. Examples include gabapentin (Neurontin) for postherpetic neuralgia, pregabalin (Lyrica) for postherpetic neuralgia and diabetic neuropathy, and carbamazepine (Tegretol), oxcarbazepine (Trileptal) and lamotrigine (Lamictal) help control episodes of facial pain in trigeminal neuralgia. These medications are given at similar doses as for seizure management. Side effects include drowsiness, dizziness, fatigue, and nausea.

Anti-Depressants (SSRIs, TCAs) Antidepressants may be used to treat chronic pain, although not all antidepressants are effective at reducing pain. These medications can increase the availability of these neurotransmitters by blocking the reuptake of serotonin and norepinephrine, thus enhancing pain inhibition. The drugs work only if used consistently and effects take several weeks.

The FDA has approved some tricyclic antidepressants (TCAs) (e.g., amitriptyline, doxepin, nortriptyline), selective serotonin reuptake inhibitors (SSRIs) (e.g., citalopram, fluoxetine, paroxetine, sertraline), and selective serotonin norepinephrine reuptake inhibitors (SSNRIs) (e.g., duloxetine, venlafaxine) to treat pain. SSRIs and SSNRIs have fewer side effects than tricyclic antidepressants but may not be as effective at treating neuropathic pain as TCAs. The most common side effects with antidepressants are blurry vision, constipation, difficulty urinating, dry mouth, fatigue, headache and nausea.

Oral Corticosteroids Oral corticosteroids have very powerful anti-inflammatory effects and can be an effective treatment for pain flare-ups. Side effects include weight gain, blood glucose alterations, nausea, headache, mood changes, difficulty sleeping, and a weakened immune system. Steroids should not be used by patients with an active infection, due to the potential to exacerbate the infection. Steroids can mask symptoms that would lead to an untreated complication or disease.

Topical Analgesics Analgesics that are applied directly to the skin, such as EMLA cream and lidocaine patch (Lidoderm) can numb the skin and reduce pain by decreasing nerve stimulation. Lidocaine topical patches have proven effective in treating neuropathic pain. Capsaicin is a naturally occurring substance found in chili peppers used as a topical analgesic cream. Cooling spray such as Biofreeze™ applied directly on the skin can also help to relieve pain.

Combination Therapy The combination of opioid and non-opioid analgesics often results in superior analgesia to that produced by either agent alone. Lower doses and reduced side effects occur when combining different agents. Compound or combined analgesics usually contain a small amount of a mild opioid and a simple analgesic such as aspirin or acetaminophen.

Bisphosphonates can be used to treat bone pain. Bisphosphonates can also help reduce bone loss in other chronic pain conditions improving the quality of life.

Hormone therapy can be used to relieve pain due to tumors. By reducing the size of the tumor, pain can be relieved.

Antiarrhythmics slow the electrical conduction of the heart and along nerve pathways, and can be effective for relieving neuropathic pain. Examples of antiarrhythmics include lidocaine, mexiletine (oral form of lidocaine) and tocainide. There are a number of drug interactions associated with antiarrhythmic including concomitant use of opioids, caffeine, antiplatelet medications, cigarette smoking, etc. Contraindications include second or third degree heart block.

Beta-blockers prevent norepinephrine (fight or flight response) from binding to beta-receptors, decreasing heart rate, force of cardiac contractions, relief of migraines, and decreased tremor. Some beta-blockers are absorbed by brain better than others. Propanolol (Inderal) crosses the blood brain barrier well and therefore, causes more central nervous system side effects (hallucinations, nightmares, and depression) but may be more effective in treating migraines. Some beta-blockers are contraindicated for asthmatics as they can block bronchodilation. Cardiology consultation is recommended before prescribing these.

Interventional /Surgical Treatment Methods
The nurse life care planner should include the health care provider cost, cost of the assistant (if there is one) fluoroscopy cost, outpatient surgery room, medications and supplies, and recovery (if needed) when completing the section of the life care plan concerning interventional or surgical treatments.

Facet Joint Injections
Most injection procedures involve placing local anesthetics and steroids into a muscle, around a nerve, or into a joint. The small joints of the spine (facet joints) can cause pain. When arthritis or injury damages these small joints, pain in the midline, arm, or leg is common.

Facet joint injections are diagnostic to determine the cause of the pain and may not provide long-term relief from the pain. During the facet joint injection, the tip of a small needle is placed inside the joint and the joint is filled with anesthetic medication to numb the joint and a steroid to reduce inflammation.

The nurse life care planner uses the knowledge of how a procedure is completed to be able to predict the costs for all levels of the procedure. This procedure would need the cost of the fluoroscope, assistant (if used), outpatient surgery room (based on time blocks), medications and supplies, and post-procedure care. This information is also used by the nurse life care planner in developing questions for the patient and/or medical provider to have a clear focus for the plan. Questions such as:

- How long are these types of injections used before changing to different modalities?
- In most cases, how long are these injections effective?
- Do you have references to support the usage of these modalities with this type of injury?

The information is used to provide and support the rationale in the life care plan.

These injections can be performed no more than three or four times per year because of the risks related to the steroid medications and the possibility of scar tissue formation. The procedure is performed in either an inpatient or outpatient surgical center under local anesthesia and fluoroscopic guidance. This is not performed in a private medical office.

Joint Injections
A mixture of corticosteroid and local anesthetic is injected into a joint or bursa. Lubricants may also be injected in osteoarthritic joints. Repeated injections into a joint every three months has been shown to be safe. Hyaluronan is injected

in three injections over three weeks. Hylan G-F 20 (Synvisc) can be injected as a one-time injection and has shown to be equal to or better than the multiple dosing schedules in clinical trials.

Injections give demonstrable relief in the short term. Recurrence of symptoms is common, such as in bursitis and tendinopathy. The ideal outcome is total relief of pain with normal power and full range of motion. The anti-inflammatory effect of the corticosteroid is apparent in 24 to 48 hours after the injection and may continue for three weeks to three months.

Nerve Root Blocks
When adding nerve root blocks to the life care plan, the nurse considers provisions for the health care provider, assistant, surgical center, fluoroscopy, supplies and medications, and recovery.

Nerve blocks Injections of medication into the nerve can be used to alleviate pain. Selective nerve root blocks are similar to epidural injections; however, medication is injected around just a few damaged nerve roots. Sympathetic nerve blocks are injections into the nerve ganglia to control pain deep within the body. Nerve root blocks are used for diagnostic and therapeutic purposes for chronic regional pain syndrome, spinal stenosis, nerve root entrapment, and sciatica. Corticosteroids are used with a short and/or long acting local anesthetic to reduce inflammation and cause analgesic effect.

Bier block anesthesia involves the intravenous injection of sympathetic blocking agents (e.g., guanethidine, bretyllium, clonidine) into an extremity and limiting the spread of the agent to the entire body by applying a tourniquet to the extremity. Since the medication is trapped in the limb, it numbs the entire limb below the tourniquet. This is a day surgery procedure.

These injections can be performed no more than three or four times per year because of the risks related to the steroid medications. Steroid medications may or may not be used with all blocks; therefore, the block frequency is at the discretion of the provider. The maximum sustained benefit from a series of sympathetic blocks is usually apparent after a series of three to six blocks. Future exacerbations of symptoms may be responsive to one to three blocks. Bier Blocks can be performed every month or two.

Incidental recurrent laryngeal nerve block or superior laryngeal nerve block resulting in hoarseness and shortness of breath may occur with stellate ganglion block. Numbness around the vocal cords temporarily places the patient at risk of aspiration and adequate precautions should be enforced; Horner's sign (temporary drooping of the upper eye lid) is a short-term side effect. Back pain, hematuria, hypotension secondary to vasodilation are complications of lumbar sympathetic blocks. Bleeding and hematoma at the injection site is also a potential risk. Side effects from the steroid medications include headaches, mild fluid retention, increased blood sugar levels, flushing, palpitations and sleeping difficulties.

Relief may be achieved for hours to days or weeks. If 50% pain relief is achieved from the nerve root block, a repeat block is performed. A nurse life care planner may use the resources provided by the American Pain Association, who has specific guidelines for all injections, types of pain modalities. These include supportive studies and articles for reference.

Radiofrequency Ablation
The procedure is performed in an outpatient surgical center, or in a medical facility, under a local anesthetic so the patient will be awake during the procedure. X-ray or fluoroscopic guidance is necessary. When adding radiofrequency ablations to the life care plan, the nurse includes the health care provider, the assistant, surgical center, fluoroscopy, supplies and medications, and recovery.

Radiofrequency ablation is a procedure used to reduce pain by using radio waves or electrical current to produce heat to destroy a small area of nerve tissue. Radiofrequency can be used to treat chronic low back and neck pain and pain related to degenerative joint pain from arthritis, and for CRPS to interrupt the sympathetic nerve supply to the involved arm or leg. Pain relief duration varies depending on the cause and location of the pain. Pain relief can range from three to 12 months or longer. The nurse life care planner may add other types of injections to resolve pain issues if the ablations do not last the entire year.

Epidural Steroid Injection (ESI)
ESI is done with fluoroscopic guidance, usually with local anesthesia, in a suitably equipped health care provider office, an outpatient surgical center, or in a medical facility (if a patient is admitted with intractable pain). When ESI is considered for the life care plan, the nurse includes as the health care provider, the assistant, surgical center, fluoroscopy, supplies and medications, and recovery.

An epidural steroid injection including a long lasting corticosteroid and a local anesthetic is administered into the epidural space. The goal of this treatment is to reduce local inflammation of nerves in or surrounding the epidural space, thereby reducing pain, numbness, tingling and other symptoms attributable to inflammation or swelling in the local area of the injection.

The effects of the steroid begin in 3-5 days post injection, and may last several days to several months. This procedure may be repeated one or two times if the first injection does not help reduce pain symptoms. The three injections are administered two weeks apart. If pain is relieved after one injection, a second or third injection may not be necessary. Alternatively, lack of pain relief will generally be an indicator for a second, and possibly a third, trial of this procedure. The interval between injections depends upon the type of steroid used. Spinal headache, infection and bleeding into the epidural space are also risks associated with the procedure.

Spinal Cord Stimulator

The spinal cord stimulator (SCS) is an implantable device used as a method of pain control for chronic intractable pain. A psychological evaluation will be required prior to temporary trial implantation procedure.

The procedure is performed in an outpatient surgical center under a general anesthetic. X-ray or fluoroscopic guidance is necessary to guide the placement of the leads. When adding a spinal cord stimulator to a life care plan, the nurse includes the cost of the health care provider, the assistant, surgical center, fluoroscopy, supplies and medications, and recovery for temporary lead placement, and, if successful, permanent lead placement and follow-up care. Due to the cost and invasive nature of the spinal cord stimulator, the patient should have tried and failed other methods of pain relief including physical therapy, oral medications, and injections prior to consideration of the device.

An initial trial is performed and continues for three to seven days depending on the patient needs and response. The permanent implantation occurs one to four weeks following successful outcome of the trial (greater than 50% pain relief).

The patient returns to the provider every two months for evaluation and device reprogramming. Some patients find the spinal cord find it is not working as effectively after several years. Leads can then be revised or repositioned and reconnected to the battery back and effectiveness is resumed.

The battery pack requires replacement at frequencies depending on manufacture warranty (typically every five to seven years). Studies conducted comparing non-rechargeable to rechargeable units have demonstrated 4.2 fewer re-implantations per typical patient (e.g., age 46 years) in the rechargeable units (Hornberger, Kumar, Verhulst, Clark and Hernandez, 2008). All units have an external control unit. A SCS (IPG) cannot be implanted in patients with demand pacemakers.

Recent well-controlled studies show that with careful selection of patients and successful temporary trial and test stimulation, spinal cord stimulation is safe, reduces pain, and improves the quality of life in patients with intractable pain. Selected patients with chronic pain, refractory to other treatments have benefited from SCS. Surgical revision rates are high primarily due to hardware battery depletion, lead migration particularly in the cervical region and surgical complications (9% infection rate). Post-operative antibiotics were not used in the study reporting 9% infection rate but wound infections treated with antibiotics were successful (Kay, McIntyre, Macrae, and Varma, 2001).

Overall, patient reported pain relief was categorized as substantial (60%) and clinician reported pain relief was categorized as substantial (67%) in questionnaire responders. Of the patient questionnaire responders 81% required daily analgesics and 33% reported being able to undertake activities of daily living not previously achievable prior to the SCS (Kay, McIntyre, Macrae, and Varma, 2001).

Intrathecal Pump

The intrathecal pump can produce profound pain relief when maximum conservative therapy has failed. A temporary trial is performed prior to implanting a permanent system. Psychological screening is recommended prior to the trial. A provider experienced in the technique, such as a neurosurgeon or pain management specialist, should perform pump placement.

The procedure is performed in a hospital or outpatient surgical center with fluoroscopy under a general anesthetic. Some health care providers discharge the patient same day; others require a 23-hour stay, and others require an overnight stay. The decision on length of stay depends on health care provider preference and patient comorbid diagnoses. Refills can be performed during an office visit.

The trial is performed as an inpatient hospital stay and may last for 24 hours, up to three days. During the first 24 hours, any oral opioids medications are slowly titrated down, while the intrathecal infusion is gradually increased. The goal is to receive all opioids via the intrathecal route. Non-opioid medication such as NSAIDS, tricyclic antidepressants, neuroleptic medications may still be necessary and continued during the trial period. Adjustments are through the physician's office or, in an emergency, the emergency department.

If the temporary trial is successful (50% reduction in pain) the permanent system is implanted using fluoroscopy on an outpatient or inpatient setting. The pump is inserted just below the rib margin in the abdomen with the catheter tubing tunneled around the abdomen toward the spine and into the intrathecal space. The pump is placed in the lower quadrant of the abdomen for ease of refilling. Over time, fibroblasts will form a tight fibrous capsule around the pump, anchoring it in place.

Intrathecal drug delivery is an option for people who have failed conservative therapy, would not benefit from additional aggressive surgery, is dependent on pain medications, and do not have psychological problems. It also includes patients without a medical condition that would contraindicate the placement of a pump, is not allergic to any medication used in the pump, and has had a positive response to the trial implantation.

Medications used include opioids, local anesthetics, adrenergic agonists, N-methyl-D-asparate receptor agonists, and other agents. The first line of treatment includes morphine and hydromorphone. There is clinical evidence that morphine provides good analgesia in patients with chronic refractory pain. Another study demonstrated that hydromorphone after treatment with morphine resulted in decreased nausea and drowsiness. Pain scores were comparable after switching from morphine to hydromorphone (Anderson, Cooke, Burchiel, 2001). Second line treatment may be selected for patients with neuropathic symptoms. The medication may consist of either hydromorphone or morphine and the addition of either bupivacaine or clonidine. Ziconotide is a non-opioid medication with several studies demonstrating its efficacy in the intrathecal space.

The concentration of the medication determines refill frequency. Morphine is stable in solution for approximately 90 days; therefore a morphine pump refill should occur about once every three months, again, depending on the concentration of the medication. The pump battery will need replacement between three and six years after placement.

Intrathecal pumps are invasive and costly procedures. Surgical complications can include bleeding, neurological injury, infection, cerebral spinal leads, and malposition of the subcutaneous pockets. Successful temporary trial does not always ensure successful permanent placement. Catheter migration may require further operations for repositioning. Infections may result requiring the removal of the pump; and there is always a possibility of damage to the spinal cord or the spinal nerves. Additional complications may include post-dural puncture headaches, drug side effects, respiratory depression, withdrawal, and urinary retention and hesitancy.

Pump malfunction is very rare. Usually the pump stops working causing sudden onset of pain and morphine withdrawal symptoms. However, there is a theoretical risk that the pump could go out of control, injecting excessive dosages. This situation is potentially lethal if not detected in time. Inadvertent subcutaneous injection of concentrated morphine solution while attempting to refill the pump can result in severe respiratory depression and death.

Other side effects are related to the medication itself. In one retrospective study, patients receiving intrathecal opioids demonstrated changes in their neuroendocrine function such as hypogonadotropic hypogonadism. Some patients developed central hypocortisolism and 95% reported decreased libido (Verhelst et al., 2000). Laboratory studies should be considered in the plan to monitor endocrine function for this reason.

Implantation of the intrathecal morphine pump is contraindicated:
- In the presence of infection
- When the pump cannot be implanted 2.5 cm or less from the surface of the skin
- In patients whose body size is not sufficient to accept the pump bulk and weight

Pricing / Life Care Plan Guidelines.
When including an intrathecal pump in a life care plan, consider the following components for both trial and permanent placement and replacement every three to six years:
- Psychological evaluation (before trial only)
- Health care provider CPT Code
- Anesthesiology
- Fluoroscopy
- Surgical Suite (procedure time, supplies, medications, etc.)
- Hardware cost
- Recovery costs include assistance for ADL's, driving
- Possible need for assistance with ADLs during adjustment period and when replacement pumps are implanted

- Office visits for system analysis and refill every three months or sooner for as long as the intrathecal pump is implanted

Recent well-controlled studies show that with careful selection of patients and successful temporary trial and test stimulation, intrathecal pump placement for medication administration reduces pain and improves quality of life. (See also *Chapter 1, Spinal Cord Injury*, for more information on pricing implanted medication pumps.)

Conditions Associated with Long Term Opioid Treatment
There is general controversy surrounding the long-term use of opioid therapy for non-cancer pain. The definition of addiction does not necessarily fit a patient with physical dependence upon a drug or drugs. Individuals with chronic pain should be evaluated on a case-by-case basis. Below are definitions of tolerance, physical dependence, and addiction.

- *Tolerance* is a physiologic state resulting from regular use of a drug, development of need for higher dose of the specific drug to obtain the same pain relief effect, or reduced effect of drug noticed over time if dosage is not altered.

- *Dependence* is a state of normal physiologic adaptation to a drug that develops over time. When the drug dose is abruptly discontinued, withdrawal signs and symptoms occur.

- *Addiction*, as defined in The Free Medical Dictionary by Farlex, is a persistent, compulsive dependence on a behavior or substance. The term has been partially replaced by the word *dependence* for substance abuse. Addiction has been extended, however, to include mood-altering behaviors or activities. Some researchers speak of two types of addictions: substance addictions (for example, alcoholism, drug abuse, and smoking); and process addictions (for example, gambling, spending, shopping, eating, and sexual activity). There is a growing recognition that many addicts, such as polydrug abusers, are addicted to more than one substance or process.

Opioids are the current mainstay of treatment for moderate to severe pain. Opioids are effective, have a good risk/benefit ratio, and are easily titrated for therapeutic effect. However, opioids have adverse side effects, drug interactions, or dosing requirements that need consideration. A good understanding of the different classes of opioid, opioids with special safety concerns (e.g., hydromorphone, tramadol, meperidine, methadone), opioid titration, interactions and abuse is important when considering long term opioid use (Prescriber's Letter, 2010).

Many side effects of opioids are well known and include:

- Respiratory depression
- Nausea/vomiting
- Sedation / reduced psychomotor performance
- Constipation
- Bladder dysfunction
- Itching
- Physical dependence
- Tolerance

Less well-known effects include:

- Hormonal effects
- Immune effects
- Hyperalgesia
- Cardiac complications

Summary description of side effects of opioid treatment

Respiratory Depression: As opioid doses are increased, the respiratory center in the brain becomes less responsive to carbon dioxide, causing progressive respiratory depression. This effect is not as pronounced in patients being treated for severe or chronic pain. Respiratory depression is rarely seen during chronic opioid therapy (Ballantyne, 2006). Respiratory depression often manifests as a decrease in respiratory rate and is made worse because the cough reflex is also depressed. Respiratory depression can be potentiated by other respiratory depressants (e.g., benzodiazepines). The combination of, for example, methadone and alprazolam has been fatal, despite low methadone levels. Methadone has also caused fatalities when combined with other opioids or alcohol due to respiratory depression (DiPiro, 2008). In patients with underlying pulmonary dysfunction, it is especially important to be cautious because of their already-compromised respiratory mechanisms.

Nausea / Vomiting: Opioids decrease peristalsis of the gastrointestinal tract and reduce biliary and pancreatic secretions, resulting in slowed motility, nausea, vomiting and constipation. Nausea and vomiting are common side effects of regular opioid therapy and usually resolve with continued use (DiPiro, 2008). Anti-nausea medications can be tried to reduce this side effect in the initial titration phase of treatment.

Sedation: Opioids' sedating effects are well known. Drowsiness, lethargy, apathy, and decreased ability to concentrate, especially in opioid-naive patients, are thought to be caused by anticholinergic effects. This is typically apparent at the beginning of opioid therapy, but it is also seen on dose increases.

Initially, when opioids are added to a pain regimen, ability to drive or operate heavy machinery may be diminished. However, once a stable dose is achieved, patients without cognitive or psychomotor impairment should be able to drive normally. Psychostimulants may counteract the sedating effects of opioids and may improve psychomotor performance (Benyamin, 2008). Other medications can potentiate central nervous system depression (e.g., antidepressants, muscle relaxants).

A recent study demonstrated significantly improved neuropsychological test scores in long-term opioid users with low back pain when taking opioids for pain. The conclusion is that long-term use of opioids does not impair cognitive ability or psychomotor functioning. Rather, pain itself can have an adverse effect on cognitive function that is improved with opioid analgesia (Jamison, 2003).

Opioids do not directly affect cerebral circulation. Nevertheless, drug-induced respiratory depression can increase intracranial pressure. Caution is advised in head trauma patients who are not ventilated, because opioids may exaggerate this pressure and cloud the neurological status (DiPiro, 2008).

Constipation: Constipation is the most common side effect and does not resolve with opioid tolerance. Chronic constipation can result in hemorrhoids, rectal pain, bowel obstruction, megacolon, potential bowel rupture and death. Constipation should be anticipated, monitored, and treated early, aggressively, and effectively throughout opioid therapy (Benyamin, 2008).

Bladder dysfunction: Difficulty voiding or urinary retention are significant problems. Many other factors may play a role in bladder dysfunction and, as a consequence, few studies pertaining to opioid use and bladder dysfunction are available. Opioids decrease detrusor tone and the force of contraction, decrease the sensation of bladder fullness and the urge to void and inhibit the voiding reflex (Benyamin, 2008).

Itching: Pruritis is a typical side effect of opioid use due to histamine release from cutaneous mast cells. Hives, increased heart rate, and low blood pressure can also result from histamine release. These symptoms may be a sign of a pseudoallergy or a true allergy to opioids. Most allergic-type reactions to opioids involve codeine, morphine, or meperidine (Prescriber's Letter, 2006). Histamine release can exacerbate bronchospasms in patients with a history of asthma.

Hormonal Effects: Long-term opioid use results in suppression of both the hypothalamic-pituitary-adrenal and the gonadal axes. The effects of opioids on hormonal function are well understood and are called opioid endocrinopathy or opioid-induced androgen deficiency (Ballantyne, 2006). The effects can be found whether opioids are administered transdermally, intravenously, intrathecally or orally.

Numerous studies have documented that luteinizing hormone; the effects of opioids (Ballantyne, 2006) suppress follicle stimulating hormone, testosterone, estrogen and cortisol. Gonadotrophin releasing hormone, dehydroepiandrosterone and dehydroepiandrosterone sulfates, adrenocorticotropin, corticotropin-releasing hormone and cortisol have also been affected by opioids. Infertility and decreased libido, and aggression may result. Testosterone deficiency is the most frequently noted side effect when blood levels are tested. Testosterone replacement can help correct the deficiency (Ballantyne, 2006).

Women experience similar hormonally-linked side effects of opioids including depression, dysmenorrhea, sexual dysfunction, and reduced bone mineral density. Testosterone and estrogen levels are also reduced in women taking opioids (Benyamin, 2008). The reduction in estrogen may have serious implications for osteoporosis and fractures in women. This may support scheduled DEXA scans and early initiation of bisphosphonates in this population.

Immune system effects: The potential mechanism by which central opioid receptors mediate peripheral immunosuppression involves the autonomic nervous system in addition to the hypothalamic-pituitary-adrenal axes (Benyamin, 2008).

Preclinical research shows that opioids alter the development, differentiation and function of immune cells. Research is limited, but opioids have been shown to exacerbate immunosuppression in HIV patients. Direct evidence that opioids impair immune function in susceptible individuals is concerning, but no studies of immune function in patients receiving long-term opioid therapy for chronic pain has been done. Pain itself can suppress immune function so patients receiving prolonged opioid therapy without good pain relief make them more vulnerable to immune system deficiencies (Benyamin, 2008).

Hyperalgesia: There are limited studies on this newly-recognized side effect. Nevertheless, sensitization and increasing pain despite increasing doses of opioids may be related to opioid metabolites, and enhanced by the release of excitatory neurotransmitters. Ketamine is one of the few treatment options for hyperalgesia. Calcium channel blockers have been studied and shown to relax smooth muscle tone and reduce muscle spasms (e.g., its use in treating angina), thereby reducing pain and preventing hyperalgesia (DiPiro, 2008).

Cardiac Complications: Parasympathetic stimulation may also contribute to bradycardia and hypotension seen with histamine release (as above) (Benyamin, 2008). Recently research has shown QT prolongation associated with methadone (Prescriber's Letter, 2006). Therefore EKGs be monitored during methadone treatment. When other medications that cause hypokalemia are taken concurrently, it is especially important to monitor cardiac response. Risk factors for this side effect include heart failure, structural heart disease, hypokalemia, and family history of sudden cardiac death. Dosage increases, high methadone use, liver dysfunction, and the use of other QT prolonging drugs (e.g., antipsychotics such as quetiapine, Seroquel) may also increase the risk (Benyamin, 2008).

Geriatric Considerations

Opioids have particular precautions in the elderly. Methadone is not recommended in the elderly because of the slower metabolism and difficulty to titrate. Caution should be taken with initiation of therapy and dosage increases because severe toxicities may not become apparent for two to five days. Methadone has numerous drug interactions and can be clinically important in an elderly person with comorbid diagnoses and taking other medications. Side effects such as sedation and respiratory depression are increased when methadone is combined with alcohol or other drugs (Prescriber's Letter, 2006).

Tramadol came on the market as an unscheduled drug, but many pharmacists and prescribers are seeing cases of tramadol abuse. Tramadol does have addictive properties. The FDA added strong warnings about tramadol abuse due to its opioid effects in 2010. The FDA also cautions about deaths due to overdose and suicide, especially in patients with preexisting addiction, emotional problems, or taking other CNS depressants (e.g., benzodiazepines, sedatives).

Tramadol should be avoided in patients with a history of seizures as it may increase the risk of seizures. Concomitant use with serotonin reuptake inhibitors, opioids, tricyclic antidepressants, monoamine oxidase inhibitors, neuroleptics or other drugs can reduce the seizure threshold and, therefore, increase the risk of seizures (DiPiro, 2008).

Questions To Consider During Client Assessment

All of these issues have implications for life care planning.

- Are current medications (or treatments) controlling pain?
- Is the current treatment plan expected to remain in place long-term?
- Are current medications or treatments possibly causing side effects?
- Has prescribing provider given any other medications or treatments to help counteract the side effect(s)?
- Has prescribing provider mentioned any long term plan for other treatment to help counteract side effect(s)?
- Does patient drive after taking narcotic pain medication? Does the prescribing health care provider recommend against driving because of medication regimen?
- Is there any history of drug seeking behavior?
- Is there any history of problems with law enforcement associated with drug use?

Medical Supplies And Durable Medical Equipment
TENS - Transcutanous Electric Nerve Stimulation

Transcutaneous electrical nerve stimulation is one of the most commonly used forms of electro-analgesia. There is ongoing debate about efficacy. The currently proposed mechanisms of action include:

- Inhibition in the dorsal horn of the spinal cord
- Endogenous pain control via endorphins
- Direct inhibition of an abnormally excited nerve
- Restoration of afferent input

The TENS unit provides electrical stimulation. Frequency and strength can be adjusted according to patient response. The stimulation theoretically helps to limit or block transmission of pain signals to the central nervous system.

Product Specifics The TENS unit includes a signal unit, a battery, and a set of electrodes. Electrode supply should be replaced regularly. The average life of a TENS unit varies depending upon model and frequency of use. Electrode replacements should be calculated when considering projected cost. The patient should be trained by the physical therapist on the use of the TENS according to the expected use or pain centers of the patient.

Newer electrical stimulation devices similar to TENS include:

- The IFC (Interferential current therapy) a device that delivers alternating current signals with different frequency.
- The PENS (Percutaneous electrical nerve stimulation)— uses combination of electro-acupuncture and TENS approach. An acupuncture-like needle is used instead of an electrode and placed at a dermatome level consistent with pain symptoms.
- A TENS unit is generally used for analgesia based upon the patient controlling the device. The patient adjusts frequencies and intensities of signal to determine what will work best.

Side Effects/Complications Skin irritation can occur, usually associated with electrode gel or tape used to secure the electrodes.

Contraindications
- Pacemaker
- Pregnancy
- Do not use over anterior neck due to risk of laryngospasm
- Do not place in area with reduced sensitivity to avoid possibility of burn
- Use cautiously with spinal cord stimulator or intrathecal pump.

Independence and Mobility Aids: Various familiar aids for independence may be useful for a debilitated chronic pain patient, and considered after nurse life care planner assessment. Preservation of independence is the ultimate goal of chronic pain management, and a justifiable rationale for recommendation for aids. PT or OT consult is may be helpful.

- Reachers and grab bars
- Vehicle adaptations
- Specialty mattress or seating surface
- Bathroom safety: safe access, tub transfer bench, hand held shower head
- Modified home entry/egress
- Wheelchair or scooter
- Cane, walker
- Consider frequency of use when estimating replacement frequency

Nursing Diagnoses To Consider

- *Activity Intolerance:* Insufficient physiological or psychological energy to endure or complete required or desired daily activities
- *Impaired Physical Mobility:* Limitation in independent purposeful physical movement of one or more extremities
- *Sleep Deprivation:* Prolonged periods without sleep (sustained natural, periodic suspension of relative consciousness)
- *Constipation:* Decrease in normal frequency of defecation accompanied by difficult or incomplete passage of stool and/or excessively hard, dry stool.
- *Chronic Pain:* Unpleasant sensory or emotional experience arising from actual or potential tissue damage or described in terms of such damage (International Association for the Study of Pain); sudden or slow onset of any intensity from mild to severe with an anticipated or predictable end and a duration of greater than 6 months

- *Acute Pain:* Unpleasant sensory or emotional experience arising from actual or potential tissue damage or described in terms of such damage (International Association for the Study of Pain); sudden or slow onset of any intensity from mild to severe with an anticipated or predictable end and a duration of less than 6 months
- *Fatigue:* An overwhelming sense of exhaustion and decreased capacity for physical and mental work at the usual level.
- *Impaired Social Interaction:* Insufficient or excessive quantity or ineffective quality of social exchange.
- *Post-Trauma Syndrome:* Sustained maladaptive response to a traumatic, overwhelming event.

References

Aetna. (2012). Clinical Policy Bulletin: Quantitative Sensory Testing Methods. From http://www.aetna.com/cpb/medical/data/300_399/0357.html

Anderson, V, Cooke, B, Burchiel, K. (2001). Intrathecal hydromorphone for chronic nonmalignant pain: A retrospective study. *Pain Medicine.* 2. p. 287-97

Ballantyne, J. (2006). Opioids for chronic nonterminal pain. Retrieved from www.medscape.com

Benyamin, R, Trescot, A, Datta, S, et al.(2008). Opioid complications and side effects. Retrieved from www.painhealth care providerjournal.com. *Pain Physician* 2008: Opioid Special Issue

California Department of Workers' compensation. (2007), Workers' compensation final regulations, Medical treatment utilization schedule, Title 8-California Code of Regulations, Sections 9792.20-9792.23, Industrial Relations, Division 1., Department of Industrial Relations, Chapter 4.5, Subchapter 1., Administrative Director, Administrative Rules, Section 9792.2, retrieved from http://www.dir.ca.gov/dwc/DWCPropRegs/MedicalTreatmentUtilizationSchedule/MTUS_regulations.htm

Chronic Pain: Assessment and Management Guidelines (2011). Retrieved from http://www.icsi.org/guidelines_ and_more/gl_os_prot/musculo-skeletal/pain_ chronic_assessment_and_management_of_14399/ pain_chronic_assessment_and_management_of_14400. html

DiPiro, J, Talbert, et al. (2008). Pharmacotherapy: A pathophysiological approach (7th ed). New York, NY:McGraw-Hill

Gatchel R, Ricard M, et al. (2009) The Comprehensive Muscular Activity Profile (CMAP): Its High Sensitivity, Specificity and Overall Classificiation Rate for Detecting submaximal Effort on Functional Capacity Testing. Journal of Occupational Rehabilitation 19:1 p. 49-52

Gerber (2009). Chronic Pain Medical Treatment Guidelines. Retrieved from http://www.dir.ca.gov/dwc

Gray RP. (2001). Adjunctive Agents in the Management of Chronic Pain: Local anesthetic and antiarrhythmic agents. Retrieved from http://www.medscape.com/ viewarticle/409782_4

Hornberger J, Kumar K et al. (2008) Rechargeable spinal cord stimulation versus nonrechargeable system for patients with failed back surgery syndrome: A cost-consequence analysis. Clinical Journal of Pain 2008; 24 p.244-252.

International Association for the Study of Pain (2009), http:// www.iasp-pain.org/AM/Template.cfm?Section=Fact_ Sheets1andTemplate=/CM/ContentDisplay. cfmandContentID=7187.Global Year Against Cancer Pain: October 2008-October 2009.

Kay A, McIntyre M et al. (2001). Spinal cord stimulation - a long-term evaluation in patients with chronic pain. British Journal of Neurosurgery 2001; 15:4 p.335-341

Knight K, Brand F et al. (2006). Implantable intrathecal pumps for chronic pain: Highlights and updates. Retrieved from http://www.ncbi.nlm.nih.gov/pmc/articles/ PMC2080496/

Kumar K, Toth C, et al. (1998). Epidural spinal cord stimulation for treatment of chronic pain - some predictors of success. Surgical Neurology 1998; 50: p. 110-120.

Mezey M, Berkman BJ et al. (2001). The Encyclopedia of Elder Care. New York, NY: Springer Publishing Company

NCCAM (2009). Acupuncture for Pain. National Institute of Health, retrieved from http://nccam.nih.gov/health/acupuncture/acupuncture-for-pain.htm

NCCAM (2007), Acupuncture: An Introduction, National Institute of Health, retrieved from http://nccam.nih.gov/health/acupuncture/acupuncture-for-pain.htm#introduction

Prescriber's letter. Opioid Dosing: Focus on safety. 2010;26(5):260712

Robbins J. (2008). A Symphony in the Brain. The Evolution of the New Brain Wave Biofeedback. New York, NY: Grove Press

Saunders S and Longworth S. (2009). Injection Techniques in Orthopaedics and Sports Medicine. New York; NY:Elsevier

Seems M (2007). Acupuncture Clinical Practice Guidelines, Tri-state College of Acupuncture. retrieved from http://www.tsca.edu/site/alumni/c/acupuncture-clinical-practice-guidelines/

Stanton-Hicks M (2011). The Future of peripheral nerve stimulation. Progressive Neurology Surgery. 24 p.210-217

Swingle P, (2008). Biofeedback for the brain; how neurotherapy effectively treats depression, ADHD, autism and more. Piscataway, NJ: Rutgers University Press.

The National Certification Commission for Acupuncture and Oriental Medicine (NCCAOM). (2010) State Licensing Information, 2010, retrieved from http://www.nccaom.org/regulatory-affairs/state-licensure-map

Toombs J, Kral L. (2005) Methadone treatment for pain. American Family Physician Web. Retrieved from www.aafp.org/afp 2005

Turk D and Melzack R. (2001). Handbook of pain assessment (2nd ed.) New York, NY: Guilford Press

Verhelst J, Maeyaert J et al. (2000) Endocrine consequences of long term intrathecal administration of opioids. Journal of Clinical Endocrinology, 85: P. 2215-2222.

CHAPTER 4

Amputation

Terri Brandley, BSN, RN, CCM
Shelly Kinney, MSN, RN, CCM, CNLCP
Karen Yates RN, LNC, NLCP
Jean Beaubien, BSN, RN, CRRN, CDMS, CCM,
CNLCP, contributor

Introduction

Since ancient times, amputations have been common in war. Some cultures used amputation as a form of punishment. Disease and accidents caused many others. Treatment options were limited to minimizing blood loss and preventing infection. Rehabilitation services, either medical or psychological, were nonexistent (Kirkup, 2010).

Today, the causes of amputation are unchanged. However, amputation treatment and rehabilitation are now complex, multidisciplinary, comprehensive, and individualized. Medical knowledge, surgical techniques, and prosthetic technology are vastly improved, involving a wide array of disciplines. Infection rates are reduced. Rehabilitation programs maximize functionality and overall health to help prevent complications. Terminology has also evolved, such as referring to the "residual limb" rather than "stump" or "stub."

Amputation is the surgical removal of all or part of a body part that is enclosed by skin (*Webster's New World Medical Dictionary*, 2013). Traumatic amputation is an accidental severing of a body part.

Amputation may be performed at any level in the upper extremities (digits, hand, arm) or in the lower extremities (toes, foot, leg). Division through a long bone is considered to be a true amputation. The point at which the limb or digit is incised or removed is known as the *amputation level*.

Surgeons determine amputation level by measuring blood flow in the area, determining where complete healing is most likely to occur with least risk of complications, to permit greatest function and most efficient prosthesis use. Optimum function may be gained with a more distal amputation, while risk of complications is reduced when the amputation level is more proximal. Amputation levels are referred to by site as upper extremity (UE), above elbow (AE), below elbow (BE), lower extremity (LE), above the knee (AK), below the knee (BK), or through the knee (TK). More recent terminology classes amputation by the major bone transected, e.g., transtibial (below the knee), transradial (below the elbow), or transfemoral (above the knee). *Disarticulation* is amputation through a joint (Medical Disability Advisor, 2012).

The same general principles and treatment goals, i.e., removing damaged tissue, relieving pain, and preparing a site for prosthesis, and helping the client return to the most comfortable and functional life possible, apply to all forms of amputation.

Role of the Nurse Life Care Planner

Clients with amputations can lead fully productive lives. Media coverage on returning war veterans and trauma victims has brought considerable attention to amputations and prosthetics. The importance of a multidisciplinary, individualized rehabilitation plan with not only the physical and psychological aspects of amputation but social functioning (work, school, leisure activities, family role) is essential to life care plan development (Santiago and Coyle, 2004).

Amputation causes triple losses: loss of function, loss of sensation, and loss of body image (Racy, 1989). These issues require a holistic approach, including medical, psychological, societal, and other appropriate interventions. Nurse life care planners specifically consider these aspects in the individualized life care plan, reviewing records, evaluating the individuals, interviewing providers, and documenting all pertinent data. The nurse life care plan is based on assessment of these data.

Ideally, rehabilitation begins before amputation. Loss of a body part affects endurance, function, and strength of the other extremities. With planned amputation, the client should be educated about the surgical process and expectations following amputation, including the psychological aspects and post-amputation quality of life and, if possible, optimizing physical condition (Kurichi, 2013).

The nurse life care planner is uniquely qualified to develop a plan with nursing diagnoses as the foundation. It is important to include recommendations by all providers on the multidisciplinary team: surgeon, rehabilitation physician, pain management physician, nursing staff, clinical nurse specialist, occupational therapist, physical therapist, social worker, home health, prosthetist, psychologist, and psychiatrist. It is also important to consider the client's occupation and leisure or sports activities, age, and role in the family and support system (Santiago and Coyle, 2004).

The life care plan should be holistic and individualized. The client's overall health, whether the dominant side is affected, and developmental stage are important considerations. Work or school concerns should be addressed by including qualified vocational or educational counselors or coaches. Family therapy is often overlooked in life care plans for amputees. If there are significant body image issues affecting the amputee, sexuality therapy might be beneficial. Sleep evaluation and pain management are also integral to a comprehensive life care plan. Weight management, fitness, and smoking cessation may also need to be included (DiGiacomo et al., 2004).

The life care planner should not assume that all individuals with amputation will want or need a prosthesis, and individuals with multiple amputations may not desire or benefit from prosthetic replacement at every amputation site.

Even those who wear prostheses perform some activities such as bathing and donning undergarments without the device. Some individuals, particularly those with very proximal or very distal amputations, may choose to forego prostheses altogether . . . the patient, family, and clinicians may decide not to proceed with definitive fitting. Other clients, particularly those with multiple disorders, cannot cope with the physical demands of prostheses. A few individuals do not wear prostheses simply because they are unaware of current componentry and funding sources (Edelstein, 2002).

Incidence and Causation (Amputee Coalition of America [ACA], 2012)
Each year, over 185,000 people in the United States lose a limb or portion of a limb to accident or disease. There are over two million amputees in the United States today. The leading cause of amputations is peripheral vascular disease due to diabetes and peripheral arterial disease. In 2009, hospital costs with amputations were over $18.3 billion. The mortality rate associated with peripheral vascular disease is high. Nearly half of persons with peripheral vascular disease die within five years of amputation. Of diabetes patients with lower extremity amputations, up to 55% will require amputation of the second limb within two to three years.

Peripheral Vascular Disease (PVD)
Peripheral vascular disease is the most common cause of lower extremity amputation in adults (Miller, S. 2010). Classical indicators of PVD are intermittent claudication and the loss of one or more lower extremity pulses. Comprehensive, holistic consideration of overall health concerns and prevention of complications from any underlying disease state, e.g., diabetes, ongoing vascular disease, or hypertension is critical.

Trauma

Trauma is the second most common cause of an amputation in adults (Zeigler-Graham et al., 2008). Controlling hemorrhage and preventing additional tissue damage are immediate priorities. Although any amputation can cause emotional issues, the sudden circumstances of traumatic amputation may cause significant psychological and interpersonal issues (Racy, 2002).

Burns

Burns can cause a great deal of tissue loss leading to amputation, particularly of fingers and toes. In the case of severe lower extremity burns, there are "high rates of cellulitis, deep vein thrombosis, and bacteremia. Fourth-degree lower-extremity burns require multistage reconstructive procedures but limb salvage is possible in a majority of cases" (Parrett et al., 2006). Preserving remaining healthy tissue and preventing infection are priorities; scarring can pose challenges for prosthetic fit and use, and increased skin fragility must be considered. Cosmetic issues can be significant, and often involve not only the area of the amputation but other areas of the body as well.

Frostbite

Frostbite is partially or completely frozen body tissue. Maintenance of healthy remaining tissue and mobility are priorities to maximize functional abilities. Parts of the body most often affected by frostbite are the hands, feet, nose, and ears. Tetanus immunization is recommended. Triple phase technetium bone scan can assess viability of remaining bony tissue. Surgical amputation may be necessary; cosmetic losses can be significant (Medical Disability Advisor, 2012).

Infections

Localized infections require treatment with antibiotics. More systemic infections (i.e., osteomyelitis) require more aggressive intravenous antibiotics and other treatments to prevent further tissue damage and loss. Necrotic areas of tissue may require surgical debridement and resultant residual limb revision in certain locations. This will ultimately affect the fit and replacement schedule of the prosthesis if the affected residual limb is involved (Bowker, 2002).

Tumors

For many years amputation was the conventional treatment of malignant bone and soft-tissue tumors. With the advent of new cancer therapies, it is no longer (Mnaymneh, 2002). When necessary, amputation due to cancer (most often osteosarcoma) typically occurs near the epiphyses of long bones. The treatment team and nurse life care planner must consider need for future diagnostic and systemic treatments as well as future functional capabilities (Moore, 2002).

Nonunion of Bone

Fracture nonunion is an indication for amputation. It will likely require additional interventions to improve bone health, healing, stability, and recovery time. Consultation with healthcare providers is essential. Bone growth stimulation, additional surgery options, and therapies should be considered. Smoking delays bone healing; consideration should be given to smoking cessation classes during this time. A healed fracture may prevent the need for amputation surgery.

Pediatric Considerations

Surgery and management of amputations in children is very different from adults. With children and young adults, continuing growth will affect prosthesis fit and functionality. Multiple revision surgeries are common in the pediatric population, as bone growth continues in the residual limb (Osebold et al., 2001). Phantom pain is experienced in nearly 100% of pediatric traumatic amputees (Krane and Heller, 1995). Principles of amputation in children include preservation of as much residual limb length as possible, preservation of the growth plates, disarticulation when possible, preservation of the knee joint when possible, and stabilization of the proximal residual limb (Pediatric Orthopedic Society of America, 2013).

As with adults, assessment and care for psychological factors are important to include in the life care plan (Clerici et al., 2004). Those factors may include mutilating surgery, the impact of prosthetic and skin issues on school and work attendance, coping with body image, and dealing with the cruelties and curiosity of other children.

Functional demands of a prosthesis are very different in an active, growing child than an adult. A young child may find a prosthesis cumbersome and become functionally independent without one. Therapy can help to optimize a child's independent functional ability with prosthetic training with an age-appropriate prosthesis for the child's weight and usual physical activity. The life care planner should provide for periodic follow-up by pediatric physiatrists and other specialists to assess the child's needs and response to treatment. A school counselor and school nurse can also assist with school modifications during this time.

The life care planner will consider needs for frequent follow-up and updated equipment during childhood for the timeframe recommended by the treating providers of care until adult growth is achieved. At age eighteen, almost ¾ inch (2.5 cm) of growth remains for boys and slightly less for girls, for whom growth is 99% complete (Doyle, 2009).

Congenital

Birth defects are the most common cause of amputations in children. There are multiple adaptive surgical techniques to maximize bony functional abilities. The procedures may give the child more mobility and prosthetic options; however, the resulting deformities can be difficult socially. In all of these procedures, existing bones and tissues are moved and reformed to improve function (Pediatric Orthopedic Society of America, 2013).

Trauma

Trauma is the most common cause of acquired amputations in children (Pediatric Orthopedic Society of America, 2013).

Tumors

Cancers of the bone, typically osteosarcoma, are more common in children than in adults. Management may include chemotherapy and radiation and frequent bone and body scans. These children can miss a great deal of school and social peer activities. Depending upon the area amputated and the age of the child, the nurse life care planner must consider client and family wishes, function, cosmetic appearance, and weight of the prosthesis and growth of the child (Edelstein, 2002).

Burns

Significant burns and tissue injury can lead to amputation and, as with adults, pose special challenges for rehabilitation and long-term follow-up. Prevention and safety measures are important to preserve the integrity of the healthy tissue. Please see also the chapter on Burns for more information.

Infections

As with adults, localized infections require treatment with antibiotics. More systemic infections (e.g., osteomyelitis) require more aggressive intravenous antibiotics and other treatments to prevent further tissue damage and loss. Necrotic tissue may require surgical debridement and residual limb revision. This will ultimately affect the fit of a prosthesis and replacement schedule for devices if the affected residual limb is involved.

Amputation Terminology

The nurse life care planner should be knowledgeable about general amputation terminology. Common types of amputations include the following (Bulstrede et al., 2002):

- Open amputation: wound is left open for drainage
- Closed amputation: wound is closed during surgery
- Cineplastic amputation: a flap is formed with inclusion of the implanted prosthesis, which innervates the muscle directly
- Guillotine amputation: straight cut through the limb
- Disarticulation: limb is severed through the joint
- Circular: circular incision with a single flap
- Stump revision: revision of the shape or scar of a residual limb
- Syme amputation: below the ankle amputation

Principles of surgical options include the following (Nelson and Blauvelt, 2007):
- Choose as distal a site as possible.
- Preserve joints (especially the elbow and knee).
- Preservation of adequate blood supply for healing is the first priority

Function, site, and appearance are important considerations in comprehensive rehabilitation. With any amputation, the life care planner should provide for training and function to the highest level attainable based on the evaluation and recommendations of the treating team. Additionally, the prosthesis should fit the expectations of the client. The client will require evaluations by the prosthetist on a regular basis until the fit and function have been fully established.

The nurse life care planner must be aware of the client's psychological coping with functional loss. Actions such as anger, hostility, blame, refusal, or body image problems are symptoms of grief. Mental health care should be included to develop and facilitate coping skills, assess for and treat anxiety, and to screen for and treat post-traumatic stress syndrome.

Psychological sequelae can interfere with recovery and rehabilitation, prolonging recovery and delaying or preventing return to normal life activities. The Amputee Coalition of America (ACA) is an excellent resource for amputees and their significant others in the rehabilitation and reintegration process. These services are typically provided at no charge.

Classifications

Amputation levels have been classified for uniformity. The nurse life care planner will need to understand these classification systems to understand recovery, tissue healing, function, cosmetic and prosthetics as they are important in planning for a client's needs and collaboration with prosthetist and rehabilitation team. This information is essential to develop an individualized life care plan.

The International Organization for Standardization (ISO) classification is generalized for all medical clientele. Please refer to the article by Day (1991) for details. Table 1 gives abbreviations for *limb prosthetics* and is very specific for the prosthetist. It describes the site with more accuracy.

Table 1. Limb Prosthetics Abbreviations.

Shoulder, complete	SH	Forequarter
Arm, complete	Arm	Shoulder disarticulation
Arm, Partial (upper 1/3)	AE	Short
Arm, Partial (middle 1/3)	AE	Medium
Arm, Partial (lower 1/3)	AE	Long
Forearm, complete	FO	Elbow disarticulation
Forearm, partial (upper 1/3)	BE	Short
Forearm, partial (middle 1/3)	BE	Medium
Upper Extremity		
Forearm, partial (lower 1/3)	BE	Long

Carpal, complete	WD	Wrist disarticulation
Carpal, partial		WD with some carpal
Metacarpal, complete	MC	
Metacarpal, partial	MC	Partial hand
Phalangeal, complete	Ph	By joint of finger
Hip, complete		Hemi-pelvectomy
Thigh, complete		Hip disarticulation
Thigh, partial (upper 1/3)	AK	Short
Thigh, partial (middle 1/3)	AK	Medium
Thigh, partial (lower 1/3)	AK	Long
Leg, complete		Knee disarticulation
Leg, partial (upper 1/3)	BK	Short
Leg, partial (middle 1/3)	BK	Medium
Leg, partial (lower 1/3)	BK	Long
Tarsal, complete	Ta	Ankle disarticulation
Tarsal, partial	Ta	Some of heel bones
Metatarsal, complete	MT	All of the metatarsals
Metatarsal, partial	MT	Some of the metatarsals
Phalangeal, complete	Ph	All of the toes
Phalangeal, partial	Ph	Part of a toe
Pelvis		Complete hemicorporectomy

Enneking Classification In the 1970s and 1980s, Dr. Enneking developed the principles of surgical resection and established a Surgical Staging System for musculoskeletal tumors based on specific muscle groups to prevent amputation. A basic understanding of the tumor staging system can guide the life care planner in knowledgeable discussion with treating providers. Today, the Musculo-Skeletal Tumor Society uses the Enneking Classification to define muscle amputation for cancer removal. The Enneking Classification includes the following stages (Jawad and Scully, 2010):

- **Intra-compartmental**: within a muscle or group of muscles, with the removal of a portion of the muscle

- **Extra-compartmental** - removal of the entire muscle group from insertion to origin and possible other surrounding tissue such as skin and bone. This is equivalent biologically to an amputation one joint above the lesion

    These two stages are further categorized as benign or malignant.

- **Benign tumors** are
    - o Latent
    - o Active
    - o Aggressive

    Malignant tumor staging is determined by three subcategories:
- **Grade:**
    - o G 1: Low grade, uniform cell type without atypia, few mitoses
    - o G 2: High grade, atypical nuclei, mitoses pronounced

- **Site:**
    - o T 1: Intracompartmental (Confined within limits of periosteum
    - o T 2: Extracompartmental (Breach in an adjacent joint cartilage, bone cortex (or periosteum), fascia lata, quadriceps, and joint capsule)

- **Metastasis**
  o   M 0: No identifiable skip lesions or distant metastases
  o   M 1: Any skip lesions, regional lymph nodes, or distant metastases

Replantation

Replantation is the surgical procedure in which an amputated body part is reattached to the rest of the body, including nerve, arterial, and venous anastomoses. The quality of nerve repair and subsequent nerve regeneration largely determines the functional outcome of a replanted extremity (Meyer, 2003). Replantations can be attempted in any traumatic amputation if assessment indicates that function of the amputated body part may be restored. However, these procedures can be associated with prolonged hospitalization, secondary operations, complications, and prolonged aggressive rehabilitation (Yaffe et al., 2009).

The mechanism of injury will determine whether a replantation can be attempted. *Crush* injury typically results in extensive tissue damage and possible infection. *Avulsion* injury is also associated with significant tissue damage. Damage from these two types of injury is typically irreversible. *Guillotine* (clean and sharp) injury is more likely to be successfully replanted than a crush or avulsion injury (Clontz, 2004).

Factors influencing whether replantation is successful include the patient's overall condition, existence of other serious injuries, how long the body part has been detached, and how the body part has been salvaged and stored. No body part is too small to be salvaged, even a fingertip (Clontz, 2004).

Ischemic time is a critical factor in successful reattachment of severed body parts. Limbs with significant amounts of soft tissue loss are less tolerant to ischemia. Crush injuries require reattachment of the limb or part within six to eight hours. Most digits must be reattached within eight hours, or twenty-four hours if kept cooled (Blank-Reid, 2003).

In the case of hand replantation, four hours is the maximum window of time allowable for the replantation to be successful (Fayerman, 2006).

Replantations are almost always attempted for amputations to the hands, thumbs, fingertips, and arms below the elbow, or for any body part of a child. However, due to the increased risk of potentially life-threatening complications, replantations are almost never attempted for a severely crushed, mangled, or contaminated body part. Clients with a history of hypertension, diabetes, peripheral vascular disease, or psychiatric illness are carefully evaluated for replantations (Clontz, 2004).

Children who are otherwise healthy have a high success rate for replantations of all types. In addition to an optimum cosmetic outcome, children typically achieve an excellent long-term functional outcome. However, limbs lost by children in farm machinery-related accidents only had a 20% success rate for reattachment (McClure, 2005), because these often involve crush injury with a contaminated object.

In a study by the Mayo Clinic, two of twelve patients studied were able to undergo successful replantation with continued function and some sensation at the eight-year follow-up (Edwards, 2005). Some body parts, such as the ear, have been successfully replanted even after more than ten hours of detachment before surgery.

Microvascular anastomosis by a microvascular surgeon is very important for successful blood flow after reattachment. The establishment of effective venous return, postoperative treatment, observation, and appropriate nursing care are also vital to a successful outcome (Liang, 2004).

The first successful arm replantation was performed in 1962; the first successful digit replantation in 1965 (Cheng, 2004). These were followed by scores of successful upper extremity replantations. However, attempts at lower extremity replantation have met with less success. The Mangled Extremity Severity Score (Helfet et al., 1990) is used to rate lower extremity trauma and is based on skeletal and soft tissue damage, limb ischemia, shock, and patient age. Scores range from two to fourteen and successful limb salvage is most likely to occur with a score of 6 or lower. The functional outcome of lower extremity replantation is often poor, and the muscle of the lower limb requires rapid revascularization. Often lower limb sensory recovery is never established, resulting in lifelong increased risk of foot ulceration. Subsequent reamputation due to complications of reperfusion, muscle necrosis, and need for complex reconstructive surgery is common after lower extremity replantation attempts (Webb, 2005).

In upper extremity replantation, the more distal the injury, the better the prognosis for recovery. More proximal upper extremity replantation success is less predictable (Webb, 2005). Fingertips should be always be aggressively replanted, which can cause a minimal loss in function and improved cosmesis in most instances (Matsuzaki, 2004). Those clients who have not had joint injury will typically also have better movement than those with joint injury. Physicians typically consider a 60% to 80% return of function as an excellent outcome (Czerne, 2006).

Transpositional replantation may be considered in those cases in which replantation is not feasible, such as in multiple digit amputations; it can be beneficial to reattach severed body parts to other positions than their original biological placement. A finger reattached to the thumb position may provide a more positive functional outcome of the hand (Schwahegger, 1999). Basic hand function can be restored by transpositional digital replantations without additional reconstructive procedures, reducing the need for secondary operations (Cheng, 2004).

Long-term complications can progress for some time beyond the immediate post-operative period. Even successful replantations rarely restore normal function and sensation completely. One long-term complication of replantation is intolerance to cold temperatures. This may improve after approximately two years. Stiffness, decreased range of motion, and decreased sensation are also common complications. Some complications, such as contractures, can be avoided with appropriate postoperative care and positioning. Temporary braces can protect newly repaired tendons while allowing some limited movement of the extremity.

Rejection and failure of the replantation is another possible complication. This is typically caused by vascular problems and can only be improved by a second (revision) surgery.

Patients who undergo replantation surgery typically can expect lengthy rehabilitation. Some will require additional surgery to free up tendons from scar tissue, release stiff joints, reposition muscles or replace damaged nerve tissue (Czerne, 2006). In the case of hand injuries, rehabilitation will focus on grasping, strengthening, and digit flexibility.

Phantom pain, often described as crushing, grinding, or burning, pain, can be a common problem. Although phantom pain may occur in the immediate postoperative period, it can continue indefinitely. Since pain can affect sleep, and the literature suggests that poor sleep can cause increased pain, the nurse life care planner should consider the need for a sleep evaluation and therapy if indicated (Smith and Haythornthwaite, 2004).

Physical and occupational therapy is typically provided to minimize contractures and improve mobility to the greatest extent possible. A supervised rehabilitation program consisting of orthotics, physical therapy, and dynamic splinting to minimize flexion contractures may be required. Passive range of motion exercises by a therapist can begin several weeks after surgery.

Late failures due to tendon adhesion, stiffness, joint inadequacy, flexor tendon adherence, or delayed or nonunion of the bone ends can complicate a complete recovery. Return of sensation may take up to four to six months. The full extent of neurologic recovery is not known until approximately one year. Some permanent functional limitations can be anticipated, including decreased range of motion, decreased sensation, cold intolerance, and reduced strength. These limitations may impair the ability to perform independent activities of daily living with adaptive equipment. Work and school activities may require modifications (Czerne, 2006).

Upper Extremity Amputation

The loss of a hand or arm requires more extensive rehabilitation than the loss of a lower extremity. The complexity of the function of the hand and fingers is difficult to replicate. Improving functional status is the priority for rehabilitation considerations. Modern prosthetics have progressed beyond the hook device; myoelectric arms are very sophisticated and are much more functional and cosmetic than older prostheses. Considerations of the dominant versus non-dominant side are important. Rehabilitation with the non-dominant upper extremity is a much more complex and protracted recovery process. Consideration should be provided for multiple prostheses to address different functions. A variety of prosthetic attachments should also be explored with the amputee and the prosthetist.

Fingers

A loss of one or two fingers normally does not hinder hand function; however, the client may choose to have a cosmetic prosthesis for them. These prostheses are very lifelike and match the individual's skin and nails. It is important to discuss replacement intervals for the prosthesis with the prosthetist. Consider the client's age, lifestyle, occupation, schooling, and social and psychological factors.

Typically, hand function is more limited if more fingers are lost. Grasping objects with just the thumb is very difficult. If this is a dominant hand, consider alternate hand therapy for writing, eating, self-care, dressing, hobbies, work, school, and other activities. The life care planner should provide for assistive devices to improve functional abilities. Considerations may include a tape recorder, Dictaphone™, voice recognition computer software or a dictation / transcription app for notes, adaptive activities of daily living (ADL) items for tying shoes, fastening clothes, driving, cooking, using the computer, and other needs for work, school, and leisure. Occupational, physical, psychological, and other therapies should be included in the plan as indicated. If a recent occupational therapy (OT) assessment has not been completed, a good assessment can help guide recommendations for adaptive equipment and technologies.

Thumb
The thumb is critical for effective grasp. Extensive physical and occupational therapies and adaptive devices should be provided to maximize functional ability. Surgical interventions can create a semi-functional thumb prosthesis or device to mimic thumb function using the next digit or toe transplant. Some prostheses are available. These services and items may be addressed as with finger amputation.

Hand
Hand amputation typically occurs from some sort of trauma. Loss of the wrist joint and grasp cause difficulties with ADLs and personal care. School or work accommodations should be specific to the client's needs. If this is a dominant hand, the client will require training to use the non-dominant hand for ADLs, writing, and tasks.

Hand prostheses are most often cosmetic, but can serve to balance or hold items with both hands. However, progress in developing myoelectric prostheses controlled with upper muscle groups is continuing. These devices now have mechanisms to open and close the hand so the client can hold or grasp an item. The nurse life care planner should collaborate with the OT regarding the client's functional wishes. Occupational and physical therapy and a driving evaluation should be considered.

Forearm

This is an amputation between the wrist and the elbow. Preserving the elbow joint, if possible, allows more function. Occupational, physical, and other therapies and the prosthetist's involvement should be provided throughout recovery and rehabilitation. A driving evaluation should be considered.

Arm

This is amputation between the elbow and the shoulder, with loss of elbow and wrist joints. The prosthesis is strapped around the shoulder and is controlled by the shoulder muscles. Occupational, physical, and other therapies will and prosthetist involvement should be provided throughout recovery and rehabilitation. A driving evaluation should be considered.

Shoulder

In shoulder-level arm loss, functionality and prosthetic function are already complicated. Even with the rare congenital limb deficiencies, surgical revision is generally avoided to preserve as much native tissue as possible. Consultation and care from specialized upper extremity/shoulder therapists and prosthetists are necessary. Myoelectric prostheses or functional shoulder harness type prostheses are generally used.

Extensive physical and occupational therapies should be expected. All activities of daily living will need to be accomplished one-handed. If the dominant arm is involved, this will require additional rehabilitation training to maximize independence. This type of limb loss affects life choices regarding occupations, physical activity, and social activities. Psychology, psychiatry, and possibly family therapy services are important for clients and their families to integrate limb loss into their lives.

Lower Extremity Amputation

Resulting gait disturbances can require assistive devices and physical/occupational therapies. Effective ambulation for short and long distances and leisure/hobby activities are also important. The prosthetist is an integral part of this process. Weight-bearing shifts may place additional stresses on the contralateral lower extremity that should be considered in rehabilitation and long term needs. Alternative forms of mobility, e.g., crutches, walker, wheelchair, scooter, or I-BOT™, should be provided for times when the client is unable to wear the prosthesis, such as nighttime or when the primary prosthesis is undergoing repair. Consider multiple prosthetic devices depending on the activities of the client (VA/DOD Clinical Practice Guideline for Rehabilitation of Lower Limb Amputation, 2007).

Toes

Amputation of one or two toes typically does not affect the function of the foot and leg significantly. Loss of the great toe will usually affect balance. Physical therapy may be required. The shoe will require adjustment or an insert placed into the toe. If three to five toes are amputated, more difficulties with balance are anticipated. An ankle-foot orthotic (AFO) may be needed to stabilize balance. Additional surgeries may improve balance and decrease tissue stress (Wagner, 2002).

Foot-metatarsals

The two most commonly performed amputations of the mid-foot are tarsometatarsal disarticulation (Lisfranc procedure) and midtarsal disarticulation (Chopart procedure). As long as the heel remains, there is a portion of the foot for balance. As with multiple toe amputation, an AFO may be needed. Ambulation aids, e.g., a walker or cane, may be beneficial. Physical therapy and additional surgeries may be required (Wagner, 2002). The prosthetist will also actively participate in the patient's therapy. A driver safety evaluation should also be included in the plan.

Ankle
The most commonly performed amputation involving the rear foot is the Syme procedure, removal of the talus and calcaneus. This leaves the fatty portion of the heel to allow some weight bearing, protecting the tibia and fibula and cushioning the prosthetic device (Wagner, 2002).

Contralateral extremity strength, activity levels, and age are important considerations for prosthetic choice. Since this joint is needed for a smooth gait, the foot prosthesis typically compensates with limited motion at the foot, mimicking normal foot function and weight bearing.

Knee
This is an amputation at the knee itself. Loss of knee and ankle joints makes walking more complicated. Prosthesis fitting is more difficult; energy expenditure with ambulation is greater. This level of amputation will begin to have the biggest impact on the work setting and work day and adjustment should be considered.

Above the Knee (AKA)
Above-the-knee prosthesis fit is more complex; suction socket may be helpful. Additional strapping may be indicated to keep the prosthesis from coming loose and rubbing to prevent additional skin irritation. Multiple types and layers of stump socks will be required to protect the skin and ensure adequate fit.

Hip

Hip disarticulation is only done to preserve the life of the client. This may be due to infection, crush injury, accident, shrapnel, or pressure ulcer. The prosthetic unit straps onto the waist and comprises many components. It is very important to consider alternative methods of mobility such as a wheelchair or scooter, with this type of amputation.

Hemipelvectomy

This is an aggressive and invasive surgery that leaves the client without a bony case to support the abdominal contents on one side of the body (Lusardi and Nielsen, 2006). This is a complex injury, affecting not only ambulation due to the loss of a limb but also the adjustment of the urinary and gastrointestinal systems. Ileus is a significant risk, and the client initially may require nasogastric feeding until the body is able to adjust. Once healing occurs, the client can be fitted with a prosthesis, which comprises many parts and straps to the waist.

This type of injury requires support from multidisciplinary team with physiatry, prosthetists, physical and occupational therapy, mental health, nutrition services, rehabilitation, case management, and possibly gastrointestinal and urological specialists. Sexual therapy might also be a consideration.

Bilateral Amputation

Bilateral amputation greatly complicates recovery. It is more difficult to compensate for two missing limbs than one, particularly upper extremities, despite the advances in modern prostheses. Double and triple amputations are more common in recent war veterans than in past wars. A multidisciplinary team approach is required, including physical, occupational, vocational, mental health, prosthetic, rehabilitation therapies, pain management, and sexual therapy. Workplace and school accommodations may also be necessary.

Some multiple amputees find that they prefer not to use a prosthesis for one remaining residual limb. Alternative forms of mobility are essential to these patients. I-BOTS™, Segways™, standing wheelchairs, and other mobility devices greatly improve quality of life. Driving evaluation and adaptive vehicles should also be considered in the plan (VA/DOD Clinical Practice Guideline for Rehabilitation of Lower Limb Amputation, 2007).

Mastectomy

From many years, mastectomy, originally called "radical mastectomy," was the only treatment available for patients with breast cancer regardless of stage or location. Currently, a surgeon may recommend that only the malignant areas and margins surrounding them (lumpectomy) be removed. For more extensive disease, surgical mastectomy techniques have also improved, with less disfiguring scars than in past years. The muscles of the breast are left intact as much as possible.

A simple or total mastectomy is the removal of breast tissue, which can include the nipple, leaving the lymph nodes intact. A simple mastectomy can be recommended if cancer is found in more than one part of the breast or for other medical considerations.

However, surgeons will recommend radical mastectomy when the cancer has spread to the chest muscles under the breast. A modified radical mastectomy procedure involves removal of the entire breast (breast tissue, nipple, and lymph nodes, leaving the breast muscles intact) and axillary dissection, removal of axillary lymph nodes. Today, most clients who have mastectomies opt for the modified radical mastectomy. Life care plan considerations include mental health therapies for the individual and her support system for re-integration and dealing with a cancer diagnosis. Sexual therapy for body image changes can also be considered. Lymphedema resulting from removal of lymph nodes may require occupational therapy for mobilization and chronic edema management with compression garments and other devices. Pain management may also be a concern (Susan G. Komen for the Cure, 2013).

Ear and Nose

Prostheses are generally not needed for functional status. However, reconstruction can have beneficial psychological effects and improve function of the organs allowing improved smell, taste, vision and hearing.

Once the surrounding tissue has healed, the plastic surgeon will perform surgeries to replicate the ear or nose. The cartilage and skin tissue used for the procedure is usually autologous but can be an allograft or synthetic graft as well. These grafts can be costly and involve several revision surgeries over the life expectancy (Bhattacharya, 2012).

Prosthetic cosmetic reconstruction, called anaplastology, replaces the missing part with a carefully constructed prosthesis. These may be attached with magnets implanted in the subcutaneous tissue, adhesives, or mounted on eyeglasses. These can be life altering for persons with significant facial deformity resulting from surgical or traumatic losses, allowing reintegration into society (Tanner and Mobley, 2006).

Of growing interest and incidence is facial transplantation in the case of severe burns or facial trauma. "Facial transplantation may reduce the risk of depressive and anxiety disorders other than post-traumatic stress disorder. . . . it may be a surgical intervention with the potential to reduce the psychiatric suffering associated with pediatric burns. Furthermore, patients with pediatric burns may experience the stigma of disfigurement and psychiatric conditions" (Hanson et al., 2008). The first facial transplants have been performed and this option is a future consideration in both adult and pediatric clients.

The life care planner should pay close attention to inclusion of psychological support for all amputees, but especially in the case of facial disfigurement.

Revisions

Amputation is often the prelude to a long rehabilitation process aimed at overcoming the disability of the tissue loss, whether an extremity, part of an extremity, or another body part. During amputation, a residual limb is prepared for suitable fitting of prosthesis. A residual limb must be shaped over time with compression stockings and progressive movement for proper prosthesis fit.

Appropriate use and fit of any prosthetic device is very important to decrease risk of mechanical complications that may cause an injury requiring revision. Delayed fitting of prosthesis has also been associated with an increased risk for re-amputation or revision.

Even minor fluctuations in weight can affect prosthesis fit. Nutritional counseling and exercise therapies to maintain a healthy weight and diet might be considerations in the life care plan. Smoking should also be avoided, as this decreases oxygen levels in the blood and can impair healing. Smoking cessation classes should be a considered. Sleep is another often-overlooked issue, generally related to chronic phantom or other pain. Pain also needs to be managed for the client's quality of life over the life expectancy.

Revisions can be prevented in many cases if greater attention is paid to skin care and overall health promotion. Excellent skin care is integral to successful prosthesis fitting and to prevent further tissue loss. Proper prosthesis fit and skin care with moisture barriers and emollients will prevent or minimize skin breakdown due to friction or moisture.

Several complications may result in need to revise a primary amputation. These include infection, contractures, neuroma, pain in the residual limb, skin breakdown, or an ill-fitting prosthetic device. Progression of peripheral vascular disease, diabetes, or other conditions can also make additional amputations necessary. Children and young adults may require additional surgeries if continued residual limb bone growth affects prosthesis fit.

Complications must be recognized and addressed promptly to avoid further surgery and prolonged rehabilitation (Sherman, 1995). When anticipating the cost of possible complications, future amputation revision, or surgical intervention, the life care planner should obtain all information available from the treating physician, prosthetist, physical and occupational therapists, case manager, psychologist/counselor, mental health, and any other treating provider(s).

Prosthetic Options
A prosthetist has specialized knowledge and certification in prosthetics and fitting the amputee. When determining whether a client should use a prosthesis, a hands-on prosthetic assessment is crucial. The prosthetist will consider the following:

- Independence with ADLs
- Independence with ambulation
- Self-care activities
- Family activities
- Work/school accommodations
- Leisure/hobby activities
- Sports activity accommodations
- Outdoor activities
- Cosmetic
- Self-esteem and body image concerns
- Relationship concerns with childcare and other family activities
- Sexuality

The following graph (Figure 1) shows an optimal prosthetic rehabilitation timeline and milestones (Lang M, 2009).

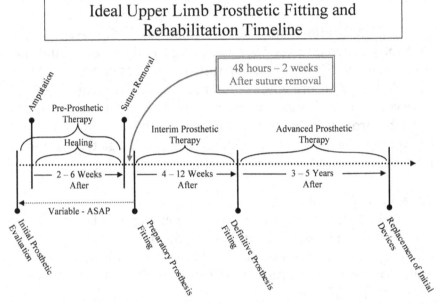

Figure 1. Used with permission from JNLCP.

Types of Prostheses

Prosthetics may be *endoskeletal* (components of the prosthesis are internal and the prosthesis simulates a natural looking limb) or *exoskeletal* (components of the prosthesis are visible). Modern lower limb prosthetics are often exoskeletal, though some may be covered in material colored to match the client's own skin tone.

Prosthetic components include hydraulic, suction, electrical, and other options to optimize function. Flexible articulating ankles, knees, elbows, and wrists ease mobility on uneven terrains and improve dexterity with ADLs. The hydraulic knee may help prevent falls by improving balance and providing more adjustability for sudden body movements. A weight-activated safety knee is commonly used in weaker or older clients, as it has as a mechanical brake to help prevent falls. The older and less functional manual locking knee, with a switch to lock and unlock the knee, requires the client to consciously lock or unlock the knee to sit or stand.

Myoelectric arms are usually endoskeletal, with simulated cosmetic skin to match the client's skin. Skin electrodes are placed on the arm inside of the socket for the muscles to generate electrical stimulation of the hand or elbow. The arm can be myoelectric or switch-controlled, or a combination, e.g., a switch-controlled elbow with a myoelectric wrist and fingers. The traditional hand hooks can be used with a cable-controlled harness strapped around the shoulders and powered by shoulder movement; others are electronically powered.

Replacing the Prosthesis

The replacement period for an individual prosthesis can vary according to the age, activity level, location, and functional requirements. The best guideline for replacement is the past history of the patient's own past prosthetic replacement needs, obtained from treating prosthetists and therapists and the client's own account. The product warranty can provide some guidelines.

Liner(s), socks, individual components, and other related prosthetic items require more frequent replacements than the entire prosthesis. Replacements are more frequent with younger, more active clients. The location of the amputation also makes a difference: more adjustments and replacements are necessary where there is less functional tissue present (e.g., above the knee, above the elbow).

There are a number of components to a custom-made prosthesis that makes it difficult to obtain an absolute cost for a particular prosthesis. Fluctuations in weight also affect the fit of the prosthesis. Prosthetic and physical therapy needs with prostheses should be considered for the life care plan.

Pediatric Prosthetic Considerations

As the children and young adults grow, they often require additional surgical revisions and prosthetic replacements. The Oklahoma Infant Leg, a prosthesis for infants from three months to one year of age, uses expanded polyethylene to form a one piece, ultra-light jointed leg. It provides flexibility in the socket as well as the joints of the child.

Diagnostic Tests

The nurse life care planner should be knowledgeable about diagnostic tests anticipated for the amputee client (Table 2). Consultation with the multidisciplinary team about the anticipated diagnostic tests, frequency and costs over the client's life expectancy is important information for the life care plan.

Table 2. Diagnostic Tests

Diagnostic Tests	Purpose of Test
C-reactive protein	Indicator of infection <1 no infection; >8 significant infection
Hemoglobin	Must be >10 g/dL as oxygenated blood is required for proper wound healing
Absolute lymphocyte count	<1,500/mL indicates immune deficiency and increased possibility of infection
Serum albumin levels	A level of ≤ 3.5 g/dL indicates malnutrition and diminished abilityto heal the wound
Radiography	Anteroposterior and lateral radiography of the extremity
Magnetic resonance imaging	Determine surgical margins, particularly in osteomyelitis or tumors
Technetium Tc-99m pyrophosphate bone scanning	Assist in predicting the need for amputation in electrical burns and frostbite by distinguishing viable and nonviable tissues
Doppler ultrasound	Determine arterial tissue perfusion. A minimum measurement of 70 mmHg is believed to be necessary for wound healing
Ischemic index (II)	A ratio of the Doppler pressure at the level being tested to the brachial systolic pressure. ≥0.5 at the surgical level is necessary to support wound healing.
Ankle-brachial index	Believed to be the best indicator for assessing adequate flow to the ischemic limb. An index<0.45 indicates incisions distal to the ankle will not heal.

Nursing Diagnoses To Consider:

- *Impaired Physical Mobility*: Limitation in independent purposeful physical movement of one or more extremities

- *Risk for Infection:* At increased risk for being invaded by pathogenic organisms
- *Risk for Falls:* At risk of increased susceptibility to falling that may cause physical harm
- *Risk for Injury:* At risk of injury as a result of environmental conditions interacting with the individual's adaptive and defensive resources
- *Risk for Peripheral Neurovascular Dysfunction:* At risk for disruption in the circulation, sensation, or motion of an extremity
- *Impaired Skin Integrity:* Altered epidermis and/or dermis
- *Risk for Impaired Skin Integrity:* Risk for altered epidermis and/or dermis
- *Chronic Pain:* Unpleasant sensory or emotional experience arising from actual or potential tissue damage or described in terms of such damage (International Association for the Study of Pain); sudden or slow onset of any intensity from mild to severe with an anticipated or predictable end and a duration of greater than 6 months
- *Impaired Bed Mobility:* Limitation of independent movement from one bed position to another
- *Impaired Wheelchair Mobility:* Limitation of independent operation of wheelchair within environment
- *Impaired Walking:* Limitation of independent movement within the environment on foot
- *Fatigue:* An overwhelming sense of exhaustion and decreased capacity for physical and mental work at the usual level
- *Risk for Activity Intolerance:* At risk for experiencing insufficient physiological or psychological energy to endure complete required or desired daily activities
- *Impaired Home Maintenance:* Inability to independently maintain a safe growth-promoting immediate environment

- *Readiness for Enhanced Self-Care:* A pattern or performing activities for oneself that helps to meet health-related goals and can be strengthened (
- *Self-Care Deficit:* A constellation of culturally framed behaviors involving one or more self-care activities in which there is a failure to maintain a socially accepted standard of health and well-being

Team Members

Surgeons Important considerations in the shaping of the prosthesis and anticipated future revision surgeries may involve orthopedic, vascular, and plastic surgeons.

Physiatrist Physiatrists work well with life care planners, as they are used to working in the team setting with mutual goals set by team members and looking at the patient holistically. Physiatrists can provide valuable information regarding life expectancy, expected functional outcomes, future anticipated medical care and other related needs, including architectural modifications, psychosocial issues, disability or maximum medical improvement status, medications, pain management, therapies, and work and school accommodations. Health maintenance, preventive care, and potential or anticipated amputation-related needs are all important considerations (American Academy of Physical Medicine and Rehabilitation, 2013).

Nursing Rehabilitation nursing staff plays an important role in giving feedback regarding medication response, providing psychosocial, family, and support system information, and integrating the client into a holistic system for discharge to home. Nursing staff work with all members of the team to develop a plan of care with goals for discharge planning and goal attainment and ensure the patient and family receive necessary teaching to follow through with the nursing and medical plan of care.

Therapy Consider two major types of therapies for the amputee: functional and emotional. Both are needed to assist the amputee to reach maximum medical improvement and independence. Therapies may be provided by many professional disciplines.

Physical Therapist The PT provides the life care planner valuable input regarding therapy and equipment to treat current and future functional limitations and mobility issues.

Occupational Therapist Occupational therapists (OT) often focus on fine motor skills such as grasping, writing, and ADLs such as grooming, cooking, toileting, and bathing. The OT teaches wheelchair and adaptive aid use, recommends ways to improve functional status, and performs home evaluation assessments.

Accurate estimates for adaptive aids to promote independence, wheelchairs, driving adaptation, and other items, appropriate therapy and equipment selection and replacement in future years are fundamental in life care planning. Some occupational therapists specialize in hand therapy, driving evaluations, and wheelchair fitting and customization (seating evaluation), and are very good sources of information for current, future and replacement equipment needs.

Initial daily inpatient and outpatient therapy can be intense. If a major portion of one or more extremities is involved, therapy will begin in an inpatient acute hospital setting. As healing occurs, the amputee may be transferred to a subacute rehabilitation facility. If a subacute facility is not required, the amputee will participate in outpatient therapies, and the life care planner should consider providing for transportation to and from the facility.

The life care planner should consider provisions for periodic additional therapies expected for the rest of the amputee's life. These will include costs for therapy, transportation, services, and supplies. The life care planner should anticipate episodic increases at times of growth spurts for children up to age 21 years, and at the other end of the age spectrum, as the body loses muscle bulk and tone with the effects of aging. Every time a new prosthetic device is necessary, additional therapy is likely. Surgical intervention is another event warranting therapy. The following should trigger the assessment for further therapy (Gailey, 2008):

- Change in body weight, height, or body mass
- Surgical intervention around the site
- Irritation or pain at the site
- New prosthesis, for replacement or for growth, complications, or other changes complicating fit
- Body changes due to aging

Mental Health (*Psychiatrist, psychologist, social worker, licensed counselor, sexual therapist, family therapist*) The mental health specialist's assessment can be very helpful to the life care planner in developing a plan for psychosocial adaptation to amputation, providing resources for current and future assessment, coping skills, support systems, and social re-integration. Amputations affect body image and self-esteem. Issues such as dating, marriage, childbearing, and parental milestones (e.g., walking a daughter down the aisle, coaching a child's team) are important client-centered considerations. Specific therapy and medications may be indicated.

Peer Support Support groups are available at little or no charge through national organizations and local rehabilitation hospital facilities. These groups can be helpful to the client and family members as peer support. Mental health providers, social workers, and rehabilitation case managers can be a resource to the life care planner seeking these supports.

Vocational Consultant The vocational counselor can help find workplaces that can provide work accommodations identified by OT. A vocational skills assessment can be helpful in searching for educational and career options. Some rehabilitation counselors have special expertise in technology and adaptions to the work environment. Revision surgeries and complications from the amputation may also require career changes for which the vocational consultant's expertise may be needed.

Education Specialist (academic coach) Children and young adults may find academic activities often interrupted by medical care. Physical accommodations may be necessary at school, such as extra time for travel between classes, access to facilities, and other issues. Working with school nurses, teachers, and coaches might help address missing assignments, other educational type of needs, and accommodations.

Driving Evaluator A certified driver rehabilitation specialist (CDRS) can assess the ability of the client to drive safely and make recommendations for appropriate assistive aids, such as hand controls or other devices for safe driving (Association for Driver Rehabilitation, 2007).

Prosthetist The prosthetist gives the life care planner important information regarding the appropriate type of prosthetic device, costs, replacement schedules, and, most importantly, proper fit to prevent complications. Prosthetic training is important for preventing complications and maximizing functional abilities. The prosthetist should be certified and have obtained additional education in orthotics and prosthetics for amputees. Orthotics such as shoe inserts or braces may also be required and need to be included in the life care plan for balance, safe mobility, and ADL skills.

Nurse Case Manager Nurse case managers can be internal, in the facility with overlapping roles with the social worker for discharge planning, or external. Case managers can be valuable sources of information about psychosocial status, support systems, job situation, and other information. The life care planner should provide for case management by an experienced nurse case manager to coordinate the care and services recommended in the life care plan (AANLCP, 2013).

Spiritual Counselor Spiritual leaders or counselors provide a great deal of psychological support during any crisis such as adaptation to a disability for the client and their families. Religious counseling may be more acceptable in some cultures than counseling with a mental health professional.

Support Team

Family The importance of the family and significant others in rehabilitation has been recognized in the professional literature for many years and should not be underestimated. Their level of support, encouragement, and involvement directly influences the client's attitude and motivation to return to the community, work, and home setting. Relationships are affected and psychosocial adaptations made by those closest to the client as well as the client.

Breadwinners for a young family will be concerned about caregiving needs and educational needs for children; those who care for elderly or disabled family members will need assistance with future planning. Providing for education through support groups for families and significant others is an important component of any health plan of care, including the life care plan. The life care planner must carefully consider the family's role in the client's future care planning needs and willingness or ability to meet needs psychosocially as well as physically, and consider alternative options for families requiring assistance in these areas.

Employer Financial security and stability are universal concerns. A client cannot concentrate on necessary rehabilitation while worried about whether he will lose his job and home. Working to obtain an employer's willingness to modify a current job or identify a different position is important to rehabilitation. Vocational and/or educational counseling may need to be provided over the client's life expectancy.

Community During rehabilitation, a recreational therapist will often work with the rehabilitation team to take patients on community outings. These can be safe, protected trial runs to identify community barriers and demonstrate to client and family how to handle others' reactions to the disability. Social reintegration into the community and family is critical to successful rehabilitation of any amputation client, enhancing the client's quality of life to the fullest extent possible.

Equipment
Function

Assistive aids are essential in improving the client's functional ability, self-care activities and independence. Clients can use adaptive aids (e.g., a reacher or dressing/ toileting aids) to promote independence. Improving the client's independence with self-care skills, life activities, and reintegration into society are critical to the client's self-esteem. Functional aids address ADLs with fine motor skills such as reaching, dressing, toileting, eating, bathing, and other self-care skills. Functional aids for the lower extremities assist with mobility.

The life care planner should consult with the OT, PT, and prosthetist regarding appropriate assistive aids, prosthetics, braces, splints, and other items needed currently and anticipated over the life expectancy. Other items to consider are health maintenance items such as adaptive swimming equipment, swim prosthesis, adapted weight system for lifting weights, or other leisure time activity adaptive equipment. Amputee and disabled organized sports activities also promote fitness. Prevention of health complications to improve endurance and decreased complications over the life expectancy is part of the client's life care plan.

ADLs

As the general population ages, vendors have rushed to service an expanded market for tools to assist disabled people with ADLs. There are dressing kits to aid with pulling up pants, buttoning, bra hooks, and zippers; adapted toothbrush or toothpaste holders, hair dryer holders, long-handled sponges for bathing; and many, many others. One item often not considered is a flexible mirror for use with dressing, grooming, and toileting. One can purchase adapted eating utensils, cooking handles, cooking tools, and other devices for kitchen independence. The OT can be very helpful in providing this type of information, products, catalogs, and websites for adaptive items and their appropriate replacement schedules.

Mobility

Wheelchair technology has come a long way, and scooters are now commonplace. Wheelchairs that raise a client to standing and adapt for changes in elevation have greatly improved mobility for the disabled. OT and PT providers can be a wealth of information regarding vendors, options, and replacement schedules.

Cosmetic

Artificial skin and devices to match the client's own skin have greatly improved and are developed and refined daily. Some clients may desire a helper artificial arm made with cosmetic skin for work or social purposes. For some, the appearance of a device is just as important as its function and for others function is the key. The importance of a properly fitting prosthesis cannot be underestimated, as it will not only affect the appearance but the functionality of the equipment. These items should be considered in the context of the client's medical, psychological and other needs in the individualized client-specific life care plan.

Medical Complications

Edema control and shaping of the residual limb for prosthetic fit should occur early in the recovery period. These two problems cause the majority of problems with a prosthesis and the affected limb (Gailey and Clark, 2002). These are treated preemptively with a shrinker, applied as soon as the surgeon observes that healing is progressing. Some possible complications are listed below:

- Ischemia: delayed healing, tethering of scar
- Infection
- Residual limb shrinkage: pain and skin breakdown in prosthesis
- Neuroma formation: pain and can affect fit of prosthesis
- Heterotopic ossification
- Sexuality issues
- Hematomas
- Contractures
- Dermatological issues: skin breakdown, allergies to prosthetic material
- Phantom limb pain
- Degenerative changes

Medications are commonly given for the following conditions or symptoms.

Edema Edema is common in the residual limb, particularly in the early postoperative period, due to inflammation from surgery, altered neurovascular pathways, and neuroma formation. Medications commonly used depend upon the cause. Diuretics are commonly prescribed.

Pain Neuropathic pain, or phantom pain, is caused by tissue injury where the nerve fibers are damaged, dysfunctional, or otherwise injured. These damaged nerve fibers send incorrect signals to the other pain centers. Typical complaints include shooting, burning, tingling, numbness, and electrical-type sensations of pain (Gailey and Clark, 2002). These conditions may improve in time or persist. Medication agents typically include anticonvulsants, antidepressant medications, and medications for neuropathic pain. These medications are more effective than opioids due to the mechanism of action on the nerve endings. (*See also Chapter 6, Pain*)

Neuroma scar formation at the residual limb is not uncommon and often responds to desensitization therapies and medications. Anti-inflammatories are also beneficial with inflammation or arthritic changes. Spinal cord stimulators can be used. (*See also Chapter 6, Pain*)

Sleep Medications to improve sleep can also help with pain management. Impaired sleep, pain, and mood disturbance can become a vicious cycle requiring the intervention of the multidisciplinary team.

Circulation Treatment can include external continuous motion pumps, pharmacological agents for anticoagulation and red blood cell flexibility, statin usage independent of cholesterol levels, surgical approaches, and arterial bypass surgical procedures.

Outcomes The goal for any intervention is optimized function and independence. This is cost-effective and improves quality of life. The nurse life care planner should obtain information from all members of the rehabilitation team, and consider all side effects, replacement schedules, and other needs to prevent or minimize future complications.

Sexuality
A client's sexuality may be greatly affected by a change in his or her body image. (Racy, 2002), hindering desire to initiate or complete a sexual relationship. An amputee in a relationship faces a number of obstacles and may be concerned about the following questions:

- Will I hurt my partner?
- Will my partner hurt me?
- Will the sight of the amputation repulse my partner?

- Do I need to use certain positions or use positioning aids?
- What happens if I cannot perform?
- Will my partner still love me?

An amputee who has not yet found a partner may have the following concerns:
- Who would want to be with me?
- How do I go about disclosing my amputation?
- What do I do with my prosthesis?
- What about dating and sexuality?

These questions and concerns should be addressed with professional assistance or with another amputee at the same level and status. Consider providing for a sexual therapist in the life care plan, depending upon the client's assessment. (*See also Chapter 1, Spinal Cord Injury, on information on the PLISSIT Model for sexuality issues.*)

Nursing Diagnoses To Consider:
- *Sexual Dysfunction*: The state in which an individual experiences a change in sexual function during the sexual response phases of desire, excited in, and/or orgasm, which is viewed is unsatisfying, and rewarding, or inadequate
- *Ineffective Sexuality Pattern*: Expressions of concern regarding own sexuality
- *Spiritual Distress:* Impaired ability to experience and integrate meaning and purpose in life through connectedness with self, others, art, music, literature, nature, and /or a power greater than oneself.
- *Post-Trauma Syndrome:* Sustained maladaptive response to a traumatic, overwhelming event.
- *Ineffective Coping:* Inability to form a valid appraisal of the stressors, inadequate choices of practiced responses, and/or inability to use available resources.
- *Grieving*: A normal, complex process that includes emotional, physical, spiritual, social and intellectual

responses and behaviors by which individuals, families and communities incorporate an actual, anticipated, or perceived loss into their daily lives.

- *Situational Low Self-Esteem:* Development of a negative perception of self-worth in response to a current situation
- *Powerlessness:* The lived experience of lack of control over a situation, including a perception that one's actions do not significantly affect an outcome.
- *Disturbed Body Image:* Confusion in mental picture of one's physical self.

Resources

- Able data/ National Institute for Disability and Developmental Research (NIDDR).
- www2.ed.gov/about/offices/list/osers/nid
- AANLCP. www.aanlcp.org
- Active Living. www.activeliving.com
- AgrAbility Project. www.agrability.org
- Alliance for Technology Access. www.ataccess.org
- American Occupational Therapy Association. www.aota.org
- American Orthotic and Prosthetic Association. www.aopanet.org
- American Physical Therapy Association. www.apta.org
- American Pediatric Surgical Nurses Association. www.apsna.org
- American Rehabilitation Nurses Association. www.rehabnurse.org
- Amputee Coalition of America. www.amputee-coalition.org
- Army Times. www.armytimes.com
- Association for Driver Rehabilitation Specialists. www.aded.net
- Care for International Rehabilitation. www.cirnetwork.org
- Department of Defense. www.defense.gov
- Disabled Sports USA. www.dsusa.org

- Express Medical Supply, Inc. www.exmed.net
- Hanger Prosthetics and Orthotics. www.hanger.com
- Life Like Laboratory. www.lifelikelab.com
- Living Skin. www.livingskin.com
- Maxi-aid. www.maxiaids.com
- National Association for the Advancement of Orthotics and Prosthetics. www.naaop.org
- National Center on Physical Activity and Disability. www.ncpad.org
- National Amputation Foundation. www. nationalamputation.org
- National Limb Loss Information Center (Amputee Coalition). www.amputee-coalition.org
- and P Digital Technologies. www.oandp.com
- Otto Bock Healthcare. www.ottobockus.com
- Pediatric Orthopedic Surgeons of America, www.posna. org
- Pillet Hand Prosthesis. www.pillet.com
- PMSI, www.pmsionline.com
- Prosthetic University of Michigan. www.med.umich.edu
- Sammons and Preston. www.sammonspreston.com
- Society of Pediatric Nurses. www.pedsnurses.org
- US Army Amputee Patient Care Program and Amputee Coalition of America www.amputee-coalition.org
- Veterans Administration. www.va.gov

References

American Association of Nurse Life Care Planners (2013) Scope and Standards of Practice, Standard 11, Communication.

American Occupational Therapy Association. (2013). About occupational therapy: what is occupational therapy? Retrieved 6/22/13. http://www.aota.org/Consumers. aspx

American Physical Therapy Association. (2011). Today's physical therapist: a comprehensive review of a 21st century health care profession.

Amputee Coalition of America. (2012.). Healthcare providers. Retrieved from http://www.amputee-coalition.org/healthcare-providers/

Association for Driver Rehabilitation Specialists. (2007). Driving after a limb amputation: fact sheet. Ruston, LA: 2007. http://www.driver-ed.org/i4a/pages/index.cfm?pageid=507

Bhattacharya V. (2012). Management of soft tissue wounds of the face. Indian journal of plastic surgery. 45(3): 436-443.

Blank-Reid C. (2003, July). Traumatic amputations, unkind cuts. Nursing 2003, 49-51.

Bowden G. (Ed.). (2002). Oxford textbook of orthopedics and trauma. New York, NY: Oxford University Press.

Bowker JH. (2002). The choice between limb salvage and amputation: infection. Atlas of Limb Prosthetics: Surgical, Prosthetic, and Rehabilitation Principles. Rosemont, IL. American Academy of Orthopedic Surgeons, edition 2, 1992, Reprinted 2002. Retrieved 6/20/13 http://www.oandplibrary.org/alp/

Bulstrode C, Buckwalter J, et al. (2006). Orthotics and prosthetics in rehabilitation (2nd ed.). St. Louis, MO: Saunders/Elsevier.

Burger, H. and Marincek, C. (1997). The lifestyle of young client after lower limb amputation caused by injury. Prosthetics and Orthotics International Journal, 21 (1), 35-9.

Canale, S. T., Daugherty, K., and Jones, L. (Eds.). (2003). Campbell's Operative Orthopaedics (10th ed.). (Vols. 1-2). St Louis, MO: Mosby/Elsevier.

Carroll, K. (2001). Adaptive prosthetics for the lower extremity. Foot and Ankle Clinic, 6(2), 371-86.

Case Management Resource Guide. (2002): Philadelphia, PA: Dorland Health Care Information.

Cavanaugh SR, Shin LM, and Karamouz N. (2006). Psychiatric and emotional sequelae of surgical amputation. Psychosomatics, 47(6), 459-64.

Center for Assistive Technology and Environmental Access. (2007). Retrieved from Assistivetech.net: National Public Website on Assistive Technology: http://assistivetech.net

Chadderton HC. (2007). Reintegration and adjustment as seen by the amputee. Retrieved from National Amputee Centre, The War Amps website: http://www.waramps.ca/nac/life/ adjust.html

Cheng, N. C. (2004, June 13). Double transpositional replantation feasible for five digit amputation. Medical Devices and Surgical Technology Week, 215.

Clerici CA, Ferrari A et al. (2004). Clinical experience with psychological aspects in pediatric patients amputated for malignancies. Tumori. 90: 399-404.

Clonitz AS, Annonio D, and Walker L. (2004). Trauma nursing: Amputation. RN, 67(7), 38-43.

Cook A. (2002). Assistive Technologies, Principles and Practice (2nd ed.). St. Louis, MO: Mosby/Elsevier.

Day, HJB. (1991). The ISO/ISPO classification of congenital limb deficiency. Prosthetics and Orthotics International. 15. 67-69.

Czerne MR. (2006, April 1). Reattaching hand, complex, difficult. Knight Rider Tribune Business News

DeBakey, M, Chaudry A, and Woods K. (2007). Open Label Study of Duloxetine for the Treatment of Phantom Limb Pain. (Baylor College of Medicine, No. NCT00425230). Retrieved from ClinicalTrials.gov

DiGiacomo R, et al. (2004). The rehabilitation of people with amputations. World Health Organization.

Doyle DA. (2009). Physical Growth of Infants and Children. The Merck Manual for Healthcare Professionals. Retrieved from www.merckmanuals.com/professional.

Dudek NL, Dehaan MN, and Marks MB. (2003). Bone Overgrowth in the Adult Traumatic Amputee. American Journal of Physical Medicine and Rehabilitation, 82(11), 897-900.

Edelstein J. (2002). Special considerations-rehabilitation without prostheses: functional skills training.

Atlas of Limb Prosthetics: Surgical, Prosthetic, and Rehabilitation Principles. Retrieved 6/21/13. www. oandplibrary.org.

Edwards AR. (2005, April 7). Replantation benefits few children who lose limbs in farm accidents. Information Week, (1204), 19. Retrieved from http://www. informationweek.com/news/160502506

Ferri FF. (2004). Ferri's Clinical Advisor 2004: Instant Diagnosis and Treatment. St. Louis, MO: Mosby/Elsevier.

Ferryman P. (2000). Sewing a hand back on: Takes time and a team. The Vancouver Sun, p. C-6.

Flor H, Nikolajsen L, and Staehelin JT. (2006). Phantom limb pain: a case of maladaptive CNS plasticity? Nature Reviews Neuroscience, 7(11), 873-81.

Frieden RA. (2005). The geriatric amputee. Physical Medicine and Rehabilitation Clinics of North America, 16(1), 179-95.

Gailey R, Allen K, et al. (2008). Review of secondary conditions associated with lower-limb amputation and long term prosthesis use. Journal of Rehabilitation Research and Development. 45(1): 15-30.

Gailey R, Clark CR. (2002). Physical therapy management of adult lower limb amputees. Atlas of Limb Prosthetics: Surgical, Prosthetic and Rehabilitation Principles. Retrieved 6/21/13. www.oandplibrary.org

Giannoudis P V. (Ed.) (2012). Practical Procedures in Orthopaedic Surgery: Joint Aspiration/ Injection, Bone Graft Harvesting and Lower Limb Amputations. London, England: Springer.

Green G, Short K, and Easle, M. (2001). Trans-tibial amputation: Prosthetic use and functional outcome. Foot and Ankle Clinic, 6(2), 315-327.

Ham R, Regan JM, and Roberts VC. (1987). Evaluation of introducing the team approach to the care of the amputee: The Dulwich study. Prosthetics and Orthotics International, 11(1), 25-30.

Hanson MD, Zuker RM, Shaul ZR. (2008). Pediatric facial burns: Is facial transplantation the new reconstructive psychosurgery? Canadian Journal of Plastic Surgery. 16(4):205-210.

Heim M, Wershavski D and Arazi-Margalit MA. (1998). The will to walk—a partnership involving dual dynamics. Disability Rehabilitation, 20(2), 74-7.

Helfet DL, Howey T, Sanders R. Limb salvage versus amputation. Preliminary results of the Mangled Extremity Severity Score. Clin Orthop Relat Res. 1990;256:80-6

Herdman TH (2012)(Ed.) NANDA International Nursing Diagnosis: Definitions and Classification, 2012-2014. Oxford: Wiley-Blackwell

Highsmith M, and Kahle J (2006, March/April). Prosthetic socks. inMotion,16(2), Hogg, M. (2007, February). Electromagnetic radiation blocking fabric reduces fibromyalgia and amputee pain. Retrieved from The Environmental Illness Resource website: http://www. ei-resource.org

Howerton PS. (1988). Vocational rehabilitation and replantation: A dynamic relationship. Journal of Rehabilitation. October-December, 16-19.

Jacobs JC. (2002). Accessible Bathroom Design: Tearing Down the Barriers. Tuscaloosa, AL: Jireh Publishing.

Jacobsen JM. (1998). Nursing's role with amputee support groups. Journal of Vascular Nursing, 16 (2), 31-34.

Jawad MU, Scully SP. (2010). In Brief: Enneking Classification: Benign and Malignant Tumors of the Musculoskeletal System. Clinical Orthopaedics and Related Research, 2010 July; 468(7): 2000-2002.

Jeffries GE. (1998, March-April). Pain management post-amputation pain. In Motion, (8)2,. Johnson, K. (Ed.). (1997). Advanced Practice Nursing in Rehabilitation: A Core Curriculum. Glenview, IL: Rehabilitation Nursing Foundation.

Karacoloff LA. (1986). Lower extremity amputation: A guide to functional outcomes in physical therapy management. F. J. Schneider (Ed). Rockville, MD: Aspen Systems.

Kerr M. (2013). Identity and gender development: self development: definitions. Lecture notes. Retrieved 6/23/13. http://faculty.txwes.edu/mskerr/ files/3304/3304_ch4.htm

Kirkup JR. (2010). A History of Limb Amputation. London, England: Springer.

Krane EJ, Heller LB. (1995). The prevalence of phantom sensation and pain in pediatric amputees. Journal of Pain Symptom Management. 1995 Jan;10(1):21-9.

Kuiken TA, Schechtman L, and Harden RN. (2005). Phantom limb pain treatment with Mirtazapine: A case series. Pain Practice, 5(4), 356-60.

Kurichi JE, Bates BE, Stineman MG. 2013. Amputation. In: JH Stone, M Blouin, editors. International Encyclopedia of Rehabilitation. Available online: http://cirrie.buffalo. edu/encyclopedia/en/article/251/

Lang M (2009) Upper limb prosthetic rehabilitation: what and when. Journal of Nurse Life Care Planning 2009: vol. 9, no. 4, 134-9

Lange C and Heuft G. (2001). Coping with illness and psychotherapy for patients after amputation. Orthopade, 30(3), 155-60.

Liang Y, Li X, et al. (2004). Successful auricle replantation via microvascular anastomosis 10 hours after complete avulsion. Acta Oto Laryngologica, 124(5), 645-648.

Matsuzaki H. (2004, December 19). Fingertip replantation feasible after digital artery anastomosis alone. Medical Devices and Surgical Technology Week, 252.

McAuliffe JA. (2010). Shoulder disarticulation and forequarter amputation: Surgical principles. In Atlas of Limb Prosthetics: Surgical, Prosthetic, and Rehabilitation Principles. Retrieved from www.oandplibrary.org/alp/ chap10-01.asp

McClure SK, and Shaughnessy WJ. (2005). Farm-related limb amputations in children. Journal of Pediatric Orthopedics, 25(2), 133-137.

McDermott MM, Guralnick JM.et al. (2003). Statin use and leg functioning in patients with and without lower extremity peripheral arterial disease. Circulation, 107(5), 757-761.

Meyer VE. (2003). Upper extremity replantation, a review. European Surgery, 35(4), 67- 173.

Miller S. (2010). Arterial disease: lower extremity implications. Lower extremity review. Retrieved 6/20/13. http://lowerextremityreview.com/article/ arterial-disease-lower-extremity-implications

Mills EJ. (2006). Amputation. In Handbook of Medical-Surgical Nursing, 4th Edition. Hagerstown, MD. Lippincott, Williams, and Wilkins.

Moore TJ. (2002). planning for optimal function in amputation surgery. Atlas of Limb Prosthetics: Surgical, Prosthetic, and Rehabilitation Principles. Rosemont, IL. American Academy of Orthopedic Surgeons, edition 2, 1992, Reprinted 2002. Retrieved 6/20/13 http://www. oandplibrary.org/alp/

Murdock G. (1996). Amputations, surgical practice and patient management. Atlanta, Ga. Elsevier.

Murray C. (2010). Amputation, prosthesis use, and phantom limb pain: an interdisciplinary perspective. New York, NY: Springer.

National AgrAbility Project. Assistive technologies: Fact sheet. (2007). http://www.agrability.org/Resources/at/index. cfm

National Institute for Disability and Developmental Research (NIDDR) (2007). Aids for daily living: Fact sheet. retrieved from http://www2.ed.gov/about/offices/list/ osers/nidrr/ index.html

National Limb Loss Information Center (2006). Financial assistance for prostheses and other assistive devices: fact sheet. Retrieved from the Amputee Coalition website: http:// www.amputee-coalition.org/fact_ sheets/assist_orgs.html

Nelson FRT and Blauvelt CT. (2007). A manual of orthopaedic terminology (7th ed.). St. Louis, MO: Mosby/Elsevier.

O'Brien JG, Chennubhotla SA, and Chennubhotla RV. (2005). Treatment of edema. American Family Physician, 71(11), 2111-2117.

Osterman H. (1997). The process of amputation and rehabilitation. Clinics In Podiatric Medicine and Surgery, 14(4), 585-597.

Pagana KD and Pagana TJ. (2001). Mosby's Diagnostic and Laboratory Test Reference (6th ed.). St Louis, MO: Mosby/Elsevier.

Pandian G and Kowalske K. (1999). Daily functioning of patients with an amputated lower extremity. Clinical Orthopaedics and Related Research, (361), 91-97.

Parratt BM, Pomahac B, Demling RH, and Orgill DP. (2006). Journal of Burn Care Research, 27:1, 34-39.

Pediatric Orthopedic Society of North America. (2013). Physician education. Retrieved from http://www.posna.org/education/education.asp

Physicians' Desk Reference (2005) Physicians' Desk Reference 59th ed Montvale NJ: Mosby/ Elsevier.

Pinzur M. (2010). Infection, ischemia, and amputation, an issue of foot and ankle clinics. Philadelphia, PA: Saunders/ Elsevier.

Porter RS and Kaplan JL. (Eds). (2012). The Merck Manual for Healthcare Professionals. http://www.merckmanuals.com/professional/index.html

Potter BK, and Scoville CR. (2006). Amputation is not isolated: an overview of the US Army amputee patient care program and associated amputee injuries [Special issue]. Journal of the American Academy of Orthopedic Surgeons, 14(10 Spec No), S188-190.

Prendergast J, Scarborough P., and Burke TJ. (2006). Monochromatic infrared energy: New hope for painful, numb feet? Diabetes Self-Management. 2:52, p.54-6

Racy JC (2002). Psychological adaption to amputation. Atlas of Limb Prosthetics: Surgical, Prosthetic, and Rehabilitation Principles. Rosemont, IL. American Academy of Orthopedic Surgeons, edition 2, 1992,

Reprinted 2002. Retrieved 6/20/13 http://www. oandplibrary.org/alp/

Reed Group (2012). Amputation. Medical Disability Advisor. Retrieved 6/20/2013

Richardson JP, Daly MP., and Adelman, AM. (1989). Rehabilitation in the elderly. Maryland Medical Journal, 38(2),149-153.

Rogers JL. (1998). Serving amputee patients in rural settings. Caring, 17(9), p. 32-35

Rossbach P. (2004). When to replace a prosthesis: Fact sheet. Retrieved from the Amputee Coalition website: http://www.amputee-coalition.org/fact_sheets/ prosreplacprof.html

Sabolich J. and Sabolich S. (1997). You're not alone. Austin, TX: Hanger Prosthetics and Orthotics.

Santiago MC, and Coyle CP. (2004, April). Leisure-time physical activity and secondary conditions in women with physical disabilities. Disability and Rehabilitation, 26(8), 485-494.

Shoski C. (1998). Pain management: A discussion of the various techniques and types of drugs currently available for pain control with medications. inMotion, 8(5).

Sherman RA, and Casey Jones DE. (1995). The Amputee's Guide to the Amputation and Recovery Processes (2nd ed.). Suquamish, WA: Author.

Smith GD and Michael JW. (2004). Atlas of Amputations and Limb Deficiencies: Surgical, Prosthetic and Rehabilitation Principles (3rd ed.). J. H. Bowker, Ed. Rosemont, IL: American Academy of Orthopaedic Surgeons.

Smith MT and Haythornthwaite JA. (2004). How do sleep disturbance and chronic pain inter-relate? Insights from the longitudinal and cognitive-behavioral clinical trials literature. Sleep Medicine Reviews. 8(2):119-32.

Susan G. Komen for the Cure. (2011). Facts for life: treatment choices, and overview. Retrieved 6/22/13. http://ww5. komen.org/uploadedFiles/Content_Binaries/806-386. pdf

Tanner PB and Mobley SR. (2006). Extermal auricular and facial prosthetics: a collaborative effort of the plastic surgeon and anaplastologist. Facial Plastic Surgery Clinics of North America. 14(2):137-45. Retrieved 6/22/13. http://www.ncbi.nlm.nih.gov/pubmed/16750771

Transpositional replantation of digits. Case reports. Scandinavian Journal of Plastic and Reconstructive Surgery and Hand Surgery, 33(2), 243-249.

Tyner TR, Parks, N et al. (2007). Effects of collagen nerve guide on neuroma formation and neuropathic pain in a rat model. American Journal of Surgery, 193(1), e1-6.

US Army Amputee Patient Care Program and Amputee Coalition of America. (2006,). Managing pain related to amputation: wound pain and phantom limb pain. Military In-Step. Retrieved from http://www.amputee-coalition.org/military-instep/usaf-amputee-care-program.html

VA/DOD Clinical practice guideline for rehabilitation of lower limb amputation. (2007).

Van Beek AL, Lim PK, et al. (2007). Management of vasospastic disorders with botulinum toxin A. Plastic Reconstructive Surgery. 119(1), 217-226.

Wagner WF. (2002). Partial foot amputations: surgical procedures. Atlas of Limb Prosthetics: Surgical, Prosthetic and Rehabilitation Principles. Retrieved 6/22/13 www.oandplibrary.org.

Webb JB. (2005). Replantation in trauma. Trauma, 7, 1-9.

Weed RO and Berens DE. (Eds.). (2010). Life Care Planning and Case Management Handbook (3rd ed.). New York, NY: CRC Press.

Wiest J. (2002, March/ April). What's new in mobility for people with disabilities? inMotion 12(2).

Wood MR, Hunter GA, and Millstein SG. (1987). The value of revision surgery after initial amputation of an upper or lower limb. Prosthetic and Orthotics International, 11(1), 17-20

Yaffee B, Hutt D, et al. (2009). Major upper extremity
   replantations. Journal of Hand Micorsurgery. 1(2). 63-67
Zaidman B. Worker and injury characteristics of amputation
   claims. Minnesota Department of Labor and Industry,
   Winter 2002
Ziegler-Graham K, MacKenzie EJ, et al. Estimating the
   prevalence of limb loss in the United States: 2005 to
   2050. Archives of Physical Medicine and Rehabilitation.
   2008;89(3):422-9.

CHAPTER 5

Burns and Life Care Planning

Chris Ann Daniel, BSHS, RN, CCM, CNLCP, MSCC, LNC, CHC
Glenda Evans-Shaw, BSN, RN, PHN, CCM, CNLCP
Shelene Giles, MS, BSN, BA, RN, CRC, CNLCP, CLCP, MSCC, LNCC
Wendie Howland, MN, RN-BC, CRRN, CCM, CNLCP, LNCC
April Pettengill, BSN, RN, CRRN, CNLCP, MSCC
Kim Wages, BSN, RN, BBA, CRRN, CNLCP, MSCC
Barbara Bate, RN-BC, CCM, CRRN, CNLCP, LNCC, MSCC,
contributor

Introduction

The Burn Foundation reports that burns are the third leading cause of accidental deaths in the United States. Since 1995, the American Burn Association National Burn Repository has gathered statistics on burn injuries. This information has been instrumental in planning for the complicated and costly medical care of burn patients. The current statistics, compiled from 183,036 acute burn cases, which required admission to a burn center between January 2002 and June 2011. The findings showed:

- Sixty-five percent of burn injuries occurred in the home
- 8 of 10 burn cases were from flame burns and scalds
- Flame and fire burns were more common in adults
- Scald burns were most common in children under 5 years of age
- Patients between ages of 5 and 60 years old accounted for 69% of cases
- The majority (70%) of burn patients were men
- 96.3% of burn patients survived hospitalization
- The leading complication was pneumonia
- Seventy-two percent of patients had a burn size of less than 10% TBSA (American Burn Association, 2012).

Burn process

Skin is the largest organ in the body and serves as protection from injury, viruses, and bacteria, regulation of body temperature by adjusting blood flow and through evaporation from sweat glands, dehydration prevention, conservation of fluid, moisture control through perspiration, sensory and stimulation from the environment, and production of Vitamin D.

There are two primary layers of the skin. The epidermis is the outer layer and represents approximately 10% of the skin's total thickness. The dermis is the inner layer and represents approximately 90% of the total thickness. The dermis layer contains blood vessels, nerve fibers, lymphatic system, sweat glands, sebaceous glands, hair follicles, connective tissue, capillaries, collagen fibers, and elastic fibers. The dermis layer is the receptor for heat, cold, pain, and pressure (Kagan, Peck, and Ahrenholz, 2009).

When skin is burned, its ability to protect against invaders is lost, creating a breeding ground for bacteria. Preventing infections is a priority because infection slows healing and increases scarring. Skin also assists to determine a person's physical identity, which can be disrupted following a severe burn injury.

Classification of Burns and Total Body Surface Area

In 1800, Dupuytren developed the burn injury classification still in use (Herndon, 2012).

- A *superficial burn* (first degree) extends to the epidermis, such as sunburn. There is minimal tissue damage and the injury should heal independently within a few days.
- A *partial thickness burn* (second degree) has two classifications, depending upon the involvement of the dermis layer.

- A *superficial partial thickness burn* involves the epidermis and part of the dermis. This should heal independently with minimal medical treatment.
- A *deep partial thickness burn* involves the epidermis and most of the dermis and may require medical treatment.
- A *full thickness burn* (third degree) extends completely through the dermis.
- A *deep full thickness burn* (fourth degree) extends beyond the dermis and may include muscle, tendons, and bone. When the majority of the dermis is involved, extensive medical treatment includes inpatient care, surgical debridement, wound care, skin grafting, and consideration of reconstructive surgeries.

Partial thickness to full-thickness burns can be expected to have long-term complications. These burns cause severe scarring and lifetime medical and psychological sequelae. Clinicians determine the size of burns based on total body surface area involved (TBSA). Presently, there are two ways to quantify TBSA: *Wallace's Rule of Nines* and the *Lund and Browder Classification.*

Wallace's Rule of Nines identifies areas of the body in 9% increments (Herndon, 2012). When using Wallace's Rule of Nines, the head equals 9% (4.5% each for anterior and posterior areas), the trunk equals 18% for anterior portion and 18% for the posterior portion, each arm equals 9% (4.5% anterior and 4.5% posterior), each leg equals 9% anterior and 9% posterior, and the groin accounts for 1%. This equals a total of 100% of the total body surface. Adult TBSA differs from pediatric TBSA (for example, adult head = 9% vs. pediatric head = 18%, and adult legs = 18% vs. pediatric leg14%).

The *Lund and Browder Classification* bases the percentage of TBSA on the growth and development of the burn patient (Herndon, 2012). A burn of even 20% of total body surface can be life-threatening.

Types of Burns

There are four types of burns: thermal, scald, electrical, chemical, and inhalation, each characterized by different elements and processes. Knowing the etiology of a burn is important to plan specific treatment regimen and long-term care.

The most common burns are thermal and scald burns. A thermal burn, the most common burn in adults, is caused by exposure to high temperature, such as flame or contact with a hot surface. A scald burn, most common in children and the elderly, is caused by high-temperature liquid such as hot water, grease, or steam. Although the boiling point of water is 212 degrees Fahrenheit (100 degrees Celsius), water temperatures over 100 degrees Fahrenheit (37.8 degrees Celsius) can scald. The severity of the scald depends on temperature of the liquid and exposure time. These burns occur most frequently in the kitchen.

An electrical burn results from exposure to live electricity, classified as low-or high-output. Low electrical output is less than 1000 volts (e.g., ordinary U.S. home electrical service). High electric output is over 1000 volts (e.g., commercial or industrial service). The actual current path is the most important factor when considering the extent of the injury. Electrical current follows the path of least resistance. Clinicians can often determine the entrance and exit wounds based on the location and severity of the burns. Electrical injuries can be deceptive, presenting with only minimal external skin damage but having severe internal damage to deep tissue.

Associated conditions (e.g., electrical effects on the cardiac, pulmonary, orthopedic, neurological, ophthalmological systems) may be undiagnosed initially or develop later. Long-term complications of electrical burns are not fully understood. Research has begun to document life-long degeneration and complications associated with this complex injury (Singerman, Gomez, and Fish, Oct. 2008).

A chemical burn is the result of exposure to caustic elements that destroy skin tissue. Chemicals can include alkalis, acids, or organic compounds. Severity depends on the specific chemical, concentration, and contact time. Superficial chemical burns can be deceptive and lead to full-thickness damage in a short time. Chemical burn damage can progress until the chemical is removed or neutralized from the skin (Kagan, Peck, Ahrenholz, et al., 2009). An inhalation burn occurs when a person inhales chemicals, vapors, gases, smoke, or hot air. This causes burns to the oral and esophageal tissues and can extend into the gastrointestinal and respiratory areas. Inhalation burns are the most common cause of burn deaths in house fires. Like electrical burns, the long-term complications of inhalation burns are being considered in medical research.

Related Trauma

Burn injuries cause significant physiological changes. Depending on the severity and size of the burn, these acute systemic changes can include but are not limited to:

- Alteration and disruption in vascular and lymphatic systems
- Fluid volume deficit, proportional to depth and extent of burns
- Vascular fluid loss within first 24 to 48 hours
- Hematocrit increase due to capillary fluid loss
- Compensation for fluid loss
- Diuresis after fluid moves back into vascular system
- Decreased protein in interstitial spaces
- Capillary stasis, ischemia, and necrosis
- Altered acid-base balance
- Gastrointestinal disturbances (especially if burn exceeds 30% of TBSA)
- Caloric loss

- Decreased circulating blood volume, decreased cardiac output and increased pulse rate
- Decreased stroke volume, increased rise in peripheral resistance
- Decreased tissue perfusion, can cause acidosis, renal failure and irreversible burn shock
- Myoglobinuria: protein myoglobin released from damaged muscles can damage kidneys unless sufficient fluids are given to dilute in the renal tubules.

Secondary diagnoses can also be seen with burn-related trauma depending on the mechanism of injury. These can include but are not limited to:

- Orthopedic/musculoskeletal injuries
- Brain injury
- Traumatic amputation
- Blindness (eye injury from a chemical burn, explosion, and/or automobile fire)
- Pre-existing health issues complicate the course of burn care and treatment choices
- Curling's ulcer (involving esophagus and prepyloric area of the stomach)
- Upper airway obstruction within first 48 hours, from pharyngeal/laryngeal edema
- Restrictive pulmonary due to chest edema with circumferential chest burns and/or open lacerations
- Toxic fumes from burning items and water used to extinguish the fire, e.g.:
- Corrosive acids and alkalis
- Plastics
- Noxious gases
- Hydrogen cyanide, hydrochloric acid
- Sulfuric acid
- Halogens
- Phosgene

Carbon monoxide poisoning (causes headaches, visual changes, confusion, irritability, decreased judgment, nausea, and can lead to significant central nervous system (CNS) toxicity (Sen, Greenhalgh, and Pamieri, Nov/Dec 2010).

Medical Complications

The medical complications associated with a burn can be extensive, even with a small (but deep) burn. Several common complications will be discussed in this portion of the chapter.

Burn survivors are at a higher risk for sunburn, skin cancer, and skin sensitivity/allergies, while electrical burn survivors are at high risk for arthritis and joint dysfunction. The care and treatment of a burn survivor are life-long. Children and the elderly are at higher risk for developing complications. Early detection of complications allows early intervention to reduce their severity and effect.

Hypertrophic scarring

Burn scars can take up to two years to fully mature. The deeper the burn, the higher the risk for the injured person is for developing hypertrophic scars (Herndon, 2012). These are raised, firm, erythematous scars that form as the result of exuberant collagen synthesis and limited collagen lysis during the remodeling phase of wound healing; the result is the formation of thick, hyalinized collagen bundles of fibroblasts and fibrocytes) (Tanzi and Alster, 2004). Hypertrophic scarring is located within the boundaries of the wound or excision sites, appears irritated, and can have a rubbery, leathery feel. This fragile scar tissue can be easily damaged and is sun sensitive. Factors contributing to hypertrophic scarring include wound infection, genetics, immunologic factors, repeated harvesting of donor sites, altered ground substance, age, chronic inflammatory process, location of injury, and mechanical tension. Scar hypertrophy may be evident at 8 to 12 weeks after wound closure (Herndon, 2012).

Treatment of hypertrophic scarring includes stretching, massage, modalities (e.g., ultrasound, paraffin, continuous passive motion (CPM), electrical stimulation), compression garments, silicone gel sheets, transparent facemasks, serial casting, splints, steroid injections, and surgery. The most widely applied treatment is pressure therapy using compression garments, inserts, or orthotics. However, there is no guarantee that hypertrophic scarring will not recur. Depending on location, patients can develop secondary diagnosis at later stages (e.g., carpal tunnel syndrome, epicondylitis, and shoulder impingement).

Keloids

Keloids are raised, reddish-purple, nodular scars and occur most often for persons with darker skin pigmentation. Keloids are firmer than hypertrophic scarring (Tanzi and Alster, 2004). They result when the body continues to produce collagen after wound healing and present as thick, puckered clusters of scar tissue. They grow beyond boundaries of the wound or excision, and are more common over the breastbone, shoulders, and on ear lobes.

Treatment is similar to that for hypertrophic scarring, includes stretching, massage, modalities (e.g., ultrasound, paraffin, CPM, electrical stimulation), compression garments, silicone gel sheets, transparent facemasks, serial casting, splints, steroid injections, radiation therapy, and surgery. Keloids have a tendency to recur, sometimes larger than originally.

Contractures

A contracture is a scar that pulls the edges of the skin together. It may affect muscles and tendons and restrict normal movement. Treatment includes static splints, compression garments, occupational and physical therapy, and surgical release. Numerous surgeries may be required over several years, and extensive occupational and physical therapy should be considered after each release. Multiple surgeries may be necessary, especially in pediatric patients to allow for growth and development.

As with hypertrophic scarring and keloids, there is no guarantee that contractures will not recur. Surgical excision of hypertrophic scarring, keloids, and contractures without aggressive therapy is associated with a high rate of recurrence (McCauley, 2005).

Complex Regional Pain Syndrome (Previously Reflex Sympathetic Dystrophy [RSD])

Burn patients are at risk for developing CRPS due to the nerve damage resulting from partial thickness or full thickness burns or electrical exposure. Please refer to the CRPS section of the Pain chapter for an in-depth discussion on CRPS evaluation and treatment.

Psychological issues

Psychological care of the burn care patient may be complex and longlasting. The burn severity and TBSA cannot predict the extent of psychological trauma of the burn survivor. Regardless of size and severity, burns are considered to be the most painful traumatic injuries and can cause life-long, devastating psychological effects (Faucher, 2002).

The most significant effect on a person's long-term quality of life may not be functional impairment, but the psychological effects and impaired ability to interact normally in society (Barret-Nerin and Herndon, 2005). This should be taken into account when the nurse life care planner develops the burn life care plan. With the trauma of a burn accident, intense medical treatment, and extensive recovery, the burn survivor and family/significant others will experience significant psychological distress. Burn patients describe the loss of control during the acute phase of medical treatment in a burn center (Faucher, 2002). Myriad emotions follow a burn injury, including anxiety, fear, grief, anger, sense of loss, feelings of helplessness, and depression. Psychological symptoms that occur early during the course of rehabilitation among burn patients may also include anxiety and guilt (Faucher, 2002).

The patient and/or significant others may present as aggressive or withdrawn. Psychological and social issues are integral parts of burn treatment from the time of injury through recovery and rehabilitation; it is crucial that psychological treatment be concurrent with medical treatment in the Burn Center (Herndon, 2012). A qualified psychologist or counselor, e.g., psychiatric nurse or social worker with expertise in burns, should become involved as soon as possible. By encouraging the burn patients to make decisions regarding their medical care, the treatment team shows concerns for preserving function, regaining independence, and restoring psychological wellbeing (Herndon, 2012).

Long-term psychological symptoms include an altered body image, chronic pain, altered sensations on the burns/ scars/skin grafts, loss of independence, sleep disturbance, flashbacks, an uncertainty towards the future, difficulty with relationships and sexual intimacy, and financial concerns due to loss of income. As the burn survivor returns to social settings, society's reaction to the burns adds to the psychological trauma; this can be incapacitating. Psychological support should be provided to the patient and the family on an ongoing basis to prepare them for re-integration into the community.

Posttraumatic stress disorder (PTSD) is reported in as many as 43% of burn patients during the initial phase of hospitalization, although it often develops following discharge from the burn rehabilitation unit (Faucher, 2002). Therefore, identification of risk factors, managing pain, and reducing anxiety can help prevent patients from developing PTSD. Factors that contribute to a patient's likelihood of developing PTSD include altered self-image, poor pain control, and associated physical impairments. Other psychological diagnoses experienced by burn patients include adjustment disorder and acute stress disorder.

Pre-burn physical and psychological health, coping skills, and family and social support are closely related to the individual's behavior, distress, and recovery. Psychological distress can be manifested as generalized mood disturbance, hyper arousal related to the trauma, body image dissatisfaction, hopelessness, depression, and avoidance of aversive stimuli (Herndon, 2012). Psychological and social issues are integral parts of the burn treatment from the time of injury through recovery and rehabilitation (Herndon, 2012), the life care planner should consider provisions for continued outpatient psychological services for both patient and family. These may include short-or long-term antipsychotic medications.

Treatment Options

Treatment options for burns vary somewhat depending on the type, size, and depth and extent of the burned tissue. Some areas of the body have thicker skin and/or cartilage that assist to protect an area. Treatment options can range from simple skin protection lotions or coverings, topical treatments, to wound excision, and skin grafting. The primary concern of acute care is stabilization. However, the recovery/healing phase continues for a lengthy period after hospital discharge. The burn survivor will likely return home with dressing changes, splints, creams/ointments, and medications. Other treatment options include laser resurfacing, compression garments, therapy, injections, protective clothing, bleaching cream, as well as other topical creams and lotions. Clinicians provide close monitoring to assess the healing process.

Wound Excision

If the burned area is extensive, then wound excision is necessary. This can occur in the either the acute or chronic phases. Acutely, sloughing or dead tissue must be debrided to allow healthy tissue to form underneath. Repeated debridement may be needed for months or years to reconstruct the burned area.

Skin Grafting

Skin grafting is performed when other conservative treatment is not effective or appropriate. When there is a loss of epidermis, or sometimes dermis, skin grafts are necessary. The life care planner must provide for excellent care for graft and donor sites to optimize graft viability and donor site healing.

Two primary terms describe grafts: split thickness and full thickness. A split thickness graft is favored for larger wound surfaces. It does not include hair follicles, sweat glands and nerves. In split-thickness auto-grafting (STAG), the most common form, skin is taken from a non-burned area on the patient, meshed, and grafted to the burn site. STAG can also be in a sheet format, the gold standard for grafts. Full-thickness grafts are recommended for the smaller burns, and include all layers of the skin including blood vessels. These are appropriate for wounds of the hands, extremity creases, eyelids, nose and other facial areas. There are fewer contractures with a full thickness graft. Other surgical options include muscle flaps with a skin graft, and pedicle free-flap grafts, both of which use full thickness skin.

Temporary skin substitutes, called homografts, are used to prepare and protect a wound for autografting. They can be made of several substances: such as allografts from a cadaver; xenografts from pig skin; and biobranes from synthetic membranes. They last about 7 to 10 days before rejection by the body. Permanent skin substitutes are also available, such as cultured epithelial autograft (CEA) and Integra. These are very expensive. CEA takes about 21 days to produce. Skin grafts as a rule are performed on 20-30% of the total body surface area (TBSA) every 3 to 5 days (Kagan, Peck, and Ahrenholz, 2009).

Autograft donor sites can be full-thickness, sheet, or split-thickness. The most common donor sites for full-thickness skin are ears, upper eyelids, neck and groin. The full-thickness donor site typically provides good cosmoses, minimal care is required, has minimal pain, and has primary closure.

Donor sites for partial-thickness grafts include buttocks, back, and thighs. Partial-thickness skin is meshed (with interstices) to cover a larger burn area when a patient has minimal donor site availability. However, meshed grafts often result in more hypertrophic scarring. Sheet grafts have no interstices, so they provide better cosmesis with less scarring; these are more often used on the hands and face.

Donor sites can be harvested more than once, usually from less-visible sites such as the back, buttock, and thighs. Donor sites can be just as painful as the burn sites. They require the same care as partial thickness burns. The donor sites will be sun sensitive, may be permanently discolored, and can scar just as easily (Holavanahalli, Helm, and Kowalske, 2010).

Following the graft surgery, the injured areas are dressed with non-stick gauze and compression bandages. The grafted area is also immobilized and splinted to protect it. It is customary for the physician to make the first dressing change on the third post-operative day. Grafts are monitored for signs of infection or hematoma development. If graft appearance is satisfactory on the fifth day, the physician will change the dressing again, and subsequent dressing changes will be done once or twice daily. Depending on the area of the graft or donor site, home health may be considered for the dressing changes. In some cases a wound vacuum is used to assist with moisture control as the graft heals. A wound vacuum requires dressing changes 3-4 times per week. The vacuum container is emptied daily.

The graft site should never be placed in a dependent position. The patient with a leg graft is typically not allowed up to walk before the fifth to seventh day. Legs are double-wrapped with ACE bandages to ensure adequate compression on the graft. Inspection is required after the first ambulation to determine the level of activity permitted. The patient is usually measured for compression garments around post-operative day seven.

Precise attention to detail is always of paramount importance. If a hematoma or seroma develops at the graft site, the physician should be contacted to evaluate and treat the cause of the wound disruption. Ischemia is another common cause of graft destruction or loss. It can occur if bandages are too tight, the position inappropriate, or splints are used incorrectly.

Reconstructive Surgery

Burns take up to one year to typically heal and the injured person begins the reconstructive phase. This will include both conservative and surgical measures to lessen scarring and improve function. Some complications such as contractures, hypertrophic scarring, or keloid formation will likely lead to limited range of motion, a decline in function, difficulties with activities of daily living, and be the source of pain/discomfort. Changes in the body structure, such as growth or weight gain, can lead to complications requiring reconstructive surgeries/revisions of skin grafts in the future. The purpose of reconstructive surgery is to improve function, lessen symptoms and pain, reduce hypertrophic scars and contractures, enhance cosmesis, and prevent complications.

Examples of reconstructive surgeries include: excision and complex closure, excision and advancement flap, tissue expander insertion and removal with advancement flap, Z-plasty, Y-plasty, W-plasty, split-thickness skin graft, full-thickness skin graft, removal of lesions/tumors/neuromas, and orthopedic repair.

Skin grafts, especially over the joints (e.g., elbows, heels, fingers, behind knees) tend to deteriorate due to wear and tear, so provisions in the life care plan should be made for repeat skin grafting in the future. Just as with acute care, patients can expect extensive post-operative care with medications, dressing changes, splinting, compression garments, occupational therapy, physical therapy, and physician follow-up following reconstructive surgeries to promote the healing process, reduce scarring, and prevent complications.

The reconstructive phase can last several years beyond the initial burn. Physicians will allow for healing/recovery/rehabilitation phases as well as transition back to school or work when planning surgeries. Reconstruction postponement should not be an option due to the loss of function and increased deformities (Herndon, 2012).

Laser Resurfacing and Tattooing

Laser resurfacing may be included in the reconstructive phase to eliminate hypertrophic scarring or keloids. Facial atrophic scars can be safely and effectively resurfaced (ablative laser skin resurfacing) with high-energy, pulsed, or scanned carbon dioxide (CO2) or Erbium-Yttrium-Aluminum-Garnet (Er:YAG). (Tanzi and Alster, 2004) There are cosmetic surgery techniques used to assist with reconstructive surgery, e.g., tattooing-type surgery to areas to enhance color and naturalness, such as lips and areolar areas of the breasts.

Injections

Injections are used to treat pruritus, swelling, and deformity. The more common injections include triamcinolone (Kenalog) or botulinum (Botox). A series of three injections of Botox is completed at four-week intervals is recommended (McCauley, 2005). These injections are often performed under anesthesia related to considerations of pain and positioning of the patient.

Compression Garments

Compression garments assist to control and prevent hypertrophic scarring and contracture formation by the exertion of an external force. A wound that takes more than 21 days to heal will require the use of compression garments (Herndon, 2012). The purpose of the compression garments is to form a soft, elastic scar, allowing for improved movement and function of the area. Compression garments protect the skin from additional trauma or injury during the recovery phase when skin and nerves are extremely sensitive and fragile, usually the first six to twelve months following an injury.

These customized garments are measured to fit each individual. The patient should be evaluated and measured for refitting frequently, especially with weight changes of more than 10 pounds. New compression garments may be needed often during the healing phase, including the initial wounds and graft sites following each operation. The constricting nature of the garment mimics the pressure of healthy skin and reduces the development of irregular scarring.

Compression garments play a vital role in the proper healing of wounds and reduction of scarring, but for the garments to perform correctly, they need to be in good condition. Compression garments lose the elasticity with wearing and laundering, and should be replaced every four to six months (Hall, Kowalske, and Holvanahalli, 2011). Nurse life care planners should note that it is necessary for three pairs to be bought at each change: one to wear, one to wash, and one for accidents needing a change. Costs range from $50.00-$100.00 a pair for off-the-shelf Sigvaris or Jobst brands to $200.00 to $600.00 for custom-fitted stockings, depending on the limb being fitted.

Optimal scar management requires the compression garments be worn at all times (23 hours/day) to provide adequate, consistent and sustained pressure. Complications related to scarring may not occur for several months. Scar maturation can take up to 12 to 18 months *and up to two years to mature fully.* Most patients will need to wear the compression garments for 12-18 months (Hall, Kowalske, and Holvanahalli, 2011). Because scars in different areas of the body mature at different rates, compression garments are worn even when the peak of scar formation has passed, generally until the injured area is pliable, flat, and similar in color to adjacent uninjured skin. Skin must be soft, pliable, and elastic to allow for normal joint movement.

Another advantage of external pressure being applied by compression garments is the reduction of inflammatory responses and the amount of blood in the scar, thereby reducing itching and preventing collagen synthesis. To prevent thickening, buckling, and nodular formations seen in hypertrophic scarring the patient must be compliant with wearing compression garments.

Long Term Management of the Skin
Fragile Skin
New skin is 20% weaker than original skin, extremely sensitive, and fragile. Alternates are recommended to avoid tape or adhesive bandages. Itching (mild or severe) usually persists for one to two years on average. Itching is considered a form of pain and should be treated. Medications or creams are used to relieve irritating or bothersome itching. Medications used include oral antihistamines such as diphenhydramine (Benadryl), cetirizine (Zyrtec), or hydroxyzine (Atarax), or doxepin topical (Prudoxin) 5% cream two to three times daily. (See *Injections*, supra)

Dry Skin
As damaged skin continues to heal, the body's natural ability to lubricate the skin is lost. Moisturizers should be applied to the skin daily before application of compression garments. Moisturizers must be massaged completely into the skin. Petroleum-based creams or lotions can cause deterioration of the garment fabric. Non-petroleum-based

creams or lotions recommended for post-burn patients include Nivea cream and lotion, Eucerin cream, and Aveeno lotion. These are available over-the-counter and should be included in the life care plan.

Sun Exposure

One of the most important preventive measures a patient can utilize is to avoid the sun for the initial 18 to 24 months after the injury. After this, avoidance of the midday sun is emphasized, i.e., between the hours of 10am to 4pm when UV rays (Herndon, 2012) are the strongest. Sunglasses should be worn that block 99% to 100% of the UV radiation. These are important in the prevention of cataracts and other eye damage. For the patients whose work requires them to be outdoors a significant amount of time, a change will be necessary during the initial two years after the burn injury. An employer may be able to provide job accommodations. However, job retraining may be needed. Sunscreen of at least SPF15 must be worn at all times. Sunscreen should be applied frequently, especially following water activities or sweating. Protective clothing is also recommended for burned patients as it offers protection from the sun as well as allows for ventilation to cool the body. UV sun-protective clothing should be worn when the patient is outside for any length of time; UV clothing should be alternated and the individual should have several sets. For special areas most prone to sun exposure, such as the eyes, ears, nose, neck and the top of the head, a wide brimmed UV-treated hat is necessary. SPF clothing is available from many companies including Solumbra, Columbia, Solartex, REI, and many more. The cost for these garments should be included in the life care plan.

Compression garments

Compression garments are weaned based on healing of the skin. A sign that the scar is not truly mature indicates the person should wear compression garments for a longer period of time. Lack of pressure causes scar tissue to rapidly regenerate in an irregular pattern. Long-term routine follow-up visits should be scheduled to check the fit of the compression garments, and pressure should be discontinued only after the scar has definitively matured. Reassessment of the fit is necessary to minimize the occurrence of pressure sores from the garment or mask (Hall, Kowalske, and Holvanahalli, 2011).

Therapies

The burn survivor typically participates in extensive physical therapy, occupational therapy, and scar management in conjunction with other medical treatment (e.g., injections, splinting, compression garments, and surgeries) to increase movement and range of motion. Therapy begins in the acute phase and may commonly continue for years to give ongoing function. Physical, speech, occupational, and hand therapy are instrumental in assisting a burn patient obtain the highest level of functioning possible. These therapies occur in inpatient and outpatient settings and focus on functioning, mobility, endurance, conditioning, strengthening, scar management, and range of motion.

Scar management is a lifelong process. If a burn patient has ongoing complications of hypertrophic scarring and contractures, the physician will consider long-term physical and occupational therapies to help manage and prevent these complications. Therapy is also utilized following the numerous reconstructive surgeries many patients undergo.

The More Extensive The Burn, The Greater The Rehabilitation Challenge

Short-term rehabilitation goals are to preserve the burn patient's range of motion and functional ability. Long-term rehabilitation goals are to assist the injured person to return to independent living. This may involve training on how to compensate for functional losses in order to be as productive as possible and reintegrate into the physical environment (Herndon, 2012). Serial casting, orthotics, and splinting are essential in burn rehabilitation to promote proper positioning and reduce complications such as contractures and deformity (Herndon, 2012).

In addition to the goals of medical care and therapy above, the following treatment and rehabilitative recommendations apply to all burn patients (Hall, Kowalske, and Holvanahalli, 2011):

- Exercise to increase circulation and increase blood flow both in general and specifically to the affected area.
- Be aware of temperature and amount of energy expended to avoid overheating and exhaustion.
- Be careful in highly hot or humid areas, as the increase in body temperature can occur quickly and inadvertently.
- Avoid repeated rubbing or scratching of a sensitive area.
- Avoid dragging clothing or other objects across sensitive skin.
- Eat a healthy diet high in protein for healing, and try to avoid weight gain that can put undue pressure on new skin that has lost some or all of its elasticity.
- Avoid hot water e.g., in hot tubs, bathtub, shower, dishwater, steam rooms.
- Avoid exposure to cold temperatures since this causes a decrease of blood flow.
- Use only mild soap to protect against harmful chemicals

Outcomes

Impairments resulting from a burn are not restricted to the skin. Additional complications may affect any body system such as the following (Herndon, 2012):

- Musculoskeletal: A full thickness burn involves all layers of skin. There may be secondary damage or effects including:
  o Muscle, bone, tendon, and ligament weakness and instability
  o Chronic infection (osteomyelitis)

- o Arthritic changes
- o Ectopic calcifications (heterotopic ossification)
- o Limited range of motion or functioning
- Special senses and speech effects may include:
  - o Hearing or vision impairment resulting from thermal burns
  - o Perioral (mouth) burns interfere with mastication and result in drooling or speech impairment
  - o Loss of external ear, impairs hearing
  - o Life-threatening infections may have been treated with antibiotics that can cause deafness (aminoglycosides)
  - o Electrical injuries increase risk for cataract formation

- Respiratory system effects may include:
  - o Chronic/recurrent respiratory infections and pulmonary insufficiency due to inhalation injury or prolonged ventilator support
  - o Exacerbation of pre-existing asthma; irritant-induced asthma, reactive airway disease
- Cardiovascular system: Long-term follow-up of burn survivors of large thermal injury shows increased incidence of cardiovascular disease

- Neurological system sequelae may not become apparent up to two years following injury.

- Patients who have sustained electrical injuries:
  - o Should be closely monitored for progressive neurological deficits
  - o Are predisposed to stroke
  - o Exhibit signs of peripheral neuropathies secondary to thermal damage
  - o May develop paresis, paralysis, tremor, involuntary movement, or ataxia
  - o May have progressive degeneration of fine and gross motor coordination

o   May experience worsening neurological symptoms after return to work
o   Can have sensory deficits related to full thickness burns, including symptoms of anesthesia, dysesthesia, parasthesia, hyperesthesia, cold intolerance, intense/burning pain

- Hematologic and lymphatic: Full thickness burns, particularly of lower extremities, will also cause damage to lymphatic system. Patients may:
o   Have decreased or lack of normal lymphatic drainage (lymphedema)
o   Develop chronic edema and stasis ulcers
o   Need external support of elastic garments

- Genitourinary: Dysfunction occurs with deep perineal or buttock burns

Other Considerations
Vocational
When the burn survivor enters or re-enters employment, vocational barriers should be assessed and modifications provided to reduce the complications and allow for a successful transition into competitive employment. These barriers can include a temperature-controlled environment (too warm or too cold), sun exposure, endurance, and physical tasks, i.e., lifting, pushing/pulling, tolerance to standing, sitting, walking, hand grip, and upper extremity strength. A vocational case manager is recommended to assist in the transition and advocate for a safe work environment. If the burn survivor is unable to return to previous employment, consideration should be given for a vocational evaluation to identify appropriate employment opportunities within the burn survivor's physical capabilities.

Long Term Psychological Effects
Psychological services should be continued during transition to work, to lessen disabling psychological symptoms

and risk of developing chronic psychological diagnoses. Psychosocial issues such as family and marital support have been well known to affect patient's reports of wellbeing beyond the consequences of the injury and level of recovery. If the support system is not solid, recovery is compromised. Additionally, psychological stress must be taken into consideration in the long-term recovery of the burn victim.

Long Term Pain Control

According to an article in *Burns* (Esfahlan, Lofti, Zamanzadah, and Babapuor, 2010) burn patients have probably always been under-medicated and undertreated for pain during hospitalization for acute care. It was noted in the New England Journal of Medicine (Ballantyne and Mao, 2003) that physicians are reluctant to prescribe opioids for long-term pain control. The authors referred to this as "opiophobia," and felt that it appears to be universal among physicians.

The importance of this monumental problem is it adversely affects long-term outcome. Sustained pain can create a cycle of shock in traumatized patients, creates biochemical and metabolic disturbances, leads to tissue hypoxia in the tissue, and creates toxic products. These effects can depress the cardiovascular system. Studies have shown that adequate prompt pain relief can improve cardiovascular function.

One concern in burn care is that numerous health care professionals view pain as a transient problem. It is hard to convince them that this type of pain may result in long-term complications. More compelling evidence may be revealed by an adequate prospective study, which could provide a link between high levels of pain during hospitalization and long-term psychological stress (Patterson, Hoflund, Espey, and Sharar, 2010).

Common problems and Interventions

The most common post-burn problems reported, with suggested interventions, are:

- Dry skin: Requires frequent application of moisturizers; hot baths, soaps, and irritants should be avoided.

- Pruritus: Improves or diminishes with frequent application of moisturizers, medications, creams, and ointments.

- Hyperpigmentation and hypopigmentation: Must avoid exposure to the sun, can be easily sunburned and permanently discolored. Application of sunscreen and protective clothing is critical.

- Hypersensitive skin: Massage therapy may help to desensitize affected areas.

- Fragile skin: Easily develops friction burns and tears. Important to protect fragile skin with protective clothing or Tubigrip. Preventing infection and scarring is critical.

- Decreased sensation over grafts and donor sites: Wear protective clothing/gloves when performing tasks that are rough on the skin. Preventive care includes regular skin checks for new wounds and application of topical antibiotic ointment and dressings if necessary.

- Poor temperature regulation and inability to perspire: Dress in layers, avoid extreme temperatures, live and work in temperature-controlled work environments

- Chronic discomfort, burning, pins-and-needles sensations: Massage, lotions, medication may help; pain management referral if necessary.

- Residual scarring with poor cosmesis: May require compression garments and reconstructive surgery to correct these.

Pediatric Considerations

Burn injuries can produce overwhelming physiological and psychological challenges to a pediatric victim. The provision of medical care can induce additional trauma if developmental needs are not addressed. When young children are burned, they may experience more severe stress that exceeds their capacity to cope. Due to limited understanding and ability to express themselves, children are at high risk for development of emotional and behavioral disorders.

According to Lenore Terr's article, *What happens to early memories of trauma?* "Verbal recollections require conscious awareness but behavioral memories do not." She reported behavioral memories are stored and processed nonverbally. This is revealed through the child's play, fears, and personality changes. What Terr calls "engraved memories" may be stimulated by words or pictures, prompting the child to reenact the traumatic event. PTSD is the diagnosis most often used for children who suffer from traumatic injuries. PTSD is linked to effects on the child's social, educational and biological functioning and development (Fauerbach, Prunzinsky, and Saxe, 2007).

A pediatric burn survivor will likely have excessive absences from school due to acute and chronic medical treatment. The pediatric burn survivor will likely return to school wearing compression garments and have activity limitations. It is helpful to have the teacher(s), a guidance counselor, and a school nurse involved in the transition. Consideration should be given towards educating classmates on burns. This may lessen the child's psychological stress when returning to school.

There are many reasons to believe that survivors of severe burns, even children who appear well adjusted, will have impaired ability to develop into well-adjusted adults. Many factors may cause them to expect diminished quality of life, psychological pain, and symptoms of psychological ill health. The years of specialty treatment for the severely burned person create major family disruptions and create situations that would be expected to interfere with the survivor's normal psychological development and social integration. Years of rehabilitation and reconstructive surgeries follow the acute injury, and are not only painful physically but also separate the burn survivor from peers. Pressure garments, masks, and splints worn to combat burn scar contractures also call visual attention to the individuals who wear them, further singling them out as different from others. Even after years of work in rehabilitation, disfigurement is normal for individuals with burn scars (Barret-Nerin and Herndon, 2005).

The most obvious visible differences between adults and children are size and body proportion (Herndon, 2012). Major catastrophic illness and trauma produce both transient and permanent changes in growth patterns. In severely burned patients, nail and hair growth are attenuated during the acute post-burn period, and bone growth is slowed. Dampened height and weight gain velocities have been documented in children during the first three years post-burn, causing burned children to be slighter and shorter than their age-matched peers (Herndon, 2012).

Children may display pain through behaviors of fear, anxiety, agitation, anger, aggression, tantrums, depression, withdrawal, and regression. How the child's experience of pain from the burn injury and anxiety from the hospitalization are clinically managed will have lasting psychological effects for many months and years to come (Herndon, 2012).

Life Care Plan Considerations:
The nurse life care planner considers the medical and vocational needs of a burn survivor and identifies ways to address potential complications. Communication with the treating team is critical. Each member of the team has specialized roles. The physician can identify the medical plan of care for reconstructive surgeries and future care. The

occupational therapist and physical therapist can assist with identifying the appropriate long-term treatment modalities (scar management, compression garments, and home exercise program). Specialty consultations should be considered for assessment, diagnosis, and treatment of secondary diagnoses and associated complications. Burn life care plan components can appear costly when considering rehabilitation, reconstructive surgeries, and long-term scar management. A comprehensive nurse life care plan will clarify the rationales and value of the future medical treatment. Consideration in the life care plan should be given to:

- Medical care: burn specialist, PCP/pediatrician, dermatologist, plastic surgeon, physiatrist, ophthalmology (electrical and direct injury), psychiatrist, psychologist

- Surgeries and procedures: Triamcinolone injections, dermabrasion, excision and complex closure, excision and advancement flap, Z-plasty, split thickness skin graft, full thickness skin graft, tissue expander insertion and removal and advancement flap, bleaching cream and in extreme cases amputation of the affected limb may be necessary.

- Projected evaluations: ophthalmologist, otolaryngologist, orthopedic surgeon, neurologist, cardiologist, pulmonologist, urologist, rheumatologist, nutritionist, hand surgeon, dentist, neuropsychologist, psychologist, occupational and physical therapists, speech-language therapist, cognitive therapist; home safety evaluation

- Projected therapeutic modalities: Ongoing OT/PT for scar management, massage, conditioning, other therapies to treat and prevent complications as indicated by evaluations above

- Psychological services: episodic counseling services (individual and family) throughout life transitions (puberty, high school, college, marriage, death of family, work, medical treatment, medical complications)

- Diagnostic studies: EMG/NCV studies, venous Doppler, LE ultrasound, x-rays (heterotopic ossification), MRI (joints, spine), cardiac, pulmonary, urology, gastroenterology, pulmonary function studies

- Laboratory studies: nutritional levels, vitamin levels, general health panel, others as indicated by evaluations above

- Medications: analgesic, anti-inflammatory, gastric reflux, prescription and over-the-counter antihistamines for itching (oral/topical), sleep, psychotropic

- Influenza vaccination

- Scar management: moisturizers, sunscreen, protective clothing, protective gear for work and recreation, compression garments, OT/PT re-evaluations for measurement, splinting

- Minor skin tears: Bacitracin, over-the-counter triple antibiotic, Mepliex bandages

- Medical supplies: dressing supplies, nutritional supplements

- Pulmonary care (if inhalation injury): breathing treatments, humidifier, air cleaner

- Electrical injury: support hose, lymphedema garments

- Durable medical equipment

- Aids for independent function

- UV-protective clothing, thermo-regulated clothing

- Mobility: wheelchair, scooter, walker, age-related mobility needs, home accessibility, e.g., bathroom, kitchen, ramps, doorknobs

- Home health care (after surgeries)

- Home health assistance for ADLs

- Respite care for family/significant other caregivers

- Home health, assisted living, nursing home; consider age related services regarding burns

- Transportation or mileage reimbursement

- Educational, vocational: home bound, tutoring, vocational evaluation, vocational case manager, vocational retraining

Other Considerations:
- Nurse case manager (CCM with burn experience)
- Recreational therapy
- Gym membership or home exercise equipment
- Burn Camp for individual and family
- Cosmetic make-up: Zinc-based mineral make-up (Jane Iredale, GloMineral, Dermablend).
- Community support and burn survivor groups: American Burn Association, Phoenix Foundation, Knapp Foundation; VA Support Groups for handyman, housekeeping, yard maintenance

Potential Late Complications:
Complications can develop at later phases of a case making it extremely important for the nurse life care planner

to consider ongoing medical care to monitor and assess each case for late complications and provide for these in the life care plan. Many life care planners commonly list these items in a *Potential Complications* section, separate from *Routine Care*.

These complications are more probable than potential with major burns (greater than second degree).

- Dry skin: Sebaceous glands destroyed in partial and deep thickness burns, inability to moisturize
- Itching: inflammatory process during wound healing, changes in blood flow, collagen, nerve regeneration
- Pigmentation: Melanocytes are destroyed, lose protection from UV rays
- Sensitivity: Damaged nerve endings, neuropathic pain
- Decreased sensation: Skin grafting
- Fragile skin: Thinner dermis with poorly organized collagen and less elastin
- Poor temperature regulation: loss of eccrine (sweat) glands, loss of subcutaneous fat
- Chronic discomfort: pins and needles, burning, tingling, itching, pain, hypersensitivity
- Marjolin's ulcer: Carcinoma, increased risk for metastasis
- Epidermal inclusion cysts
- Loss of sweat glands, loss of hair growth, loss of sebaceous glands, hot and cold intolerance, psychological factors related to disfigurement, psychosocial aspects
- At risk for injury related to temperature sensitivity, risk of injury to donor and graft sites
- Orthopedic: arthritis, joint ankylosis, bilateral carpal tunnel syndrome (CTS), neuromuscular defects, muscle contractures
- Neurological: Sympathetic over-activity with changes in bowel habits, urinary, and sexual function (electricity), progressive degeneration (electricity), neuromas, skin contractures, cataracts

- Psychological: Educational/vocational barriers related to visible differences and medical condition, side effects of long term medications, exacerbation of psychological symptoms in developmental stages, difficulty with intimate relationships
- Endocrine: Pancreatitis, breast development, weight gain
- Pregnancy and breast feeding

Nursing Diagnoses To Consider:
- *Activity Intolerance:* Insufficient physiological or psychological energy to endure or complete required or desired daily activities.
- *Anxiety*: Vague uneasy feeling of discomfort or dread accompanied by an autonomic response (the source often nonspecific or unknown to the individual); a feeling of apprehension caused by anticipation of danger. It is an alerting signal that warns of impending danger and enables the individual to take measures to deal with threat.
- *Caregiver Role Strain:* Difficulty in performing family/ significant other caregiver role.
- *Chronic Pain:* Unpleasant sensory and emotional experience arising from actual or potential tissue damage or described in terms of such damage (International Association for the Study of Pain); sudden or slow onset of any intensity from mild to severe, constant or recurring without an anticipated or predictable end and with a duration of >6 months.
- *Compromised Family Coping:* An usually supportive primary person (family member, significant other, or close (friend) provides insufficient, ineffective, or compromised support, comfort, assistance, or encouragement that may be needed by the client to manage or master adaptive tasks related to his or her health challenge.
- *Delayed Growth and Development:* Deviation from age-group norms

- *Disturbed Body Image:* Confusion in mental picture of one's physical self.
- *Fatigue*: An overwhelming sustained sense of exhaustion and decreased capacity for physical and mental work at the usual level.
- *Grieving*: A normal complex process that includes emotional, physical, spiritual, social, and intellectual responses and behaviors by which individuals, families, and communities incorporate an actual, anticipated, or perceived loss into their daily lives.
- *Impaired Tissue Integrity*: Damage to mucous membrane, corneal, integumentary, or subcutaneous tissues.
- *Impaired Physical Mobility:* Limitation in independent, purposeful physical movement of the body or of one or more extremities.
- *Impaired Skin Integrity*: Altered epidermis and/or dermis.
- *Impaired Social Interaction:* Insufficient or excessive quantity or ineffective quality of social exchange.
- *Ineffective Protection:* Decrease in ability to guard self from internal or external threats such as illness or injury.
- *Post-Trauma Syndrome:* Sustained maladaptive response to a traumatic, overwhelming event.
- *Bathing Self-Care Deficit:* Impaired ability to perform or complete bathing activities of self.
- *Dressing Self-Care Deficit:* Impaired ability to perform or complete dressing activities for self.
- *Feeding Self-Care Deficit:* Impaired ability to perform or complete self-feeding activities.
- *Toileting Self-Care Deficit:* Impaired ability to perform or complete toileting activities for self.
- *Risk for Trauma:* At risk of accidental tissue injury (e.g., wound, burn, fracture).
- *Risk for Imbalanced Body Temperature:* At risk for failure to maintain body temperature within normal range.

- *Risk for Infection:* At risk for being invaded by pathogenic organisms.
- *Risk for Injury:* At risk for injury as a result of environmental conditions interacting with the individual's adaptive and defensive resources.
- *Risk for Falls:* At risk for increased susceptibility to falling that may cause physical harm.
- *Risk for Peripheral Neurovascular Dysfunction:* At risk for disruption in the circulation, sensation, or motion of an extremity.
- *Risk for Impaired Skin Integrity*: At risk for alteration in epidermis and/or dermis.

References:

Allison KP (2003,). Pulsed dye laser treatment of burn scars: alleviation or irritation. Burns 29:3 207-13.

American Burn Association. (2012). National Burn Repository. Retrieved from NBR annual report: http://www. ameriburn.org/2011NBRAnnualreport.pdf

Ballantyne J and Mao E. (2003,). Abstract for Opioid Therapy for Chronic Pain. New England Journal of Medicine, 349:22.

Barret-Nerin JP, (2005). Principles and Practices of Burn Surgery. Washington, DC: Marcel Dekker.

Beers M and Berkow R. (1999). Merck Manual 17th Ed. Washington, DC: Merck Research Laboratories.

Burn Injury Model System. (2011). Wound Care and Scar Management. Seattle: University Of Washington.

Burns/Pre-conference (2011). Journal of Nurse Life Care Planning, 11:3.

Cushing, M., Louri, G., Miller, D., and Hohn, J. (2001). Heterotopic ossification after lateral epicondylectomy. Journal of South Orthopedic Association, 10:1, 53-56.

DeSanti L and Demling RH. (2001). Topical doxepin cream is effective in relieving severe pruritis caused by burn injury: a preliminary study. Wounds, 13:6, 210-215.

Dirckx J (2001). Stedman's Concise Medical Dictionary for Health Professionals, 4th ed. Baltimore, MD: Williams and Wilkins.

Disa J (2002,). Open wound reconstruction. Retrieved from ACS Surgery Online: http://www.acssurgery.com

Esfahlan A, (2010). Burn pain and patients' responses. Burns, 36:7, 1129-1133.

Faucher, LD. (2002). Rehabilitation of the burn patient. Retrieved from ACS Surgery Online: http://www.acssurgery.com

Fauerbach J, Prunzinsky T, and Saxe G. (2007). Psychological health and function after burn injury. Journal of Burn Care and Research 28:4.

Herndon, D. (2012). Total Burn Care (2nd ed.). New York, NY: Saunder.

Holavanahalli R, Helm P, and Kowalske K. (2010,). Long-term outcomes in patients surviving large burns: The skin. Journal of Burn Care and Research, 31:4).

Kagan R, (2009). Surgical management of the burn wound and use of skin substitutes. Chicago, IL: American Burn Association.

McCauley R. (2005). Functional and aesthetic reconstruction of burn patients. Chicago: Taylor and Francis.

McCollom P. (2002). Restoration after burn injury. In S. Hoeman, Rehabilitation nursing, process, application, and outcomes (5th ed.). Glenview, IL: ARN.

Naylor MH. (2010, March). Medscape.com. Retrieved from http:www.medscape.com/viewprogram/3129.index

Patterson D, Hoflund H, Espey K, and Sharar S. (2010). Pain management. International Society of Burn Injuries.

Sen S, Greenhalgh D, and Pamieri T. (2010). Review of burn injury research for 2009. Journal of Burn Care and Research 31:6

Singerman J, Gomez M, and Fish J. (2008). Long-term sequelae of low-voltage electrical injury. Journal of Burn Care and Research; 29:5

Stouffer DJ. (1995). Journeys through hell: stories of burn survivors's reconstruction of self and identity. Boulder, CO: Rowman and Littlefield Publishers.

Tanzi E and Alster T. (2004). Laser Treatment of Scars. Skin Therapy.

The Peoples Burn Foundation. (2005). To hell and back: an education program on the reality of burn injury. VideoIndiana, Inc.

Thomas C. (2005). Taber's cyclopedic medical dictionary. Philadelphia, PA: F.A. Davis. Various. (2011).

Wardrope, J., and Smith, J. (1992). The management of wounds and burns. Oxford: Oxford University Press.

Wasserman. (2012). Physician fee reference, 23 Ed. Milwaukee, WI: Wasserman Medical Publishers, Ltd.

CHAPTER 6

Cerebral Palsy

Lynne P. Trautwein, MSN, RN, CCM, CMAC, CNLCP
Nancy J. Bond, M.Ed., CCM, CLCP

Introduction

The American Academy of Pediatrics (2012) defines cerebral palsy (CP) as "a group of permanent disorders of the development of movement and posture that cause activity limitations that are attributed to non-progressive disturbances that occurred in the developing fetal or infant brain." These disorders often occur along with disturbances of sensation, perception, cognition, communication, and behavior. Epilepsy and secondary musculoskeletal problems are also common.

The first medical descriptions of CP were written in the 1860s by English orthopedic surgeon William Little, who noted a puzzling disorder that affected children in the first years of life, which caused stiff, spastic muscles in the legs and, to a lesser degree, the arms (MyChild, 2012a). These children were noted to have difficulty grasping objects, crawling, and walking, and did not improve over time. The condition became known as *Little's disease* and is now known specifically as *spastic diplegia*, one of several disorders than affect control of movement due to developmental brain injury under the umbrella term of CP. These early reports suggested the condition resulted from a lack of oxygen during birth.

Sigmund Freud disagreed with the oxygen deprivation theory and postulated that since other conditions were often present (cognitive impairment, visual disturbances, and seizures), the onset of the disorder may have occurred earlier in life, during the brain's development in utero (MyChild, 2012). He suggested that difficult birth was merely a symptom of some other source of developmental stress. Despite little acceptance by most in the medical community, Freud's theory gained more attention in the mid-1980s, when an extensive analysis was conducted from a government study of more than 35,000 births. Researchers found that birth trauma could be attributed to only 10% of children with a diagnosis of CP. In most cases of CP, no cause of the factors explored could be found. This finding has led to further research regarding alternative causes. This chapter will discuss CP in more detail including its incidence and causes as well as options for care. The psychological impact of CP and the effects of aging are also addressed. Interview questions are included to assist the nurse life care planner with development of a life care plan as well as a methodology for identification of pediatric considerations.

Incidence

An estimated 764,000 children and adults in the United States are living with CP. Although studies vary, the number of new children diagnosed with CP is estimated to be approximately 8,000 to 10,000 per year (MyChild, 2012a). Of these new cases, around 70% occurs prior to birth, 20% occurs during the birthing process, and 10% occurs during the first two years of life (March of Dimes, 2007).

The clinical diagnosis of CP consists of the clinical history of both the mother and infant and the pediatric and neurological examination of the infant. The diagnosis is dependent upon two key findings: 1) evidence of non-progressive damage to the developing brain and 2) the presence of a resulting impairment of the neuromuscular control system of the body (United Cerebral Palsy, 2012). The latter is usually accompanied by a physiological impairment and functional disability.

Causes

Potential causes of CP can be traced to three distinct stages resulting in prenatal brain damage, perinatal brain damage, and postnatal brain damage. Each stage is discussed below.

Prenatal Brain Damage

Historically, Rh blood type incompatibility between the mother and fetus and rubella during pregnancy were common prenatal causes of CP. Both are now preventable and current research focuses on damages in the prenatal stage of brain development. Two significant areas of research are in the area of disturbance of brain cell migration and injury to the axonal myelination process.

Brain cell migration is mitigated by both genetic and environmental factors (NINDS, 2011). Alcohol, prescribed and recreational drugs, maternal infection and inflammation, environmental toxins, and radiation are factors believed to interfere with travel of the migratory cells to their destination (NINDS, 2011).

Poor myelination can occur in the fetal brain due to hemorrhage of delicate blood vessels resulting in periventricular leukomalacia (PVL). Clinical manifestations are spasticity and poor coordination of both sides of the body. Premature birth is the most common condition associated with PVL. Overall incidence of prematurity is 15% of live births, but this increases to 40% in cases involving CP (Sandkar and Mundkar, 2005). Other causes of premature birth include maternal infection, maternal and fetal immune system disturbances, maternal endocrine and metabolic disorders, placental pathology, and presence of multiple fetuses (March of Dimes, 2013).

Perinatal Brain Damage

Events during the perinatal period, the several hours immediately before and after birth including the birthing process, account for twenty percent of children with CP (MyChild, 2012b). These include compression of the infant's head in the birth canal, traumatic passage due to a large head, narrow birth canal, or poor positioning in the canal, each of which leads to increased intracranial pressure and resultant rupture of cerebral blood vessels. Diminished circulation to the brain due to pressure on the umbilical cord can result in lack of oxygen and brain cell death. Failure to breathe at birth can lead to oxygen deprivation and brain cell death.

Birth weight is also considered a factor in CP. Infants born weighing less than 3.3 pounds are considered to have very low birth weight (VLBW), and of the 40,000 infants born each year at VLBW, it is estimated that 30% are brain-injured. Multiple births are often associated VLBW, and the increased incidence of multiple births due to the use of infertility treatments may affect the incidence of CP (Wang et al., 2006).

Postnatal Brain Damage

At two years of age, the brain's basic structure has been established and its physical development is at an end. During the first two years of postnatal life, a number of factors can affect the motor control system of the brain. The most common are physical trauma due to falls or physical abuse, infection, and respiratory distress. The brain's response to such insults is often immature and nonfunctional and thus can result in CP (My Child 2012c).

Diagnosis

Making a definitive diagnosis of CP is not always easy, especially before the child's first birthday. The diagnosis may be made early in infants at high risk for CP, especially those born prematurely with complications such as intracranial bleeding and severe lung problems. Most children with CP can be diagnosed by age 18 months. Following a brain injury, such as that acquired during the birthing process or from a fall, it is important to wait and observe the child before diagnosing CP, even if the child has a lesion on brain scan and exhibits signs and symptoms consistent with CP. The lesion may not permanently impair motor activity. (Sankar and Mundkur 2005) The physician must obtain a complete prenatal and birth history before making a diagnosis of CP.

Physical Examination

The classic finding of CP is spasticity, increased muscle tone. CP classification terminology describes the number of limbs involved and type of movement disorder present.

Classification by number of limbs involved includes the following:
- Spastic hemiplegia - Affects a single limb, one side of the body
- Spastic diplegia - Affects both legs
- Spastic quadriplegia - Affects both arms and legs

Classification by movement disorder includes the following:
- Spastic - This is the most common type of CP, with hypertonic spasticity is the dominant characteristic. Contractures are common.
- Choreoathetoid - This is defined by variable muscle tone with involuntary movement that serves no purpose. Hypotonia is common, and contractures are uncommon.
- Mixed type - These children display hypertonicity displayed in spastic CP as well as involuntary, purposeless movements associated with athetoid CP.

Other signs and symptoms of CP include the following:
- Muscle tremor or spasticity, with tendency to tuck arms toward the side
- Evidence of abnormal or delayed development of motor function (most meaningful aspect)
- Persistent infantile reflexes (such as sucking and startle)
- Scissoring: a condition of the muscles in the hips and legs causing the legs to turn inward and cross or touch at the knees
- Partial or full loss of movement (paralysis)
- Sensory abnormalities
- Defects of hearing and vision
- Speech abnormalities are common
- Intellectual function: extremely bright to severe mental retardation

In addition to typical assessment questions for life care planning, the following are considerations for children with CP:

- Does the child participate in public or private education?

- If not yet in school, do the parents plan for the child to attend private or public school?

- Name of school, address, telephone number

- Name of teacher(s)

- Does the child have an IEP? An IFSP? If yes, obtain a copy of the most recent report/evaluation.

- Is the family satisfied with services offered to their child? Are there services not being provided by the school that the family believes the child needs?

- Does the child receive extended school year services? How is the child transported to and from school?

- Does the child require skilled nursing services at school? How is this funded? Does the child require assistive technology? If so, what? And how is this being funded?

- What services are being provided to the child through the educational system? Who is the provider and how is it being funded?
  - Physical therapy
  - Occupation therapy
  - Speech therapy
  - Special education services
  - Vision services
  - Hearing or audiology
  - Classroom aide

- What childcare arrangement does this family have? What are the costs? How is this funded? Does the family have respite care arrangements? How is this funded?

Diagnostic Tests

Computed tomography (CT) and magnetic resonance imaging (MRI) scans can be used to identify lesions in the brain. After 2 years of age, there is reasonable certainty for CP if the MRI confirms periventricular leukomalacia (Ashwal, 2004). Overall, brain scars, cysts, and other changes appear on scans of children with CP more frequently when compared with the general population (Ashwal and Blasco, 2004). Other diagnostic studies for CP include the following:

- Radiographs may be ordered to exclude other neurological diseases.
- Single photon emission computed tomography (SPECT) scan identifies areas of the brain in a dormant state due to a lack of oxygen.
- Blood tests to exclude metabolic or hereditary conditions (CP is not a hereditary condition).
- Hearing screening is recommended; it is estimated that over 20% of children with CP have hearing impairments.
- Visual testing is recommended as over 40% of children with CP have visual impairments.
- Gait lab analysis, or motion analysis, recording the complex walking movements of the child with spasticity, which is then compared with a normal gait.
- A complete metabolic panel and metabolic urine screen are recommended for children with CP who have normal imaging studies in order to rule out metabolic or genetic disorders (Leonard et al., 2011)

Nursing Diagnoses To Consider:
- *Risk for Disuse Syndrome:* At risk for deterioration of body systems as the result of prescribed or unavoidable musculoskeletal inactivity.

- *Impaired Bed Mobility*: Limitation of independent movement from one bed position to another
- *Impaired Physical Mobility:* Limitation in independent, purposeful physical movement of the body or of one or more extremities.
- *Impaired Wheelchair Mobility:* Limitation of independent operation of wheelchair within environment.
- *Impaired Transfer Ability:* Limitation of independent movement between two nearby surfaces.
- *Impaired Walking*: Limitation of independent movement within the environment on foot.
- *Fatigue:* An overwhelming sustained sense of exhaustion and decreased capacity for physical and mental work at the usual level.
- *Risk for Activity Intolerance:* At risk for insufficient physiological or psychological energy to complete required or desired daily activities.
- *Ineffective Breathing Pattern:* Inspiration and/or expiration that does not provide adequate ventilation.
- *Disturbed Sensory Perception* (Specify visual, auditory, kinesthetic, gustatory, tactile, olfactory): Change in the amount or patterning of incoming stimuli accompanied by diminished, distorted, or impaired response to such stimuli.
- *Risk for Impaired Skin Integrity:* Risk for altered epidermis and/or dermis.
- *Risk for Peripheral Neurovascular Dysfunction:* At risk for disruption in the circulation, sensation, or motion of an extremity.

Medical Complications
Treatment and Management

Cerebral palsy is not curable. However, much can be done to lessen its effects to allow those with CP to lead independent lives. Specific treatment is based on the child's age, overall health, and medical history; extent and type of CP; the child's tolerance for specific medications, procedures, and therapy;

expectations for the course of the disease; and the caregiver's opinion or preference. The focus of treatment or management is to prevent deformities and maximize the child's capability at home and in the community (Bond and Trautwein, 2011).

A child with CP is best treated by an interdisciplinary team of healthcare providers. That may include:

- Pediatrician or family practitioner
- Pediatric nurse practitioner
- Orthopedic surgeon
- Neurologist
- Neurosurgeon,
- Ophthalmologist
- Nurse case manager
- Dentist
- Orthotist
- Rehabilitation therapists

There are three categories of treatment: *mechanical, pharmacological,* and *functional.* Most of the mechanical therapies also improve function. It is important to note that members of the healthcare team may differ in their opinions regarding which therapy modalities are appropriate or beneficial for a given child.

Mechanical Mechanical therapies include the following:

- Physical therapy (PT): PT improves or maintains the development of the large body muscles (generally gross motor skills).
  o Corrective handling increases the range of motion (ROM) and prevents bone and joint contractures.
  o Motor skills training consists of learning better ways to move and balance and preventing weakness and deterioration of muscles.

- Occupational therapy (OT): OT improves the development of the small body muscle (generally fine motor skills). The occupational therapist designs purposeful activities to assist the patient with daily living skills.
  - o An OT or a PT may evaluate and recommend use of appropriate therapeutic and adaptive equipment.
  - o A therapist may recommend the use of adaptive equipment for use during therapy at home and at school. Adaptive equipment will assist the individual with special needs to function at an optimal level of independence.

- Speech and language therapy improves communication skills; this may include alternative communication systems. It may include oral motor therapy to improve functions of the oral cavity for oral feeding or speech (Tosi, et al., 2009).

- Music therapy may be used for the treatment of neurological mental or behavioral disorders. (Baker and Roth, 2004)

- Sensory integration therapy helps the child to overcome problems in absorbing and processing sensory information. This improves balance, steady movement, and learning sequences of movements (Wingert et al., 2008).

- Equine therapy (also known as hippotherapy or horseback riding therapy): Studies suggest that equine therapy may improve gross motor function in children with CP, which may reduce the degree of motor disability. Studies also show a significant decrease in energy expenditure when walking plus a significant increase in ability to walk, run, and jump (Williams et al., 2023).

- Constraint-induced movement (CI) therapy: CI therapy is used for children with asymmetric motor impairment. Studies demonstrated that children acquired significantly more new classes of motor skills, made significant gains in the mean amount and quality of more-affected arm use at home, and demonstrated increases in unprompted use of the more-affected upper extremity with CI therapy (Charles et al., 2007).

- Play therapy: For the child with CP, play therapy, first and foremost, develops physical skills with the additional benefits of improving emotional and social development; reducing aggression and improving cooperation with others; and assisting the child in processing a traumatic event or prepare for an upcoming event such as surgery.

- Biofeedback (gait training): Statistically significant improvements regarding tonus of plantar flexor muscles and active ROM of ankle joints have been shown (Dursun, Dursun, and Alican, 2004).

Pharmacological Systemic use of pharmacological agents is recommended to reduce spasticity. Some of the medications used include the following (MyChild, 2012c):

- *Benzodiazepines*: Primarily used to reduce muscle tone. Unfortunately, in most cases, the antispasticity component is overshadowed by the sedative effect. Diazepam (Valium) is the most well-known of the benzodiazepines.

- *Dantrolene sodium (Dantrium, Revonto)*: A unique antispasticity agent with peripheral action. It decreases the force of muscular contractions but unfortunately has the undesirable side effect of excessive sedation. This agent is contraindicated for the use in children under the age of 5 years (Skidmore-Roth, 2012).

- *Baclofen (Lioresal)*: Baclofen is typically prescribed for oral administration. It can also be administered intrathecally via an intrathecal pump (which requires surgical implantation), permitting more effective delivery of this drug. Intrathecal administration also provides a longer lasting reduction of spasticity with less risk of lethargy and confusion. Some children respond well to a combination therapy that includes oral and intrathecal baclofen. Intrathecal baclofen is administered using infusion pumps in patients with spastic CP. (*Please see Chapter 3, Pain, for more information.*)

- *Botulinum toxin (Botox)*: Botox is injected directly into the affected muscle groups and into the shortened muscle to temporarily weaken that muscle and allow it to stretch. The effects of this treatment typically last around three to six months, so injections may be required two to four times a year.

Functional

- Orthotics, casts, and splints provide stability, keep joints in position, and help stretch muscles.
- Adaptive equipment is equipment designed to help the child with CP with everyday activities. Examples may include assisted mobility devices (wheelchairs, walkers), adapted utensils, adapted toys, and computers.

Surgical Intervention

Typical growth and development is altered for children with CP, resulting in deformities of bones, joints, spine, and muscles that may result in atypical function, spasticity, and/or pain. In preschool aged children, these deformities are typically managed with non-invasive treatments, such as medication and physical therapy. As the child ages, the deformity may become more severe, cause pain, or interfere with vital body functions.

For example, severe scoliosis of the spine can impede the ability of the lungs to expand and contract normally, interfering with normal respiratory efforts.

In such cases, surgical intervention may be considered. For best outcomes, the child with CP undergoing orthopedic surgery is typically between 5 and 10 years old and has had appropriate spasticity management. The purpose of orthopedic surgery is to prevent further deformity, improve function, relieve pain, or provide for ease of care. Surgery is considered when a child has a deformity that causes pain or interferes with function that is getting worse over time, a permanent contracture, dislocated or irregularly functioning joints, a spinal deformity not improving with other treatment, or a deformity that makes caregiving difficult or impossible. Corrections made during surgery may be temporary.

Common orthopedic surgical procedures include the following:

- *Tendon lengthening:* Involves exposing the tendon and dividing it lengthwise into two halves. The two ends of the cut tendon are joined to create a longer, single tendon. The lengthened tendons reduce the tension of the muscle, thus reducing muscle tightness. It is usually done at the same time as other orthopedic procedures. Immobility is encouraged during a post-operative recovery period.

- *Adductor release:* The adductors muscles of the thigh attach the pubis to the femurs in the groin. The release involves cutting the tendon, releasing it from the bone. The procedure is done to correct scissoring, hip subluxation, or hip dislocation (Massachusetts General Hospital Orthopaedics, 2012).

- *Hamstring release:* The hamstring muscles (three muscles of the posterior thigh - semimembranous, semitendinosus, and gracilis) connect the pelvis to the back of the knee. In a hamstring release procedure, the tendons between the pelvis and the back of the knee are lengthened or cut. The procedure is done to correct contractures that prevent the child from standing straight and taking long steps when walking.

- *Achilles tendon release:* This procedure can be done percutaneously, unless done previously. The procedure can correct contractures that cause the child to walk on his or her toes, which leads to back-kneeing or a severe flat foot over time.

- *Posterior tibial tendon transfer:* This is done when the foot positions inward, causing the child to trip and fall and preventing ankle-foot orthosis (AFO) fitting. The posterior tibial tendon is split longitudinally; one half is placed on the outside of the foot and the other half remains where it normally attaches. Casting or bracing is used post-operatively to provide immobility during healing.

- *Osteotomy:* The upper end of the femur is cut and the bone is redirected to point to the hip joint in the correct direction followed by placement of a metal plate and screws or placement in a hip spica cast or both. The procedure is done to correct a persistent hip dislocation that can lead to scoliosis.

- *Spinal fusion:* This procedure is done to correct scoliosis. A fusion is done if the scoliosis is greater than 60 degrees. (A thoracolumbosacral orthosis can be used to correct scoliosis under 40 degrees.) Surgery is done in two parts: 1) straightening the spine with rigid rods and 2) adding a bone graft (bone plugs usually taken from the pelvis) to the curved area of the spine to fuse in the correct position. The spine is not completely straightened, but it is noticeably straighter. The risks associated with fusion include rod displacement, infection, pseudoarthrosis, nerve damage, and rod discomfort. The benefits of performing a fusion procedure must outweigh these risks.

Neurosurgical Procedures.

Selective dorsal rhizotomy (SDR) is often recommended (Cole et al., 2007). During this procedure, the nerve roots that cause spasticity are isolated and severed. There are established indications, contraindications, and candidate selection criteria for SDR for spastic diplegia (Cole et al., 2007).

Patient selection is a team effort. The team must confirm the diagnosis and identify spasticity as the predominant feature of the child's condition. Realistic goals must be established, and it is of utmost importance to determine the child's and family's motivation to comply consistently with therapeutic demands. The goal of SDR is to avoid the need for additional future orthopedic surgeries because spasticity has been eliminated. Studies continue to gather data to validate the end results of the surgery (Cole et al., 2007).

During SDR, the anesthesiologist uses a very short-acting muscular paralytic agent; an electromyogram (EMG) must be recorded as well (Cole et al., 2007). A physical therapist and neurophysiologist assist the neurosurgeon to examine the stimulated muscle groups before severing the related roots. Finally, a laminotomy is performed and fixation is accomplished with a plate and screws (Cole et al., 2007). Post-op care includes intensive therapy programs.

Dental Care and Treatment

Cerebral palsy itself does not cause unique oral abnormalities; however, there are several dental conditions that are more common or more severe than in the general population (So. Association of Dentists, 2001). The child with CP and the conditions listed below will benefit from regular dental visits and ongoing education in adaptive oral care techniques and medication therapy. Direct the caregivers to the National Institute of Dental and Craniofacial Research (NIDCR) for tips to assist with routine oral hygiene.

Some children with CP will require sedation for oral examinations and dental procedures. Dentists are available that specialize in the oral care of individuals with special needs; contact the American Dental Association or local dental society for more information. Common conditions include:

- *Periodontal disease:* The causes are related to inadequate oral hygiene and complications associated with oral habits, physical abilities, and malocclusion. Gingival hyperplasia may be due to certain medications, notably phenytoin (Dilantin) (So. Association of Dentists, 2001).

- *Dental caries:* Caused by inadequate oral hygiene. Other risk factors include mouth breathing, side effects of certain medications, enamel hypoplasia (incomplete calcification), and food pouching. Spasticity of the jaw may also make it difficult to open the child's mouth sufficient to provide adequate tooth brushing. In such cases, more frequent professional cleaning by a dentist or dental hygienist is indicated (So. Association of Dentists, 2001).

- *Bruxism*: Caused by spasticity of the jaw.

- *Malocclusion*: This problem is not only in the teeth being misaligned but also in the underlying musculoskeletal problem. The child with a malocclusion will require an evaluation by an orthodontist and may be a candidate for orthodontic treatment (So. Association of Dentists, 2001).

- *Dysphagia*: Difficulty with swallowing can cause food to linger longer in the mouth causing an increased risk for caries. Foods commonly prepared for children with dysphagia are semi-soft and tend to adhere to the teeth. Coughing, gagging, choking, and aspiration are other related concerns.

- *Drooling*: Those with CP may have an inability to manage saliva, causing saliva to flow outside of the mouth

- *Hyperactive bite and gag reflexes*

- *Trauma and injury*: Falls and accidents may require immediate professional attention to mouth and teeth

Nursing Diagnoses To Consider
- *Imbalanced Nutrition: Less than Body Requirements*: Intake of nutrients insufficient to meet metabolic needs.
- *Impaired Swallowing:* Abnormal functioning of the swallowing mechanism associated with deficits in oral, pharyngeal, or esophageal structure or function.
- *Deficient Fluid Volume*: Decreased intravascular, interstitial, and/or intracellular fluid.

Epilepsy

The literature indicates that 15% to 60% of the children with CP have seizures (Abdel-Hamid et al., 2011). Although epilepsy and cerebral palsy are separate disorders, seizures are not uncommon in those with severe motor problems, especially spastic CP. Some of the seizure types include the following:

- *Petit mal seizures*: These can be very subtle and may not be detected. The individual looks as if he is staring but is actually experiencing a loss of consciousness. The individual will not remember anything that occurred during this period.

- *Psychomotor seizures:* These are involuntary repetitive behaviors, such as chewing of the lips or hand rubbing. The individual may also have unusual sensory experiences or become angry or fearful during an episode.

- *Focal seizures:* Motor or sensory seizures that affect one side of the body. There may be a loss of consciousness.

- *Partial complex seizures:* Behavioral or emotional symptoms, brief loss of consciousness, or a loss of memory is experienced. Temporal lobe and frontal lobe seizures are partial complex seizures.

- *Grand mal seizures* (tonic-clonic): The most common form of seizure seen in CP, these involve the entire body. The limbs first stiffen (tonic) then jerk (clonic). This is often followed by a post-ictal period, usually five to thirty minutes, during which the individual displays drowsiness and confusion.

Epilepsy management varies but may include antiepileptic medications, surgery, vagus nerve stimulation (VNS), ketogenic diet, and other complimentary or alternative treatments (Kinney, 2012; Epilepsy Foundation, 2013). It is important that the physician (primary or specialist) is advised of any treatments used to manage the individual's seizures, including over-the-counter remedies. Management is aimed at enhancing the quality of life for the individual.

Antiepileptic Medications
Some children require medication to control their seizure activity. At times, a combination of two antiepileptics may be required in order to maintain stability. It is important to note that the U.S. Food and Drug Administration has not approved the use of all antiepileptic medications in children under sixteen years of age (FDA 2013).

It is also important to remember that as with all medications, there are potential side effects. Certain medications require routine or periodic serum level monitoring. For example, liver function tests and a complete blood count should be monitored in children on clonazepam (Klonopin) (Skidmore-Roth, 2012). Commonly used antiepileptic medications include:

- Carbamazepine (Tegretol)
- Gabapentin (Neurontin)
- Lamotrigine (Lamictal)
- Levetiracetam (Keppra)
- Oxcarbazepine (Trileptal)
- Phenytoin (Dilantin)
- Tiagabine (Gabitril)
- Topiramate (Topamax)
- Zonisamide (Zonegran)
- Felbamate (Felbatol)

Surgery

Surgery may be considered when seizures cannot be controlled with medication. There is no guarantee that surgery will be successful in controlling seizures. State-of-the-technology is applied to perform the safest and least-invasive procedure possible.

Vagus Nerve Stimulation

Vagus nerve stimulation is designed to stop seizures by sending regular, mild pulses of electrical energy to the brain via the vagus nerve, acting like a pacemaker for the brain (Fisher and Handforth, 1999). Implantation of the device is a surgical procedure that requires general anesthesia, carrying the same risks of any general anesthesia. Studies show promising results in children. In one study, six out of 19 had 90% cure of their seizures. Studies continue to determine which types of seizure are best controlled with VNS (Fisher and Handforth, 1999; Kinney, 2012).

Ketogenic Diet.

The ketogenic diet is sometimes used in conjunction with antiepileptic medications. This diet consists of a high-fat, low-carbohydrate diet. The theory as to the success of the diet on seizures is its ability to produce ketones in the body; it is not known why ketones are effective in controlling seizures. A doctor prescribes the diet, and a dietician should monitor the child. A ketogenic diet is not a long-term solution for seizure control. It is typically used for no more than one to two years (FDA, 2013).

Complementary and Alternative Medicines.

In theory, most individuals use alternative therapy along with conventional treatments. Many people, including physicians and nurses, consider complementary and alternative medicines valuable. However, caution should be taken when considering using herbal medicine to control seizures. Some reports note that some herbs may lower the seizure threshold and that individuals with epilepsy have shown untoward effects from herbal medicines when compared with other populations (Spinella, 2001). Consult with the primary physician or neurologist before considering herbal therapy.

Psychological Care and Treatment

Psychologists work with the children, families, groups, and community service systems to learn the complex issues that affect the growth and development of the child with CP. Psychological support helps to improve a sense of well-being to ease the patient's and family's worries, resolve problems and feelings of guilt, and increase the ability of the child, family, and those that connect with them to ultimately manage their own problems and make good and healthy decisions. There are many situations and emotions that an individual with CP may face; some of the most common are:

- A sense of being different
- Frustration with lack of body control

- Inability to communicate needs
- Lack of independence, especially during natural life transitions
- Embarrassment
- Feelings of inadequacy, feeling "just not good enough"
- Sexuality

All children with special needs will do their best when they form healthy attitudes towards themselves. This said, each child must be given the opportunity to speak freely with a psychologist or therapist about problems and receive guidance and tools to reach and maintain a healthy self-image.

There are many categories of therapists that can assist children with special needs and their families.

- *Counselors* tend to focus on specific current life problems, while psychotherapists usually deal with old "hurts" and personal issues in order to bring about profound changes in a current situation.
- *Psychotherapists* also encourage the development of potential.
- *Behavioral therapists* can work with physical therapists on techniques that encourage muscular and motor development.
- *Social workers* are often overlooked but are invaluable in assisting families obtain resources for care.

Many different approaches are used in therapy. Although there is a wide range of disability with the individuals with CP, remember that these individuals are no different emotionally from any other patients.

- *Humanistic* therapy addresses the growth of self through self-examination and the creative process.
- *Psychodynamic* therapy helps the individuals to understand the roots of their emotional distress.

- *Cognitive behavioral* therapy utilizes powerful tools that make connections between behavior and thinking patterns.

The category or title of the therapist is not as important as is choosing the right person, one that the child likes and can work with comfortably. The following criteria must be evaluated to seek a successful outcome in therapy: skill level of the therapist, child and family's comfort level with the therapist, and the child's and family's degree of motivation.

Family members also experience situations and feelings about a child or sibling being disabled. They also need the opportunity to work with counseling professionals to resolve issues that can cause social isolation, stress, and depression (Williams et al., 2003).

Studies reveal that while siblings of severely disabled children do not typically experience major depression, they do often manifest excess depressive affect and social isolation (Breslau and Prabucki, 1987). Studies also report that siblings of children with chronic illness or disability have a 1.6 to 2.0 times higher risk for behavioral and mental health problems (Williams, P. et al., 2003). A dose-response relationship to intervention was found and treatment gains were sustained over a period of 12 months (Williams et al., 2003).

Excess depressive symptoms were also observed in mothers of disabled children. In addition to counseling, family members, especially mothers, should be encouraged to seek formal or informal support groups (Williams et al., 2003).

Respite care is often overlooked but it is essential for the families and loved ones who often are provide continuous care without little relief. Respite care appears to result in a reduction of psychological distress.

It is important to monitor the quality of care and treatment of children with special needs as they are particularly vulnerable to abuse and neglect. For people with disabilities who require the care of others to meet their basic daily needs, neglect is as abusive as any direct physical, sexual, or verbal abuse.

Whether and how the child's emotional needs are met must also be evaluated and monitored. If the child is receiving good physical care but is no attention to emotional and psychological condition, emotional abuse is an issue. Emotional abuse and neglect can take place in any setting. Providing education and information as to how to meet the physical and emotional needs of the individual child and their disability is the most effective tool to prevent abuse (Williams et al., 2003).

If abuse is suspected, state laws require notification of Child Protective Services. Help is available from the Childhelp USA National Child Abuse Hotline at 1-800-422-4453, or visit the National Clearinghouse on Child Abuse and Neglect at https://www.childwelfare.gov.

Nursing Diagnoses To Consider:
- *Impaired Verbal Communication*: Decreased, delayed or absent ability to receive, process, transmit, and/or use a system of symbols.
- *Risk for Compromised Human Dignity:* At risk for perceived loss of respect and honor.
- *Risk for Loneliness:* At risk for experiencing discomfort associated with a desire or need for more contact with others.
- *Risk for Disturbed Personal Identity:* Risk for the inability to maintain an integrated and complete perception of self.
- *Risk for Chronic Low Self-Esteem*: At risk for longstanding negative self evaluating feelings about self or self-capabilities.

- *Disturbed Body Image:* Confusion in mental picture of one's physical self.
- *Risk for Caregiver Role Strain:* At risk for caregiver vulnerability for felt difficulty in performing the family caregiver role.
- *Dysfunctional Family Processes:* Psychosocial, spiritual, and physiological functions of the family unit are chronically disorganized, which leads to conflict, denial of problems, resistance to change, ineffective problem solving, and a series of self-perpetuating crises.
- *Sexual Dysfunction:* The state in which an individual experiences a change in sexual function during the sexual response phases of desire, excitation, and/or orgasm, which is viewed as unsatisfying, unrewarding, or inadequate.

Aging and Outcomes

Persons with CP may see an accelerated decline in functioning as they age (CPIRF, 2008). They may experience the signs of aging earlier in their lives, and to a greater degree. This is known as *secondary aging*, changes brought about by disuse or disease (*Scope UK*, 2011).

Many factors contribute to secondary aging in persons with CP. Altered posture due to contracture or spine deformity, confinement to a wheelchair, altered gait secondary to weakness or spasticity, and lack of exercise due to pain or fatigue are just a few. These conditions can contribute to decreased ability to function at an earlier age than those in the general population (*Scope UK*, 2011).

Symptoms of premature aging in persons with CP can sometimes begin in the late 20s or early 30s (Cox, Weze, and Lewis, 2005). These signs and symptoms may include:

- Increased muscle pain
- Early onset arthritis
- Osteoporosis due to decreased mobility

- Muscle wasting
- Bladder retention or incontinence
- Dental problems related to poor dental care in early life
- Pressure ulcers related to bed or wheelchair confinement
- Side effects associated with long-term use of medications

Decreased physical strength, decreased manual dexterity, and increased dysarthria can cause premature loss of achieved functional skills. This can lead to increased dependence upon caregivers and overall decreased ability to live and work independently in society. This can have even further implications such as loss of self-esteem, loss of confidence, anxiety, and depression.

Life Care Planning Considerations

Although persons with CP may experience early aging changes, life expectancy is increasing. According to the United Cerebral Palsy Foundation, except for those persons with CP who are gravely impaired at birth, life expectancy of persons with CP is approaching that of the general population (*Scope UK*, 2011).

This has great significance for the nurse preparing a life care plan for a child with CP. The focus of the initial plan may be to obtain medical care, therapy, and assistive devices to optimize independence and function. Consideration must be given, however, to the ongoing needs into and throughout adulthood. The fact that CP is not a progressive disease can lead to the misconception that motor impairments or secondary conditions will also remain static over time. This is often not the case; progressive, premature, and accelerated functional status decline is often noted.

The wide range of impairment in CP creates a unique challenge for the nurse life care planner. It would be difficult at the time of birth, early childhood, or young adolescence to determine how much secondary impairment will present in adulthood, how much these secondary conditions will influence independent function, or discern need for medical interventions far into the child's future. It is imperative, however, that the nurse life care planner consider the likelihood of secondary conditions in adulthood, and address the most probable impairment based on the areas and degree of impairment present in infancy and childhood.

For example, a child with spastic diplegic CP with significant alteration in gait during childhood can be likely to develop a decreased mobility related to pain and fatigue in adulthood. Periodic PT evaluations with short-term treatment for gait correction would be appropriate. Mobility aides such as a walker and wheelchair for longer distances would be appropriately anticipated.

Not all adults with CP will require assistance in ADLs. Some will function independently with use of adaptive aids or assistive devices. Others may require adaptive aids, assistive devices, and personal assistance. The nurse life care planner must consider the unique abilities and limitations of each person with CP when developing and updating the life care plan.

Perhaps the biggest challenges to carrying out activities of daily living in adulthood are those presented by musculoskeletal impairments. These can manifest as decreased mobility, decreased motor function, osteoporosis, increased fatigability, increased pain, and contractures (Tosi et al., 2009). Using the nursing process to assess the impairment can help the nurse life care planner choose assistive technologies to support optimum functioning.

For example, the adult may have increased pain and fatigue related to excessive wear and tear on the joints, resulting in altered gait, frequent falls, and inability to complete basic ADLs. This individual may benefit from use of a wheelchair to maintain mobility to slow further musculoskeletal compromise. Physical therapy for strengthening exercises and gait improvement may be appropriate to help reverse muscle atrophy and/or contracture, decrease weakness, and increase coordination. Psychological intervention may be appropriate to help with coping strategies. All of these interventions should be addressed in the life care plan to help slow disability progression and maximize rehabilitation, including routine interventions throughout the lifespan depending upon the nature and severity of any assessed problems.

In addition to a routine annual primary care evaluation, the adult with CP would benefit from evaluation by physiatry or specialists in cerebral palsy and other areas to identify developing problems and possibly intervene before they result in further limitation. Other specialty areas which may be appropriate, and should be addressed in the individual life care plan based on disability present, include, but are not limited to:

- Urologist
- Neurologist
- Orthopedic surgeon
- Psychologist
- Psychiatrist
- Occupational therapist
- Speech therapist
- Ophthalmologist,
- Otolaryngologist
- Vocational counselor (perhaps)

The most common problems in adults with CP include:

- *Genitourinary complaints*, e.g., incontinence in females and spasticity in both males and females. These can lead to urinary retention and kidney involvement. Urology evaluation, education in bladder management and bladder training, if possible and appropriate, could be incorporated into the life care plan.

- *Oral-motor problems* can result in difficulty chewing or swallowing. This can be compounded by secondary dental problems related to lack of early dental care.

- *Communication* can also be an issue due to decreased breath control, processing difficulties, or hearing loss.

- *Gastrointestinal problems* such as diverticulosis, constipation, and hemorrhoids may be related to neurological abnormality, decreased physical activity, or dietary influences due to oral-motor problems.

- *Medication side effects*

- *Sexuality and reproduction:* Though persons with CP can have intimate relationships, including marriage and the birth of children, physical mobility problems, spasticity, contracture, and pain can present problems.

- *Psychosocial issues* that pertain to the adult with CP can be related to loss of function, decreasing an individual's ability to perform at work, resulting in a loss of income as well as insurance benefits. Increased dependence on others for assistance can cause anxiety and depression.

Both primary impairment and secondary conditions can affect level of independence. Some persons will be able to live and work independently with little or no assistance, while others may require an assisted living environment with supportive employment. Still others may require more hands-on assistance or total care, and be unable work at all.

Programs available for the latter two categories have limited funding. The United Cerebral Palsy Association notes that waiting lists for assisted living and sheltered employment for adults with CP can be up to five years from the date of application.

Government funding through the Department of Health and Human Services may offer aid in the form of transportation, medication and case management, but again, waiting lists may be long and funding for assistance can be very difficult to procure. It is important for the life care planner to address all anticipated needs for the adult with CP (medical care and medications, assistive technologies, and living/work environments). The NLCP realistically assesses the availability of all community and government resources, which can help meet these needs in presenting a comprehensive life care plan outlining the needs and associated costs over the lifespan.

References

Abdel-Hamid HZ, et al. (2011, December 9). Cerebral palsy. Retrieved from http://emedicine.medscape.com/ article/1179555-overview

American Academy of Pediatrics. (2012). Home page. Retrieved from http://www.aap.org

Ashwal BS, Blasco PA et al. (2004) Practice Parameter: Diagnostic assessment of the child with cerebral palsy: Report of the Quality Standards Committee of the American Academy of Neurology and the Practice Committee of the Child Neurology Society. Neurology (62) 851-863

Baker F and Roth EA. (2004) Neuroplasticity and functional recovery: training models and compensatory strategies in music therapy. Nordic Journal of Music Therapy Volume 13 Issue 1.

Bond NJ and Trautwein LP. (2011) The Role of the Pediatric Care Manager in Life Care Planning. In Riddick-Grisham S and Deming LM, Editors, Pediatric Life Care Planning and Case Management. 2nd Edition. Boca Raton, FL. Taylor and Francis Group.

Breslau N and Prabucki K. (1987). Siblings of disabled children: Effects of chronic stress in the family. Archives of General Psychiatry, 44(12), 1040-1046.

Cerebral Palsy International Research Foundation. (2008, January 1). Aging and cerebral palsy. Retrieved from http://www.cpirf.org/stories/465

Charles JR, Wolf SL., et al. (2007, February). Efficacy of a child-friendly form of constraint induced movement therapy in hemoplegic cerebral palsy: a randomized control trial. Developmental Medicine and Child Neurology.

Cole GF, Farmer SE, et al. (2007). Selective dorsal rhizotomy for children with cerebral palsy: the Oswestry experience. Archives of Diseases in Childhood, 92(9), 781-785.

Cox, D., Weze, C., and Lewis, C. (2005, July). Cerebral palsy and ageing: A systematic review. London, United Kingdom: Scope. Retrieved from http://www.scope.org.uk/sites/default/files/pdfs/CP%20and%20Ageing.pdf

Dursun E, Dursun N, and Alican D. (2004). Effects of biofeedback treatment on gait in children with cerebral palsy. Disability and Rehabilitation, 26(2), 116-120.

Epilepsy Foundation (2013) Retrieved from http://www.epilepsyfoundation.org/aboutepilepsy/treatment/ketogenicdiet/index.cfm?gclid=CJDNyID117gCFUyk4Ao dT1cAYQ

Fisher RS and Handforth A. (1999). Reassessment: Vagus nerve stimulation for epilepsy. A report of the therapeutics and technology assessment subcommittee of the American Academy of Neurology. Neurology, 53, 666-669.

Kinney SK (2012) Vagus nerve therapy for seizure control. Journal of Nurse Life Care Planning, XII.2, 613-617

Leonard JM, Cozens et al. (2011). Should children with cerebral palsy and normal imaging undergo testing for inherited metabolic disorders? Developmental Medicine and Child Neurology, 53(3), 198-199.

March of Dimes. (2007, December). Cerebral palsy. Retrieved from http://www.marchofdimes.com/baby/birthdefects_cerebralpalsy.html

March of Dimes. (2013). Retrieved from http://www.marchofdimes.com/mission/what-we-know-about-prematurity.aspx

Massachusetts General Hospital Orthopaedics. (2012). Adductor release for athletic groin pain. Retrieved from http://www2.massgeneral.org/sports/protocols/Adductor%20release%20rehabilitation%0protocol.pdf

MyChild with Cerebral Palsy. (2012a). History and origin of cerebral palsy. Retrieved from http://cerebralpalsy.org/about-cerebral-palsy/history-and-origin-of-cerebral-palsy/

MyChild with Cerebral Palsy. (2012b). Prevalence and incidence of cerebral palsy. Retrieved from http://cerebralpalsy.org/about-cerebral-palsy/prevalence-of-cerebral-palsy/

MyChild with Cerebral Palsy. (2012c). Cause of cerebral palsy. Retrieved from http://cerebralpalsy.org/about-cerebral-palsy/cause/

NIND, National Institute of Neurological Disorders and Stroke. (2011, October 4). Cerebral palsy: Hope through research. Retrieved from http://www.ninds.nih.gov/disorders/cerebral_palsy/detail_cerebral_palsy.htm#179333104

Sankar C and Mundkur N. (2005). Cerebral palsy—definition, classification, etiology, and early diagnosis. Indian Journal of Pediatrics 72, 865-868.

Scope UK. (2011, April). Ageing and cerebral palsy. Retrieved from http://www.scope.org.uk/help-and-information/cerebral-palsy/ageing-and-cerebral-palsy

Skidmore-Roth, L. (2012). Nursing drug handbook 2012. Philadelphia, PA: Lippincott Williams and Wilkins

Southern Association of Institutional Dentists. (2001). Cerebral palsy: A review for dental professionals. Retrieved from http://saiddent.org/modules/12_module4.pdf

Spinella M. (2001). Herbal medicines and epilepsy: The potential for benefit and adverse effects. Epilepsy and Behavior, 2, 524-532.

Tosi LL, Maher N, et al. (2009). Adults with cerebral palsy: A workshop to define the challenges of treating and preventing secondary musculoskeletal and neuromuscular complications in this rapidly growing population. Developmental Medicine and Child Neurology, 51(Suppl 4), 2-11.

United Cerebral Palsy. (n.d.). The diagnosis of cerebral palsy. Retrieved from http://affnet.ucp.org/ucp_generaldoc. cfm/1/11654/11654/11654-11654/3968

U. S. Food and Drug Administration (2013) Retrieved from http://google2.fda.gov/search?q=children+and+anticon vulsantsandclient=FDAgovandsite=FDAgovandlr=andpr oxystylesheet=FDAgovandoutput=xml_no_dtdandgetfiel ds=*andrequiredfields=-archive%3AYes

Wang CJ, McGlynn EA et al. (2006). Quality-of-care indicators for the neurodevelopmental follow-up of very low birth weight children: Results of an expert panel process. Pediatrics, 117(6), 2080-2092.

Williams PD, Williams AR et al. (2003). A community-based intervention for siblings and parents of children with chronic illness or disability: The ISEE study. The Journal of Pediatrics, 143(3), 386-393.

Wingert, J. R., Burton, H., Sinclair, R. J., Brunstrom, J. E., and Damiano, D. L. (2008, September). Tactile sensory abilities in cerebral palsy: deficit in roughness and object discrimination. Developmental Medicine and Child Neurology.

CHAPTER 7

Age-Related Issues in Life Care Planning

Shelene Giles MS, BSN, BA, RN, CRC, CNLCP, CLCP, MSCC, LNCC
Barbara Krasa, RN, BSN, CNLCP, MSCC
Jackie Morris RN, BSN, CRRN, CNLCP
April Pettengill RN, CRRN, CDMS, CNLCP, MSCC
Anne Sambucini, RN, CCM, CDMS, CNLCP, MSC-C
Joan Schofield, BSN, MBA, RN, CNLCP
Nancy Zangmeister, RN, CRRN, CCM, CLCP, MSCC, CNLCP
Ginger Walton, MSN, RN, CNLCP, contributor

Introduction

The nurse life care planner has extensive training in nursing care across the continuum of life through nursing skills in healthcare, specialized training in case management, and life care planning education classes. Although many nurse life care planners specialize in pediatrics or elder care, all nurse life care planners consider care needs throughout the life span. This chapter discusses age-related concerns and considerations for care throughout the life span. The initial section focuses on the special needs for children and young adults. The second looks at the effect of aging on body systems and particular conditions often seen in life care planning for the adult through end of life. Nursing diagnoses will be found in other chapters of this book as noted in the individual sections.

Section One: Pediatric Considerations

Note: This section uses the words "parent" and "family" to include other family members or individuals who may be primary caregivers, parent surrogates, guardians or custodians. Many applicable nursing diagnoses may be found in the chapter on Cerebral Palsy.

Pediatric life care plans project care extending through adulthood. Therefore, preparing a life care plan for a child requires an understanding of pediatric growth and development principles and evidence-based research on aging with disability. The nurse life care planner examines the effect of a child's illness or injury on ability to function in the context of growth and achievement of developmental milestones.

Parents of a child with special needs may have just learned their child's diagnosis, relocated, or recently identified new needs to identify potential healthcare specialists. Nurse life care planners may be called upon to draft an initial life care plan within a relatively short period after the child's injury, diagnosis, or confirmation of special needs. Life care plan revisions may be requested periodically.

Effective, efficient, and coordinated healthcare service delivery is a vital component of pediatric life care planning. Various parties involved or concerned with the child's plan of care may seek out a pediatric nurse life care planner for consultative and case management services. Trust officers, estate attorneys, guardians and conservators may notice shortcomings in the existing plan of care and seek the nurse life care planner's knowledge of local and regional healthcare specialists so the child has greater opportunities to develop a meaningful life and prevent potential complications. Both child and family may benefit from a comprehensive assessment process, identification of additional interventions, updated resources and healthcare providers, or an updated care plan to allocate available financial resources more efficiently.

Designing a pediatric nurse life care plan begins with a solid understanding of pediatric rehabilitation. According to the Association of Rehabilitation Nurses, the nurse's goal is to collaborate with the child's team of healthcare providers and family to provide for a continuum of care from onset of injury or illness through adulthood.

The goal of the rehabilitation process is for children, regardless of their disability or chronic illness, to function at their maximum potential and to become contributing members to both their families and society. Physical, emotional, social, cultural, educational, developmental, and spiritual dimensions are all considered in a holistic approach to care. (ARN, 2010)

Providing for care during chronologic and developmental stages is the basis for the pediatric life care plan from childhood through adulthood. The pediatric nurse life care planner should possess a detailed knowledge of normal development and interventions to promote optimum function. Acute and chronic illnesses and developmental, acquired, and traumatic injuries can affect normal growth and development patterns. Nursing assessment skills and standardized tools can be helpful during data collection. For example, advance research on available care facilities for childhood and adult years assists with long-term planning, budgeting, and resource allocation for the time when parents as primary caregivers are no longer available and the child will need residential or facility living supports as an adult.

A good mix of case management and nurse life care planner knowledge, skills, and expertise allows for continuous care plan updates and the implementation. This chapter incorporates the concepts of growth, development, and illness or injury in the conceptual framework of Marjory Gordon's Functional Health Patterns (Gordon, Manual of Nursing Diagnostics, 2010). The nurse life care planner adds nursing diagnoses to identify functional impairments and risks for the child, combining this with knowledge of the medical diagnoses to formulate an individualized plan for the child.

Health Perception and Management
A child's ability to perceive and manage his own health is dependent on his developmental level and cognitive

ability. When appropriate, the nurse life care planner should incorporate the child's perception of his health and goals in the planning process. Including family members' perceptions, especially parents', is also critical. The parents' ability to care for their child must be identified. Do one or both parents intend to work outside the home? Does one or both of the parents intend to be the primary full-time, around-the-clock caregiver(s)? Would it be best to provide for a certain number of hours of respite per month, and/or or budget for a discrete number of weeks per year of respite? What agencies, facilities or paid trained family/friends would be available to serve in this capacity? In certain cases, hiring a home nurse or health aide may be necessary (Riddick-Grisham and Deming, 2011).

- All caregivers need to be trained about the child's complex care needs
- In addition to family caregivers, children need paid professional caregivers to participate in their care
- All family caregivers need annual hours of respite care services
- Children who are unable to maintain their own airway patency and/or have other frequent interventions around the clock need an awake and alert caregiver every night.
- Children with complex healthcare needs can attend school in the community.

Grisham and Deming (2011) recognize that "the child is an integral part of the family system in which home and family are the child's world." They further define the family-centered care philosophy as "the family and child (being) involved in all phases of care including full participation in the multi-disciplinary team." When assessing the child, the nurse life care planner will identify long-term and short-term goals for both child and family.

Health management may be affected by the psychological and physical health of the parents and primary caregivers. Families of special needs children report a number of internal and external factors contributing to high stress levels (Ergüner-Tekinalp and Akkök, 2004; Goddard, Lehr, and Lapadat, 2000; Heiman, 2002; Hensley, 2007). Internal factors include

- Shock
- Depression
- Guilt
- Anger
- Confusion
- Blaming themselves as the cause of the child's disability
- Inadequate parenting and coping skills
- Hopelessness about the future

External factors include:
- Lack of trust in providers and the healthcare system
- Limited personal time
- Stereotypes and blame expressed by others
- Expense of care and impact on family finances
- Inadequate information regarding available resources.

Professional counseling and support groups may be useful to help the family deal with the effects of the day-to-day demands.

The nurse life care planner will assess how a family manages the child's complex healthcare needs. They may be relying upon the guidance of a primary physician. Others may have set up an elaborate system of medical and therapy specialists. The degree to which there has been communication among the healthcare team members is an indicator of the extent of care coordination. The assessment visit is an opportunity to offer recommendations for accessing specialty care unknown to the family, or to provide suggestions for care coordination to facilitate communication between disciplines. The nurse can help the parents begin this process by modeling how a professional nurse institutes communication among healthcare team members to gather information and come to consensus as to needs.

Critical thinking and evidence-based standards come into play when drafting an individualized plan of care. Specialty care frequency will vary with the child's health status, disability, medical and nursing diagnoses, and physical, cognitive and developmental level. Current or past utilization frequency may or may not be indicative of future needs.

The care planner should be prepared to explain how and why the resulting home care recommendations exceed that of the child's age peers, e.g., why to provide additional toys and equipment that address the child's functional impairments and budget for respite allocations.

Nutritional-Metabolic

Feeding skills development -the ability to suck, swallow, and coordinate these processes with breathing in an organized, coordinated fashion- begins at 34 to 35 weeks gestation. By nine months of age, the child can control the movement of food in the mouth via rotary chewing. A one year old can typically chew chopped and cooked table foods. Tolerance for all food textures is usually achieved by three years of age when oral motor skills have fully matured (ASHA, 2013). Assessing where a child is at along this continuum as compared to age-peers provides useful information for future planning.

The pediatric life care planner should recognize that nutrition and feeding patterns affect health, wellness, growth and development. Assessment and identification of appropriate interventions, including referrals to consultations with therapists, dietitians/nutritionists, and medical specialists, are expected. The use of a multidisciplinary treatment team or clinic to treat feeding disorders and nutritional problems is ideal. Referral to a pediatric rehabilitation center or specialty clinic may be necessary. If the child is under three years of age, early intervention therapists may be including treatments directed towards problems with feeding.

Consider whether the child will likely have greater or less than usual metabolic needs. Children with hypotonicity, delayed mobility or immobility, and decreased physical activity often have lower caloric needs. Fevers, infection, wounds, and some movement disorders may require increased caloric intake (Kuperminc MN and Stevenson RD 2008). (*Please see Chapter 6, Cerebral Palsy, for more information.*)

Actual or potential malnutrition is a consideration and interventions should be identified if there are chronic feeding difficulties. If the child's growth chart is not available in the received medical records, plotting of height and weight on a gender specific growth chart can be a useful assessment tool. Malnutrition can impair normal brain and skeletal development as well as achievement of developmental milestones. A 2001 study by Schwarz et al. found that matching the treatment of a feeding disorder with the specific diagnosis for the feeding problem will significantly improve the child's consumption of energy, overall nutritional status, and may result in a decrease in morbidity as evidenced by a lower acute care hospitalization rate.

Many children with neurological disabilities have abnormal muscle tone, reflexes, and coordination. The resulting oral sensorimotor deficits impair normal oral processing of both liquid and solid foods. Signs of sensory neurodevelopmental feeding related dysfunction include (ASHA 2013):

- Oral hyper-and hyposensitivity,
- Excessive or absent gagging
- Oral-motor incoordination
- History of aspiration pneumonia
- Slow growth not caused by a known illness or other condition.

Consultation for swallowing evaluation, typically with a speech and language pathologist (SLP) with a specialty in feeding disorders, should be included in the plan. Children with cerebral palsy are at especially high risk for feeding difficulties, reported to be as high as an 80% prevalence rate (Rogers, et al, 1994), with aspiration occurring in about 25% of these children (Arvedson and Brodsky, 2002). Poor head, trunk, and neck control and misalignment may cause feeding difficulties.

Children diagnosed with gastroesophageal reflex (GER) often associate feedings with discomfort and therefore resist feedings. Conditions linked to GER include low birth weight, neurologic conditions causing hypo-and hypertonicity, spasticity, and chronic respiratory disease. A pediatric surgeon, gastroenterologist, or pediatrician can opine whether medications, fundoplication, or placement of a gastrostomy feeding tube is likely in the future, if not already in use.

Note whether the child is able to feed himself. A neurotypical child will start some finger foods before one year of age, progressing to utensil use and a variety of food textures. Motor, sensory, and cognitive impairments may delay self-feeding. Indeed, some children may not develop the ability to self-feed if fed by a caregiver. Medical information, therapy notes, and if available, the results of a video fluoroscopic swallow study can help the nurse life care planner to assess feeding ability, the safety of oral feedings, and the impact on the child's long term care needs.

Children who are fed orally and do not maintain steady growth or who lose weight will need an alternate form of feeding. Gastrostomy tube feeding is often recommended and is the first choice of alternative feeding for children who cannot be sustained by oral intake alone (Kleinman RE, 2004). If it is safe to feed the child orally at all, the tube feedings may serve as a supplement. The nurse life care planner should understand the goals of feeding with each child, as well as the medical likelihood of achieving those goals to anticipate equipment needs and associated costs. If a child is so neurologically impaired that complete oral nutritional intake is unlikely, his equipment and care needs will differ from one who is recovering from a temporary setback due to an acute change in condition.

If the child is to be on enteral feedings, medical supplies must be estimated over the expected duration of the therapy, perhaps for life expectancy. Feeding pumps and related supplies, bolus feeding supplies, gastronomy supplies and the cost of nutritional formulas are items for possible inclusion. Nutritionists and dieticians can offer guidelines for expected long-term caloric and nutritional needs and supplies to support childhood growth and maintenance requirements in adulthood. The cost of prepared nutritional supplements varies widely depending on caloric concentration and additives. A child could need a nutritional supplement at a higher cost temporarily until their needs are met. The nurse life care planner will need to consider whether a more routine formulation will more likely be used in later years, a factor which will alter the line item budgeting of this need over the lifetime.

Enteral feeding pumps can be rented and maintained by a rental agency or be a purchased item. The cost and benefit of rental as opposed to purchase of equipment should be assessed on an individual basis. Nursing literature, a gastroenterologist, or pediatric surgeon may be able to predict whether the typical pediatric Mic-Key button system will eventually need replacement by a conventional adult type gastrostomy system (Altman, 2003).

Consultation and regular follow-up with a SLP feeding specialist is often helpful. A feeding specialist who has worked with a child can usually answer questions and offer opinions for the long-term plan for feeding and nutritional care. Issues include (Arvedson, 1998):

- Whether the child will likely be able to acquire sufficient oral feeding skills to rely solely on table foods for nutrition
- Whether supplemental feedings will likely be necessary long-term
- What positioning aids will facilitate feeding
- What supports and resources for family education and training are available

Inclusion of specific interventional services, such as a multidisciplinary feeding clinic, speech therapist, feeding specialist, nutritionist or dietician, and gastroenterologist will depend on geographic specific practice patterns. Consider periodic diagnostics such as swallow, manometry, probe pH studies, and laboratory indices of nutrition. Examples of expected outcomes include maximized nutrition to permit growth and development, prevention of nutritional deficiencies and parental education and skills necessary for use of specific feeding equipment. Identification of expected outcomes is individualized to each child's situation and may change over time (Redstone, West. (2004).

Elimination

The development of effective bowl and bladder control is a complex physiologic process. Maturation of the sphincter muscles is usually during the toddler or early preschool years, once the child is able to stand, walk well, remove clothing, and control timing of elimination (Ball and London, 2006).

Assessment information collected by the nurse life care planner may include

- The child's developmental level and motor skills
- Behavioral functioning pattern
- Elimination patterns
- Parental perspectives and expectations regarding elimination
- Medications affecting elimination patterns

- Presence of complicating factors such as infection, kidney and gastric conditions
- The child and family's ability to follow an elimination management plan

Knowing how and when to potty-train a child with special needs is a common challenge for parents. The process of determining when the child is ready for toilet training is in part comparable to non-disabled children. However, the training period, methods and equipment are likely to differ. Children with developmental delays may be able to achieve toilet training and continence at a cognitive age of three or four (Edwards, 1999). Some may require diapering into adulthood. The risk of skin irritation and skin breakdown should be considered.

Specialists who can assist with elimination training may be available if the family lives in a metropolitan area with specialized home-based pediatric rehabilitation services. Once readiness has been determined, and if such services are available, a pediatric occupational or physical therapist can help select specialty equipment such as grab bars beside the toilet, custom or modified potty chair, adaptive toilet seats, a special footstool, and toilet back support, side-rails, or armrests. A home evaluation by a specialty nurse or therapist knowledgeable about toilet training may be appropriate and available in some regions. A pediatric rehabilitation nurse may be available to make a series of home visits to provide ongoing guidance and education regarding altered elimination patterns.

Inability to achieve toilet training can lead to shame for the child and frustration for the parent. Specialized clothing may be recommended but is not reimbursable by insurance carriers, and whether the cost of the clothing should be budgeted in litigated cases is debatable since clothing is considered a typical cost of living. This factor should not preclude educating the parents about sources for procuring specialty-clothing items.

Chronic constipation requiring stool softeners and laxatives is commonly seen with children with neurodevelopmental disabilities, pervasive developmental delays, spinal cord injury, and prescribed anti-cholinergic medications. A daily bowel plan is developed individually. Dietary measures and assuring sufficient fluid intake are the first line of management; further measures and medications may be necessary. Consider whether interventions for chronic constipation are likely to be a short-or long-term.

Children who use intermittent catheterization (IC) for neurogenic bladder will need larger catheter and supplies as they grow. Consider whether the child will be able to learn to perform safe self-catheterization. Allow for periodic urinalysis, urine culture and sensitivity studies, and episodic antibiotics due to the well-known causal link between catheterization and urinary tract/bladder infections. (*Please see Chapter 1, Spinal Cord Injury, Table 4, Medicare sterile technique catheterization guidelines, 2011*)

Skin Integrity
Children are at lower risk for alterations in skin integrity. However, skin breakdown can occur. The assessment process should include a review of medical records for past episodes of skin breakdown or skin problems and specific inquiry of the parents as to past or present skin integrity problems. As with adults, consultation with a wound care nurse or physician can be of immediate benefit to the child. Ensuring that the parents are educated regarding the risk of skin breakdown is important.

Activity and Exercise
Self-care, mobility, and play are daily activities that all children must learn. Play has been called "the work of children" (Piaget and Cook, 1952). Self-care, mobility, and play involve cognitive and physical abilities; mastery of motor skills, starting with head and later trunk control, is vital to self-care skills, mobility, exercise and play activities. Compare

the child's achievement of developmental function milestones to his age-peers. This comparison can be useful for highlighting developmental lags and how much progress is needed to acquire the motor skills needed for independent living as an adult.

Self-care

The ability to self-care and self-advocate requires cognitive, physical, and communication skills and are important co-morbidity considerations. Consider whether the services of a guardian should be put into the plan. When grown to adulthood, could the child reasonably be expected to direct caregivers to meet physical care needs in the presence of pervasive physical limitations? As an adult, will this child have the cognitive and communication abilities to self-advocate, participate in the treatment plan, and independently coordinate necessary supports to meet self-care and community integration needs?

Ferreting out the answers to these questions may be simple or complex. For instance, a child with a spinal cord injury or major burns should be assumed to have intact cognitive function unless otherwise documented. More difficult is projecting healthcare needs over time for a young child with cerebral palsy, developmental delay, or brain injury. This will likely require ongoing follow up with the treatment team over the years.

Both physical and developmental delays can hinder or prevent self-care, requiring physical, occupational, and speech language therapy for the child to achieve maximum possible independence. Typical nursing interventions include supports to optimize independence, caregiver support, adaptive and assistive equipment, physical and occupational therapy evaluations, and ongoing medical care. If the child is school-aged with a documented disability, the school systems may have physical therapy included in the child's daily program. This has changed greatly over the last few years related to decreasing budgets of the individual school system and alternate sources and options provided in the plan (Cosby and Cosby, 2013).

Mobility

A child with a traumatic brain injury who can walk independently without assistive devices yet lacks safety awareness and judgment may require safeguards. Not all assistive devices may be appropriate in all situations. A child with developmental delays or other impairments and disabilities may have long-term needs for medical and therapeutic interventions that promote fluid movement, coordination, safe gait and optimized independence. The nurse life care planner should consider effectiveness, cost, therapy frequency, interventions, equipment maintenance and replacement intervals, and caregiver preference and needs.

In choosing equipment to maximize a child's mobility, it is important to consider where it will be used. Not all equipment is appropriate in every environment; mobility needs at home, school, and in the community differ. For example, a child who can walk with a gait trainer may need a power wheelchair at school for safety and efficiency in busy hallways. The child who can ambulate short distances at home may need a wheelchair for community mobility. Other equipment needs may include leg braces, forearm crutches, walkers, trunk supporters, standard wheelchairs vs. caregiver chairs, and reverse standing walkers.

Stroller The nurse life care planner will also need to consider the family's ability to help the child with mobility. A special needs stroller or jogger may be preferable to a heavy, cumbersome wheelchair for short outings with a child who is unable to self-propel. Special needs car seats are available for those children who need more support than the traditional infant or child safety seat. These can be suggested by the physical or occupational therapist when working with the provider team.

Wheelchair considerations A child who is permanently wheelchair-bound will need a special modified van with a power lift. The van is considered a necessary family purchase; however, all adaptive changes (e.g., seating, lock-downs for wheelchairs, ramps, power lifts) are properly placed in a plan. Later as the child matures, a driving safety evaluation, driving lessons and adaptive driving devices can be included.

Some children with injuries have equipment that may be hazardous, such as a power wheelchair, if the child lacks judgment. Children with average or above-average cognitive ability may be trained to safely operate a power wheelchair at around the age of two years (Jones, McEwen, and Hansen, 2003). These chairs should include a caregiver control for times when the child is unable to control the chair.

In a child with cognitive impairment, ability to safely operate a power chair can be assessed when the child reaches a mental age of around two years. Some clinicians will use a tool such as the Pediatric Powered Wheelchair Screening Test (PPWST) to assess cognitive readiness (Furumasu, Guerette, and Tefft, 2004). Power chair manufacturers can install pre-set parameters so that a safe speed cannot be exceeded. The nurse life care planner should assess the appropriateness of recommended equipment in terms of the child's cognitive as well as physical ability.

DME In recommending durable medical equipment, especially wheelchairs and standers, the nurse life care planner should consider products with growth packages. This may be available at no additional charge or for a fee. With growth in many children, this can mean a substantial saving over complete replacement.

If needed, custom braces such as ankle foot orthoses (AFO) will not likely be adjustable and will likely require more frequent replacement for a child compared to an adult. If possible, discuss the replacement frequency of customized equipment and the child's growth pattern with the orthotist or prosthetist.

Orthopedic and physical medicine and rehabilitation notes may note the physician's goals for bracing; bracing to maintain position and prevent contractures will be significantly different from bracing for ambulation (Berker and Yalçin, 2008). The life care plan should include a general replacement frequency, which will be different in the ambulatory versus non-ambulatory child. There is usually a cost difference as well.

Exercise and play Family-based care that focuses on incorporating exercise, play, family time, and therapeutic activities into daily life can help the child achieve optimal outcomes (Ball and Bindler, 2006). Families can be taught to incorporate therapeutic methods in family time activities and still be working toward therapy goals. An example of family time that contributes to therapy goals is a membership in a facility with an indoor pool and exercise equipment. Another example of family involvement may be the use of hippotherapy as part of the physical therapy time (medical providers should agree) (Frank and McCloskey, 2011).

Family function should be considered to support the psychological and physical wellbeing of the caregivers (Raina et al., 2005). Some parents cannot provide safe therapies due to their own learning problems, social economic problems or lack of information.

Cognitive Perceptual

Cognitive perceptual functioning includes the ability to comprehend and use information, intellect, communication; and sensory function, including sight, hearing, and touch. The nurse life care planner should include questions (based on age level) concerning cognitive abilities. Assessments from pediatric neuropsychologist and other medical providers provide this information also.

Sight The preterm child is at risk for retinopathy of prematurity (ROP), which may lead to significant visual impairment (Higgins, 2006). A child with ROP will need ophthalmologic follow-up at least through early childhood. Assessment for cortical vision impairment is often needed and should be addressed in the life care plan when appropriate. A review of the pediatric ophthalmology records may indicate the expected follow-up frequency and planned treatments.

According to the American Optometric Association (2012), a child's first eye examination should be at six months. This exam identifies nearsightedness, farsightedness and astigmatism. It includes assessment of the eye movement abilities and other eye health problems. Early eye development or dysfunction can lead to the child having difficulty with communication, learning, understanding, or embarrassment with other children.

Vision problems limit personal, social economic independence, and independence. Learning disabilities are affected by visual efficiency problems (visual acuity, refractive error, ocular motility) and visual information processing problems (visual spatial orientation, analysis skills, and integration skills). The most common eye problems include (Sherman, 1973):

- Blurred vision
- Diplopia
- Asthenopia (eyestrain)
- Skipping words
- Delayed learning
- Difficulty reaching and obtaining objects

The eye care provider can determine appropriate vision needs, appliances (glasses and vision aids), surgeries, and exercises for child's age.

Sensory Deficits Some injuries, such as burns or traumatic brain injury, may result in decreased sensation or inability to perceive painful stimuli and temperature extremes (Ofek and Defrin, 2007; Malenfant, Forget et al., 1996). Safety equipment such as temperature regulators for faucets or protective clothing may be indicated, depending on the child's level of independence, mobility, and developmental age. This could include household and environmental modifications as well as constant or intermittent supervision.

Hearing Hearing impairment is not uncommon in the presence of multiple disabilities (Boyle et al., 1993). Hearing is important for language development, communication, and personal enhancement. Documentation of visual acuity and hearing is necessary to plan for care and future needs. Audiology examination can result in recommendations for adaptive hearing devices and other communication tools. This should include maintenance, supplies and replacement frequencies.

Comprehension and Intellect

Schools can play an important role in assessing the cognitive and physical abilities of a child by offering standardized testing that can provide critical information about a child's growth and development compared to his peers. Younger children may have been assessed through an early intervention program to determine the therapy treatment plan and goals prior to age three years. School-age children with special needs and disabilities have usually undergone standardized testing of intellect and cognition. The life care planner should request school records and Individualized Education Plans (IEPs) to identify the needs of the child in school (Cosby and Cosby, 2013).

Some schools administer *neuropsychological testing*, which may be especially helpful. Public school testing often focuses on educational achievement (psycho-educational testing) and may not connect the medical components to results as neuropsychological testing does. Neuropsychological testing may incur costs to the family.

Results will determine the need for future testing as the child achieves developmental milestones. School programs have specialized testing for all disabilities. The nurse life care planner should provide for these services in the life care plan.

Identified functional limitations do not always correlate with a number, e.g., intelligence quotient (IQ). In other words, a child with a lower IQ score may not necessarily have poor adaptive skills. A combination of the IQ score and level of adaptive skills will give the best estimate of the severity of mental retardation (Ball and Bindler, 2006). Considering IQ and adaptive skills together will result in better decisions on short-term and long-term care needs.

Communication
By age four months, babies will produce sounds specific to needs. At one year of age, most children have at least two or three specific words. Combining words into sentences is usually seen around age two years (Batshaw, 1997). A child with multiple disabilities may have communication disorders, such as a mixed receptive-expressive disorder, dysarthria, or may be nonverbal (Beukelman and Mirenda, 2013).

A review of standardized testing conducted by a speech and language therapist will assist the nurse life care planner in determining the type of assistive devices that may be appropriate for the individual child. The devices or needs are based on whether the child has conductive loss, sensorineural loss, or mixed loss. These are identified through audiograms. Sign language development skills for both the child and caregivers may be needed. Typical assessments for a pediatric life care plan include audiological evaluations, audiograms, tympanometry evaluations, pure tone audiometry, auditory brainstem response, and otoacoustic emissions (Jerger and Musiek, 2000). Ways of communication for the child includes oral, cued speech and manual communication such as fingerspelling (age appropriate), sign language, typing, and computerized programs. Children who are hearing impaired or nonverbal can learn sign language (Rogers, Hayden et al., 2006).

There is a vast array of assistive communication devices, from basic communication picture boards to highly technical computer systems. Understanding the underlying neurodevelopmental impairments and associated prognoses is critical; however, current developmental status may make it difficult to predict future ability to use technology. Other communication systems or methods should be age-appropriate and added at specific ages in the life care plan.

Dental Considerations

Children with disabilities often have specialized dental needs. Regular consultation with a pediatric dentist experienced with disabilities is a high priority for these children. They may need special cleaning or dental work with anesthesia, or surgery to correct malformations and bite problems (Lewis et al., 2005).

Sleep and Rest

Children who have had extended hospitalization or other disruptions to daily routine will often have disturbed sleep cycles (Owens, 2007). Pain due to gastrointestinal irritation, positioning, or other physical causes may disturb restorative sleep. The disturbed sleep pattern may affect caregivers, usually the parents, in the household. The nurse life care planner will need to assess the child's sleep to individualize the plan for appropriate care, especially in assessing the need for respite services and additional overnight awake caregivers. Aids for sleep may include, for example:

- CPAP for sleep or daily activities (including medical evaluations, frequency of replacements and needs, equipment and supplies)

- Bed protectors for incontinence
- Positioning devices
- Light-blocking window shades
- White noise generators

Information on needs can be obtained from home evaluations, medical records, and interviews with medical providers.

Self-Perception and Self-Concept
Infants begin developing a sense of self by age three months, when they begin to look at and play with their own fingers. The concept of gender and imitation of same sex behavior patterns is seen in the early preschool years (Nelms and Mullins, 1982). Children with disfigurement or obvious disabilities that are evident to others will have an awareness of their differences by preschool, or the cognitive equivalent of pre-school age (Semrud-Clikeman M, 2007).

Jean Piaget is credited with dividing intellectual development into stages (Batshaw, 1997). Children with developmental delays or mental retardation may never progress through all of the stages. An understanding of these stages, whether occurring at the chronologically typical time or not, will aid in evaluating a child's probable self-concept.

Preschool age children are *preoperational thinkers*; they engage in magical thinking, with the child assuming responsibility for events or illnesses over which they do not actually have control. As children develop more concrete thought patterns, they have more questions about their perceived differences, as they work through the stage of ordering, grouping, and classifying. They will not likely have the ability to think abstractly about their own prognosis or future care needs, as abstract thinking emerges during adolescence in the stage of formal operations (Piaget and Cook, 1952).

Early adolescents typically increase identification with their peer groups. The desire for sameness is evident in clothing styles, school supply choices, hairstyles, etc. The nurse life care planner will need to take this into account when considering equipment options, special needs camps, peer support groups, and counseling recommendations.

Role Relationships

Children with disabilities are often viewed as intellectually inferior due to their physical appearance or speech impairments. They may be placed in an unnecessarily dependent role by parents, siblings, and peers. Siblings and friends may be jealous of attention given to the child. Awareness of conflicts in role perception and relationships may support the nurse life care planner's recommendation for equipment that maximizes independence and resources that provide support services to the child and family. It is reasonable to anticipate these conflicts when developing a life care plan for a young child.

Studies have shown that children with functional limitations are more likely to live in single parent households (Newacheck, Strickland, et al., 1998). It has been reported that less than two-thirds of children with functional limitations (limitations in mobility, self-care, communication, or learning) live in a two-parent household, while three-fourths of children without functional limitations live with two parents (Hogan, Rogers, Msall, 2000). The nurse life care planner should consider living arrangements and parent involvement when addressing issues of respite care, counseling, and housing modifications.

Sexuality and Reproduction

Unless there is an interruption in normal hormone secretion, girls begin to develop primary and secondary sexual characteristics at an average age of ten years and boys at an average age of eleven years (Ball and London, 2006). Worley et al. (2002) found that Caucasian girls with cerebral palsy, having moderate to severe motor impairment, experienced menarche at a median age of fourteen years, which is 1.3 years later than those without cerebral palsy. The study also found that girls with cerebral palsy and increased body fat had more advanced sexual maturity while boys with cerebral palsy and lower body fat had more advanced sexual maturity. A caregiver will have to manage menstruation if a teen is not able to manage toileting independently. For the nurse life care planner, considerations concerning urological interventions, birth control, or safer sex practices should be included in the plan.

Coping and Stress Tolerance

Coping styles for physical discomfort, deficits in sensory integration, and awareness of differences in disabilities is unique to each individual. Children of all ages may exhibit more behaviors related to stress and inadequate coping skills than their peers. Children with an older mental age may be able express their difficulty with coping.

The nurse life care planner will need to assess the coping and stress level of not only the child, but also the family unit. In recommending intervention, consider the cognitive level of the child and consequently the appropriateness of individual counseling and support group intervention. Nearly all caregivers will need counseling at various stages of the child's life. Siblings may also require counseling at various times to deal with the disruption to family life (Seligman and Darling, 2007). The nurse life care planner may choose to include counseling in brief intervals during developmental transition times for the child and family.

Values and Beliefs

The nurse life care planner should consider a family's belief and value system. As an example, some residential care facilities for children are affiliated with a religious organization. These facilities may be recommended as an alternative to living at home if that becomes necessary. Attention to the family's beliefs will guide in selecting such a placement option.

Some families may oppose medical interventions such as placement of a gastrostomy tube or neurostimulants to increase attention, even when recommended by a medical provider (Seligman and Darling, 2007). The nurse life care planner may include these interventions, but should note the family's preferences.

The value of family time becomes significant in many families with a disabled child. Additional therapy time may provide some benefit to a child, but the benefit may not outweigh quality time taken away from the family. The Oregon Guidelines (Coolman et al., 1998), developed for children with CP, recommends episodic therapy, not year round, year-in and year-out. Therapies should be delivered when a child shows potential to advance to another functional level or in response to a change in condition (positive or negative).

School, therapies, and counseling can be overwhelming to both child and parents. The nurse life care planner should consider including a sample calendar page demonstrating the different therapy schedules to ensure the child does not do too much and has adequate time for sleep and down time.

Section Two: Aging in Adults
Note: Many applicable nursing diagnoses may be found in other chapters as mentioned.

Aging Demographics
The number of U.S. citizens age 65 and older is rising. The most rapid increase is expected between the years 2010 and 2030 when the Baby Boomer generation reaches age 65. According to the Administration on Aging (2012), the 65+ year-old population "numbered 39.6 million in 2009." This is 12.9% of the US population, one in every eight Americans. In this report, it is estimated this will increase to over 19% by the year 2030. Not including compensable injuries, it is estimated that 37% of the aging population will have some type of disability, with 16% needing some type of disability-related assistance.

Harris et al. (1975) cites three reasons for the growth of America's older population: the Baby Boom, the many young adults who immigrated to the United States during World War II, and the improvements in medical technology that have increased life expectancy.

How and when age-related changes occur are unique to each individual. Typical changes include physiological, sensory, cognitive, and personality. This chapter will review the typical changes experienced by the older adult with aging. In addition, this chapter will discuss the effects of aging on patients with amputations, traumatic brain injury, burns, cerebral palsy, chronic pain, and spinal cord injury. (*See also those chapters in this text*)

The Administration on Aging (2012) recognizes "limitations in activities because of chronic conditions with age." Four out of five older persons have at least one chronic condition, and many have more than one. The most common are arthritis, hypertension, heart disease, and hearing problems (Wolff et al., 2002).

The Physiological Effects of Aging (Poinier, 2011)
Integument

Outward signs of aging involve the *skin, hair, and nails.* Over time the skin loses underlying fat layers and oil glands causing wrinkles and reduced elasticity. Other contributing factors are nutrition, sun exposure, heredity, and hormones. These changes cause increased susceptibility to cold, bruising, and skin breakdown. Due to the atrophy of sweat glands, the individual becomes more susceptible to heat (hyperthermia). The skin develops age spots due to melanin deposits; the hair loses its pigmentation and turns gray. Reduced blood flow to the connective tissues causes the nails to thicken.

Sensorineural

General: Aging causes reduced efficiency of nerve transmission affecting response time and coordination. The brain shrinks in size, but this may not significantly affect function except in extreme cases. These changes affect sleeping patterns by decreasing the length of total sleep and rapid eye movement sleep. The lack of sleep can cause irritability and increases perceived pain. Balance and coordination may decrease.

Vision: Tear production decreases, and retinas thin. It becomes increasingly difficult for the eyes to adapt to different levels of light. Cataracts, glaucoma, and macular degeneration are the most common problems of aging eyes. Deficits can result in increased risk of falls, inability to drive or socialize, and loss of recreational activities such as reading, television, theater, or outdoor activities. Other safety issues are related to home activities such as cooking or using cleaning supplies, and ability to read medication labels or patient teaching materials. The nurse life care planner should consider adaptive equipment or assistance for these activities of daily living.

Hearing loss is one of the most common conditions affecting aging adults. It may be important to differentiate what is related to aging and what is the result of an injury;

medications can also have side effects affecting hearing. The nurse life care planner should consider provisions for hearing evaluations, hearing aids, supplies, and replacements. Safety equipment in the home could include, e.g., flashing and speaking fire and smoke detectors, lights for doorbells, and adapted telephone equipment.

Dental Health

Overall oral health depends on the individual's history of dental care. Saliva production decreases, making it difficult to wash away bacteria, and teeth and gums become more vulnerable to decay and infection. With age the gums recede.

The nurse life care planner should identify dental problems as these problems affect nutrition, coping, and communication. Normal dental evaluations are necessary for the general population; however, if the patient has been on long-term medications or has oral problems related to injuries then provisions for dental evaluations and care should be included in the life care plan.

Cardiovascular

In many studies reviewed by the Research in Action (2002) reports, the systemic effects of aging in the cardiovascular system typically become apparent in the eighth decade, the result normal cardiac muscle atrophy, valvular calcification, arteriosclerosis, and atherosclerosis. Reduced blood flow results in decreased stamina, reduced renal and hepatic function, and less cellular nourishment. This results in greater susceptibility to drug toxicity, decreased healing, and reduced response to stress.

Individuals taking medication should have periodic laboratory studies to monitor for drug levels and side effects as part of regular medical follow up; if possible, medications should be decreased. Periodic EKG and other diagnostics may be indicated. Assistance for ADLs may be needed. The individual will require more assistance through durable medical equipment and personal attendants.

Respiratory

In later life, the respiratory system loses efficiency, resulting in decreased gas exchange. Airway and lung tissue become less elastic with reduced ciliary activity. Muscles of respiration atrophy, reducing the ability to breathe deeply and cough to clear secretions. These changes are more marked if the individual smokes or lives in a polluted environment.

The result is a decreased stamina with shortness of breath and fatigue that impair ability to perform activities of daily living. The decrease in oxygen can increase anxiety. The individual will require more assistance through durable medical equipment, adaptive equipment to decrease work, and assistance. The nurse life care planner should consider provisions for regular medical follow up.

Musculoskeletal

As the body ages, general atrophy occurs in muscle groups, resulting in loss of muscle tone and strength. Regular physical exercise appears decrease the extent of these changes.

Changes in the skeletal system begin around age 35 in both men and women. Osteoporosis and reduction of weight-bearing capacity lead to reduction of height and spontaneous or compression fracture. As vertebral joints calcify, postural changes and increased rigidity make bending difficult.

The most common chronic orthopedic conditions are osteoarthritis and rheumatoid arthritis. These conditions impair mobility and performance of daily activities. The nurse life care planner should consider adaptations, medications, and assistance based on functional levels.

Gastrointestinal

According to Wells and Dumbrell (2006),

Nutrition is an important determinant of health in persons over the age of 65. . . . Because of the impact of coexisting disease on overall nutritive status, a comprehensive, multidisciplinary approach is often helpful in addressing all contributing factors in the diagnosis and treatment of compromised nutritional health in the elderly.

Over time, the gastrointestinal system experiences a reduction in the production of hydrochloric acid, digestive enzymes, and saliva and total number of taste buds. These changes result in lack of appetite, gastrointestinal distress, impaired swallowing, and gastroparesis. Absorption may be impaired, resulting in deficiencies of vitamins B, C, and K and, in extreme cases, malnutrition. If these conditions are not treated they may result in capillary weakening, easy bruising, muscle cramping, reduced appetite, weakness, mental confusion, or illness.

Endocrine

The body usually experiences approximately a 1% decrease per year in metabolic rate beginning at about the twenty-fifth year. The result is food being less well absorbed and utilized as well as a decrease in the overall metabolism of drugs. This results in decreased stamina and greater susceptibility to drug toxicity.

Sexual activity is more related to past life patterns than to age. Although frequency may diminish, sexual desire and performance may continue well into an individual's ninth decade. With age both men and women may require more stimulation to become aroused and more time to reach orgasm. The nurse life care planner should evaluate the importance of this to the involved injured person, involving the primary care or specialty provider as indicated. Medications, physical devices, and psychological treatments are often used to enhance sexual ability and are appropriate to include this into the life care plan with the appropriate nursing diagnoses.

Psychological

Longitudinal studies of personality traits have found that basic personality traits remain relatively consistent throughout one's adult life. The Baltimore Longitudinal Study of Aging (2009) found remarkable stability over periods of 10 years or more on personality inventories measuring such traits as neuroticism, extroversion, and openness to new experience. Interviews with older adults have found that self-image seems to change relatively little with age. One of the best-documented personality changes in adulthood is an increased preoccupation with one's inner self.

Many health problems common in later life can significantly affect cognitive functioning and test-taking ability. Most persons experience a modest increase in memory problems as they get older, particularly with regard to the ability to remember relatively recent experiences; learning new information, encoding it for storage, and retrieving it requires more time.

The Effects of Aging on Specific Conditions

Parkinson's disease, Alzheimer's disease, Dementia Pugilistica, Post-traumatic Dementia

The Agency for Healthcare Research and Quality (2007) the resource for evidence-based practice suggested the following considerations for medical management of dementia, Parkinson's, and related diagnoses. The practice guideline outlines the following medical treatments:

- Psychiatric management
- Psychotherapies and/or psychotherapy treatments
- General medical care to address PD, dementia, and medication management

- Treatment of agitation and psychosis
- Treatment of depression,
- Treatment of sleep disturbances

Treatment or consideration of long-term issues, including placement (www.guidelines.gov)

Please see Chapter 1, TBI, for nursing diagnoses and more information on life care planning with aging.

Burns

When developing the life care plan for the burn-injured person, age is an important consideration as it greatly affects the function, mobility, and growth of a person to be independent. The younger that injured person with the injury: the greater need for treatments, equipment, supplies, surgeries, grafts, and medical treatments including physical therapies and psychological assistance. Nursing diagnoses are important to assist the nurse life care planner to determine age appropriate diagnoses and interventions.

Please see Chapter 5, Burns, for nursing diagnoses and more information on life care planning with aging.

Aging with Chronic Pain

To understand how the chronic pain patient ages, the normal aging process and what the average person can expect in terms of pain will briefly be discussed. The development of pain in the absence of disease is not normal, yet the majority of older adults experience pain on a regular basis. Therefore, it is generally accepted both by clinicians and patients that development of acute pain or pain related to a disease process is part of the normal aging process. Chronic pain, specifically, is not part of the normal aging process (Hanks-Bell 2004). This affects the patient's discussion of pain and the clinician's treatment of pain in the aging population. There may also be gender, societal, or cultural bases for underreporting of pain (Miller 2006).

The older patient may view pain as a weakness and therefore may not discuss it with a clinician. Untreated or undertreated pain can also lead to sleep disturbances, depression, and withdrawal from society and regular activity. As pain persists untreated or undertreated, it can lead to chronic pain, which becomes harder to treat.

Please see Chapter 3, Pain, for nursing diagnoses and implications for pain management in aging.

References

AHRQ (2002) Physical activity and older Americans: Benefits and strategies. Retrieved from http://www.ahrq.gov. ppip/activity.htm

American Optometric Association (2012) The need for comprehensive vision exam of preschool school-age children. Retrieved from http://www.aoa.org/x5419. xml

Administration on Aging (2012) Aging statistics retrieved from http://www.aoa.gov/AoARoot/Aging_Statistics/index. aspx

American Pain Society (2012) What is the impact of untreated and undertreated pain? APS Press Room. Retrieved from http://www.ampainsoc.org/press/backgrounder.htm

Altman GB, editor. (2003) Feeding and medicating via a gastrostomy tube. Delmar's Fundamental and Advanced Nursing Skills. 2nd Ed, 742-749. Albany, NY: Delmar Thomson Learning.

Arvedson, JC (1998) Management of pediatric dysphagia. Otolaryngologic Clinics of North America 31:3,453-476

Arvedson, JC and Brodsky, L. (2002). Pediatric swallowing and feeding: Assessment and management (2nd ed.). Singular, Albany NY

ASHA (2013) Knowledge and skills needed by speech-language pathologists providing services to individuals with swallowing and/or feeding disorders. Dysphagia Document Review and Revision Working Group,

American Speech-Language-Hearing Association. http://www.asha.org/policy/KS2002-00079.htm

Ball J, London M, Bindler R, and Ladewig P. Maternal and child nursing care, 2nd edition. Lavoisier. Cachan Cadex, France

Baltimore Longitudinal Study of Aging (2010) Lessons from the Baltimore longitudinal study of aging. National Institute on Aging, National Institutes of Health. http://www. blsa.nih.gov/about/healthy-aging/cover

Batshaw ML (editor) (1997) Children with disabilities (4th ed.). University of Pennsylvania, Philadephia PA

Berker A and Yalçin MS (2008) Cerebral palsy: orthopedic aspects and rehabilitation. Pediatric Clinics of North America 55:5, 1209-1225

Beukelman D, Mirenda P et al. (2013) Augmentative and Alternative Communication, 4th ed. Brookes, Baltimore MD

Boyle CA, Decouflé P, Yeargin-Allsopp M. (1993) Pediatrics 93:3, 399-403

Centers for Disease Control and Prevention. (2003). Public health and aging in the United States and worldwide. Hyattsville MD.

Coolman R, Foran W, and Lee J (1998) Oregon guidelines for medically-based outpatient physical therapy and occupational therapy for children with special needs in the managed care environment. Oregon Health Sciences University, Portland OR

Cosby MF and Cosby SM (2013) Pediatric life care plan development: an overview of IDEA and Section 504. Journal of Nurse Life Care Planning XIII.1, 29-46

Ergüner-Tekinalp B and Akkök F (2004) The effect of a coping skills training program on the coping skills, hopelessness, and stress levels of mothers of children with autism. International Journal for the Advancement of Counseling, 26:3, 257 ff

Furumasu J, Guerette P, and Tefft D (2004) Relevance of the Pediatric Powered Wheelchair Screening Test for

children with cerebral palsy. Developmental Medicine
and Child Neurology 46:7, 468-474

Goddard JA, Lehr R, and Lapadat JC (2000) Parents of children
with disabilities: telling a different story. Canadian
Journal of Counselling ad Psychotherapy. 34:4, 273-289

Gordon M (2010) Manual of nursing diagnostics. Jones and
Bartlett, Sudbury MA

Hanks-Bell M, Halvey K, Paice J.(2004). Pain assessment and
management in aging. Online Journal of Issues in
Nursing. 9:4-3

Harris AR, Evans WN, and Schwab RM (1975) Education
spending in an aging America. Journal of Public
Economics. 81:3, 345-514

Heiman T (2002) Parents of children with disabilities:
resilience, coping, and future expectations. Journal of
Developmental and Physical Disabilitis 14:2, 159 ff

Hensley C (2007) Support systems for parents of children with
special needs. Association for Counselor Education
and Supervision Conference, Columbus OH. Eastern
Michigan University

Herdman TH (2012) (Ed.) NANDA-International Nursing
Diagnoses: Definitions and Classification, 2012-2014.
Oxford: Wiley-Blackwell

Hogan DP, Rogers ML, Msall ME. (2000) Functional limitations
and key indicators of well-being in children with a
disability. Archives of Pediatric and Adolescent Medicine
154:10, 1042-1048

Jerger J and Musiek F (2000) Report of the consensus
conference on the diagnosis of auditory processing
disorders in school-aged children. Journal of the
American Academy of Audiology 11 : 467-474

Jones MA, McEwen IR and Hansen L. (2003) Use of power
mobility for a young child with spinal muscular atrophy.
Physical Therapy 83:3, 253-262

Kleinman RE (Editor) Pediatric nutrition handbook, 4th
edition. American Academy of Pediatrics. Elk Grove
Village

Kuperminc MN and Stevenson RD (2008) Growth and nutrition disorders in children with cerebral palsy. Dev Disabil Res Rev. 2008; 14(2): 137-146.

Lewis C, Robertson AS, Phelps S (2005) Unmet dental care needs among children with special health care needs: Implications for the medical home. Pediatrics 116:3, 426-431

Malenfant A, Forget R, et al. (1996) Prevalence and characteristics of chronic sensory problems in burn patients. Pain 67:2-3, 493-500

Miller C and Newton S (2006). Pain perception and expression: The influence of gender, personal self-efficacy, and lifespan socialization. Pain Management Nursing 7:4 148-152.

National Institute of Neurological Disorders and Stroke (NINDS)(2006). What disabilities can result from TBI? Retrieved from http://www.ninds.nih.gov/disorders/tbi/detail_tbi.htm

Nelms BC and Mullins RG. (1982) Growth and development: a primary healthcare approach. Prentice Hall, Englewood Cliffs NJ

Newacheck PW, Strickland B, et al. (1998) An epidemiologic profile of children with special health care needs Pediatrics 102:1, 117-123

Ofek H and Defrin R (2007) The characteristics of chronic central pain after traumatic brain injury. Pain 131:3, 330-340

Owens J (2007) Classification and epidemiology of childhood sleep disorders. Sleep Medicine Clinics 2:3, 353-361

Peterson K. (2010) Managing chronic pain in the elderly. American Nurse Today. Retrieved from http://www.americannursetoday.com/article.aspx?id=7084andfid=6850

Piaget J, Cook M trans. 1952. The origins of intelligence in children. W.W.Norton and Co. New York NY

Poiner AC and Herman CJ (2011) Healthy normal aging. WebMD, Healthwise. http://www.webmd.com/healthy-aging/tc/healthy-aging-normal-aging

Raina P, O'Donnell M, et al. (2005) The health and well-being of caregivers of children with cerebral palsy. Pediatrics 115:6, 626-636

Raju TN, Higgins RD et al. (2006) Optimizing care and outcome for late-preterm (near-term) infants: A summary of the Workshop Sponsored by the National Institute of Child Health and Human Development. Pediatrics 118:1207-1214.

Redstone F, West JF. The importance of postural control for feeding. Pediatric Nursing. 2004;30:97-100.

Riddick-Graham S and Deming L. (2011) Pediatric life care planning and management, 2ⁿᵈ ed. Taylor and Francis, Boca Raton FL

Research in Action (2002) Preventing disability in the elderly with chronic disease. Research in Action. Retrieved from http://www.ahrq.gov/research/elderdis.pdf

Rogers B et al. (1994). Characteristics of dysphagia in children with cerebral palsy. Dysphagia 9:69-73

Rogers SJ, Hayden D, et al. (2006) Teaching young nonverbal children with autism useful speech: A pilot study of the Denver model and PROMPT intervention. Journal of Autism and Developmental Disorders 36: 1007-1024

Schwarz SM et al. (2001) Diagnosis and treatment of feeding disorders in children with developmental disabilities. Pediatrics 108:3, 671-676

Seligman M and Darling RB (2007) Ordinary families, special children: a systems approach to chlidhood disability, 3rd ed. The Guilford Press, New York NY

Semrud-Clikeman M (2007) Social competence in children with acquired and chronic disorders. In Social Competence in Children, p 199-226. Springer Science + Business Media, New York NY

Sherman A (1973) Relating vision disorders to learning disability. Journal of the American Optometric Association, 44:2, 140-141.

Wells JL, Dumbrell AC.(2006) Nutrition and aging: Assessment and treatment of compromised nutritional status in frail elderly patients. Clinical Interventions Aging. 1:1 67-79.

Worley G, Houlihan CM, et al. (2002) Secondary sexual characteristics in children with cerebral palsy and moderate to severe motor impairment: a cross-sectional survey. Pediatrics. 110:5. 897-902

Section III

Legal Considerations

CHAPTER 1

Legal Overview

Terri Brandley, BSN, RN, CCM
Lyn Leake, BSN, RN, CNLC

Introduction

This chapter briefly describes the legal milieu in which the nurse life care planner practices as an expert witness. The chapter begins with an initial background of the United States judicial system, followed by a discussion of some details that affect the expert witness's practice. This chapter is meant to serve as general orientation, not an all-inclusive discussion, for the nurse life care planner expert witness.

History

In the United States, federal and state legal systems are largely based on the British common law tradition of legal precedents that are continually updated, modified, and changed over time. One notable exception, however, is the state of Louisiana, which follows civil law, also known as the Napoleonic code. With this system, new legal codes are adopted, and the prior codes are voided out. Puerto Rico also has a system based on civil law. Over time, the laws of the American states have become similar, creating a commonality and forming a more nationalistic view.

With some exceptions, the American legal system is an adversarial process. Its origins are in actual physical battles between two contenders under the formerly held belief that the winner has truth on his side, so the loser must be guilty. Over time, these battles came to be closely managed by procedural rules, eventually evolving into today's litigation process. The basic premise of the adversarial system is that the truth will emerge through competition. Procedure often takes precedence over substance, so, in order to preserve the purpose of the endeavor, cross-examination and multiple actors are the mainstays of the process. Cross-examination is reminiscent of the sword fighting of old in that it is a hostile process meant to discredit the opposition (Reichel, 1999).

Federal Legal System
The United States Constitution gives specific powers to the federal (national) government. Constitutional law is an extensive field that pertains to the interpretation and implementation of the United States Constitution. Constitutional law deals with the primary relationships in our society. This type of law encompasses relationships between states, relationships between the states and federal government, and relationships between the three branches of the federal government. It also covers the rights of individuals in relation to the federal government. A central aspect of constitutional law is judicial review, the precept that the actions of the executive and legislative branches of government are subject to review, and possible invalidation, by the judicial branch.

Federal courts have exclusive jurisdiction over certain types of cases that are tried under federal statutes. Congress has the authority to establish lower federal courts below the Supreme Court. Congress controls the cases that are addressed in the federal courts. The federal court system includes 94 U.S. district courts and 13 U.S. circuit courts of appeals, as well as other specialized courts related to trade and bankruptcy. District courts are the lowest level of the federal courts. Parties dissatisfied with a decision of a U.S. district court may appeal to a U.S. court of appeals. Magistrate judges handle some district court matters. Federal judges usually serve lifetime terms.

The Supreme Court has played a critical role in interpreting the United States Constitution, and therefore, the study of constitutional law places emphasis on prior rulings made by the Supreme Court. The Supreme Court consists of the Chief Justice and eight associate justices. A party may ask the U.S. Supreme Court to review a decision from a U.S. court of appeals, but the Supreme Court is usually under no obligation to do so. The U.S. Supreme Court is the final arbiter of federal constitutional questions. The president usually consults senators or other elected officials concerning candidates to fill vacancies on the federal courts.

The cases heard in federal courts include cases that influence the constitutionality of a law and cases involving the United States government, ambassadors and public ministers, disputes between two or more states, admiralty law, and bankruptcy (Federal Judicial Center, 2012). The Department of Justice, which is responsible for prosecuting federal crimes and representing the government in civil cases, is the most frequent litigator in the federal court system (U.S. Courts, 2012). All power that is not delegated to the federal government remains with the individual states.

State Legal Systems
The structure of state court systems varies from state to state with each state having its own government structure and laws. Some states have some unique features; however, many commonalities exist among them. All states have a high-level court, usually called a state supreme court. The state constitution and laws of each state establish the state courts. Some states also have an intermediate court of appeals. Below these are the state trial courts, also referred to as circuit or district Courts. States also have designated courts to handle specific legal matters, e.g. probate court (wills and estates), juvenile court, and family court

All of the states use legal codes, or statutory laws. New York refers to its codes as *laws*, while California and Texas simply call them *codes*. Most other states use *revised statutes, compiled statutes*, or some other name for their codes. Statutes are laws passed by the U.S. Congress or state legislatures.

A statute is an act, legislation, or law. It is an expansive statement of opinion, arising from case law or an application through administrative regulations. Statutes start out as bills and are eventually passed as laws. They are published initially as slip laws or session laws, which are given public law numbers at the federal level and published in the Statutes at Large. Later, subject arranges the divided laws, allocated into a collection of laws. Each section of the original law then takes on its own identity and is signified by a new identifying number. The new law can be arranged independently from other sections of the original law. Like their federal counterparts, all state constitutions, statutes and regulations are subject to judicial interpretation.

Judges in county, parish, and state courts are elected or appointed according to systems established by each state's laws. The methods of selecting state judges vary from state to state. The most common selection systems operate by commission nomination or popular election. In the state commission system, the governor chooses the state judges from a list of candidates selected by an independent commission.

With very few exceptions, state judges serve specified, renewable terms of office as determined by state law (Federal Judicial Center, 2012). The types of cases heard in state courts include most criminal cases, probate cases (involving wills and estates), most contract cases, tort cases (personal injuries), and family law cases. State courts are the final arbiters of state laws and constitutions (U.S. Courts, 2012).

Jurisdictional Issues

Jurisdictional issues determine whether a case goes to county, state, or federal courts. Matters concerning the railroad, post office, federal agency workers, and maritime work injuries are under federal jurisdiction. Companies with offices all over the United States may seek federal jurisdiction, rather than state or local jurisdiction. Many lawsuits are settled based on the interpretation of a federal statute or regulation. Depending on the facts of the case, one or both parties involved may seek one jurisdiction over another (state versus federal court). In some cases, federal courts share jurisdiction with state courts. For example, both federal and state courts may decide cases involving patients who live in different states. State courts have exclusive jurisdiction over the vast majority of cases (Federal Judicial Center, 2012).

As the ultimate decision-making authority, the U.S. Supreme Court determines whether a ruling is constitutional or not, and its decisions are the supreme law of the land. The Supreme Court, according to the United States Constitution, can decide on two types of cases, diversity of citizenship cases and lawsuits between states:

- Diversity of citizenship cases are civil in nature, involve parties from different states, and concern amounts exceeding $75,000. Often federal courts must apply state law to these cases.
- Lawsuits between states include cases involving high-ranking figures, federal crimes, state bankruptcy, securities and banking, and those cases specified by federal statutes.

State court jurisdiction applies to cases that do not fall into the select jurisdiction of federal courts. State courts have the authority to apply and interpret the law. They also have the power to create law by way of the state legislature if there is not already an existing law to remedy a particular legal problem. Types of cases that fall under state jurisdiction include the following:

- Cases involving the state's constitution
- State criminal offenses
- Tort and personal injury law
- Contract law
- Probate (involving a decedent's will and distribution of the assets)

- Family cases, such as divorce, custody, adoption, and child support
- Municipal and zoning ordinances
- Traffic regulation

Federal and state courts share jurisdiction when a state has regulated on a matter more extensively than the federal government. They also share authority on the following types of cases:

- Diversity of citizenship
- Federal questions: A state court may interpret the U.S. Constitution if the provision has direct bearing on a case brought in state court under state law. However, interpreting the U.S. Constitution subjects the state to federal review. In these cases, the U.S. Supreme court is concerned only with the aspects of the case that involve federal matters. It does not review matters exclusively under state jurisdiction.

This brief summary of the legal system of the United States is not intended to be all-inclusive but rather to serve as a foundation for the nurse life care planner. Nurse life care planners are encouraged to use the following references to learn more detailed information about the legal system for the purpose of enhancing their understanding and furthering their own education.

References

Blackwell T. (1995). Ethical principles for life care planners. Inside Life Care Planning, 1(2), 2, 9.

Blackwell T, Havranek J. and Field T. (1996). Ethical foundation for rehabilitation professionals. NARPPS Journal, 11(3), 7-12.

Burnham W. (2002). Introduction to the Law and Legal System of the United States. Location: West Group.

Casuto D, McCollom P. (2012). Life care planning. In M.
O'Keefe (Ed.), Nursing Practice and the Law: Avoiding
Malpractice and Other Legal Risks (pp.416-430).

Chew, N. (2012). What is the nurse practice act? Retrieved
from http://www.ehow.com/about_5183011_
nurse-practice-act_.html

Comparing federal and state courts. (2012). Retrieved from:
www.uscourts.gov

Farnsworth EA. (2010). An Introduction to the Legal System of
the United States (4ᵗʰ ed.). New York, NY: Oxford Press.

Federal courts in American government. (2012). Retrieved
from: www.uscourts.gov

Federal Judicial Center (2012). The U.S. legal system: A short
description. Retrieved from: http://www.fjc.gov/
public/pdf.nsf/lookup/U.S._Legal_System_English07.
pdf/$file/U.S._Legal_System_English07.pdf

Lex and Louisiana Legal Staff. (2006). Louisiana legal-law
articles-history of Louisiana. Retrieved from: www.
la-legal.com/modules/article/view.article.php?c8

National Council of State Boards of Nursing website: www.
ncsbn.org

Nurse practice act. (2009). In Mosby's Medical Dictionary (8ᵗʰ
ed.). St. Louis, MO: Mosby /Elsevier.

Quan, K. (2011). Definitions of nursing. In The Everything New
Nurse Book: Gain Confidence, Manage Your Schedule,
and Be Ready for Anything! (2nd ed.). Avon, MA: Adams
Media.

Reichel, P. (1999). Comparative criminal justice systems
(pp.141-143). NJ: Prentice Hall.

Riddick S. and Weed R. (1996). The life care planning process
for managing catastrophically impaired patients. In
S.S.Blancett and D. L. Flarey (Eds.), Case studies in
nursing case management: health care delivery in a
world of managed care (pp. 61-91). Gaithersburg, MD:
Aspen.

Taylor S. (2012). Life care plans in court. Neurolaw Letter, 5(5),
25, 28.

Weed RO and Berens DE. (Eds.).(1999). Forensic issues for
life care planners. In Life CarePlanning and Case
Management Handbook (pp.351-369). Boca Raton, FL:
CRC Press.
Yudkoff K. (1998). The life care planning expert. In J. B. Bogart
(Ed.), Legal Nurse Consulting: Principles and Practice
(pp. 657-686). Boca Raton, FL: CRC Press.

CHAPTER 2

Litigation Processes for Life Care Planning

Barbara Bate, RN-BC, CCM, CNLCP, LNCC, MSCC

Qualifying Expert Witness

This chapter will inform the nurse life care planner of the background information needed to function as an expert witness. This includes:

- Responsibilities as an expert witness
- Tools to ensure the reports meet the criteria for expert reports
- Information for the nurse life care planner describing the role of the expert witness

Nurse life care planners functioning in the role of an expert witness should be aware of federal rules that address civil procedure, opinions, and expert testimony, in addition to important cases supporting these rules. *Federal Rules of Civil Procedure* govern the conduct of all civil actions brought in federal district courts. *Federal Rules of Evidence* rule the introduction of evidence in proceedings, both civil and criminal, in federal courts. While both do not apply to suits in state courts, the rules of many states are modeled by the federal rules.

Listed below are summaries of select Federal Rules of Evidence and Federal Rules of Civil Procedure, and information that nurse life care planners may wish to consider when working as an expert witness. As this is a general review, specific questions regarding the rules and how they affect the nurse life care planner as an expert witness are best discussed with the retaining attorney prior to acceptance of the contract to discern conflict of interest.

439

Federal Rules of Evidence (Article VII-Opinions and Expert Testimony)
Rule 702. Testimony by Experts

This rule pertains to whether expert opinions are admissible at trial. It requires that the expert opinion be pertinent and reliable. In essence, it examines whether the opinion will help the jury to decide an issue in the case, and whether the expert is qualified by education, training, and/or experience to give the opinion. It also evaluates whether the opinion is reliable. For an opinion to be permitted, the opinion should be based on documented standards and or evidenced based practice in the field of the expert (Nofsinger, personal communication, 2012).

Nurse life care planners should be aware that their reports would be reviewed closely for relevance and reliability and with the possibility of a *Daubert* hearing in front of a judge. Under the "Daubert line of cases," the judge is considered to be the gatekeeper, determining whether testimony and reports should be excluded. Several factors considered by the judge include:

- Whether the theory or technique used can be, and has been, tested (i.e., can it be challenged in an objectively vs. subjectively)
- Whether the theory or technique has been peer-reviewed and published
- Known or potential rate of error of the method used
- The existence and maintenance of standards and controls
- Whether the scientific community generally accepts the method (Babitsky, Mangraviti, 2004; Cornell, 2011).

Most state trial courts apply some variation of the *Daubert* test when determining whether expert testimony is admissible under this rule (Black, 2011).

Rule 703. Bases of Opinion Testimony by Experts

This rule permits an expert witness to express opinions based upon available facts and data, even if some of the underlying facts or data are evidence that cannot be introduced at trial. For example, an expert can use a hearsay statement as a component of reaching an opinion, even if the judge or jury would not hear that statement during the course of the trial (Nofsinger, personal communication, 2012).

Nurse life care planners frequently obtain future care recommendations and costs from providers (physical therapists, specialists, vendors, etc.) who will not be testifying at trial. This information is incorporated into the life care plan and, under this rule, can be used to support the nurse life care planner's recommendations.

Rule 704. Opinion on Ultimate Issue

Ordinarily, witnesses are not permitted to express opinions concerning the expected verdict. For example, a police officer cannot opine a criminal defendant as "guilty," and a plaintiff injured in a car accident cannot testify that the other driver was "negligent." An example of this rule in action is a physician expert testifying that the defendant physician was negligent in the care of a patient. The average judge or juror may not be able to reach an opinion without the aid of an expert because the conclusion requires expertise (Nofsinger, personal communication, 2012).

The American Nurses Association defines nursing as "the protection, promotion, and optimization of health and abilities, prevention of illness and injury, alleviation of suffering through the diagnosis and treatment of human response, and advocacy in the care of individuals, families, communities, and populations" (ANA Scope and Standards, 2010). They additionally state that "all registered nurses are educated in the art and science of nursing, with the goal of helping individuals, families, groups, communities, and populations to promote, attain, maintain, and restore health or to experience dignified death" (ANA Nursing's Social Policy and Statement, 2010). Nurse life care planners are in a unique position to aid the judge or juror in reaching an opinion regarding the plaintiff's future care needs and associated costs based upon their individual knowledge, skills, education, training and experience.

Rule 705. Disclosure of Facts or Data Underlying Expert Opinion

Experts are permitted to express their opinions without testifying as to how they arrived at those opinions. They do not have to describe all of the information that they relied on in reaching that opinion. However, if an expert expresses an opinion without testifying to all of the information that informed that opinion, the opposing attorney is free to inquire about the source information that the expert considered. As a practical matter, if an expert states a conclusory opinion, that opinion is likely to be more persuasive if the expert explains how the opinion was reached, so most attorneys will ask the expert preliminary questions about the underlying data before asking the expert to express opinions" (Nofsinger, personal communication, 2012).

The nurse life care planner may be asked to review a case and provide a verbal opinion prior to developing a report. Once developed, and the nurse life care planner has been designated as an expert, they should be prepared to share all information relied upon when forming their opinions.

Rule 706. Court Appointed Experts

A judge can choose to retain an expert in a given case. This occurs in criminal prosecutions, "rarely in civil matters" (Nofsinger, personal communication, 2012). Nevertheless, it is possible that a nurse life care planner could be asked by the court to serve as an expert witness.

Rule 26. Duty to Disclose: General Provisions Governing Discovery

This rule is broad and pertains to the sharing of information throughout the discovery period in civil proceedings in addition to outlining requirements pertaining to experts. Summary of this rule will be limited to Rule 26 (a) (2) Disclosure of Expert Testimony and Rule 26 (a)(4) Trial Preparation: Experts.

Rule 26(a)(2). Disclosure of Expert Testimony

The identity of any expert must be disclosed to the other side in the course of the litigation process prior to the disclosure deadline. If the expert was retained to complete a report, then that report must be provided to the other side. The report must reveal:

- All of the opinions held by the expert and the basis for those opinions
- Everything that was reviewed by the witness in reaching those opinions
- Any exhibits that will be used by the expert to support those opinions
- The expert's qualifications and list of any publications
- A list of any other cases that the expert has testified in during the past four years
- Disclosure of payments to the expert (J. Nofsinger, personal communication, 2012)
- Disclosure is the responsibility of the retaining party, not the nurse life care planner

26(b)(4). Trial Preparation: Experts.

After the disclosure, the opposing side has the right to depose the expert. It also states the expert does not have to disclose all communications with the retaining attorney. Draft reports and other communications do not have to be disclosed unless they reveal information about the compensation of the expert or pertain to facts/assumptions that the expert considered in reaching opinions. The rule further requires that the party taking the expert's deposition must pay the expert a reasonable fee for deposition time (Nofsinger, personal communication, 2012). The nurse life care planner should review requests for documents with the referring attorney prior to disclosing any documents as certain documents may be protected.

Rule 30. Deposition by Oral Examination

This rule governs deposition practice. Written notice to the referring attorney and witness must be given within a reasonable time and can require the witness to appear to answer questions and to produce non-privileged documents. An authorized recorder (a court reporter) must record the deposition. At a deposition, both sides can choose to ask questions for "the record." The behavior of the parties must be within certain bounds of decorum, and can include seeking information that would not necessarily be admissible at trial under the rules of evidence. Depositions may not exceed seven hours, but may be continued to a different time. After the deposition has concluded, the witness has the right to review the transcript to make corrections (Nofsinger, personal communication, 2012).

Nurse life care planners should expect to be deposed when working as experts. Many experts will take advantage of their ability to review their testimony to make sure it is correct. It is good practice for the nurse life care planner to discuss the opportunity to review with the retaining attorney and share the request for review with the court reporter and opposing party prior to leaving the deposition.

Rule 34. Producing Documents, Electronically Stored Information, and Tangible Things, or Entering onto Land, for Inspection and Other Purposes

Upon request, a party to a case must provide documents or other stored information, tangible objects, or inspection of land/tangible objects if relevant to the case. The notice must be "reasonably particular" in making such requests and specify the means by which electronically stored information should be provided. The party receiving the request may object to complying with the request and must state a reason for the objection (J. Nofsinger, personal communication, 2012). The nurse life care planner should review requests for information with the referring attorney prior to disclosure.

Legal Process

This section outlines the process for a legal proceeding along with definitions and insight into what each phase entails. An overview of the entire process assists the nurse life care planner in understanding legal procedure. As this is a general overview, specific questions regarding these processes should be discussed with the retaining attorney.

1. *Cause of action:* A group of operative facts, which give rise to one or more bases for suing; a factual situation that entitles one person to obtain a remedy in court from another person. (Black, 2011). This phase occurs following a loss or an injury. There is a limited period of time for the investigation and filing of the claim. Typically, following an injury or loss, the afflicted party (plaintiff) consults with an attorney. The attorney investigates the basis of the injury or loss and determines whether there is recovery under the law. Attempts to resolve the dispute may be made by the attorney by contacting the responsible party's insurance carrier to start settlement negotiations before the complaint is filed. (Bate, personal communication, 2012).

2. *Complaint:* The complaint is the initial pleading that starts the civil action, stating the basis for the court's jurisdiction, the basis for the plaintiff's claim, and the demand for relief (Black, 2011). The complaint defines facts and circumstances regarding the plaintiff's complaint in addition to a demand. Once filed with the

court, the complaint is delivered to the defendant (Bate, personal communication, 2012).

3. *Answer*: A defendant's first pleading that addresses the merits of the case, usually denying the plaintiff's allegations (Black, 2011). The defendant formally responds to the complaint (D. Bate, personal communication, 2012).

4. *Discovery*: "The pretrial phase of a lawsuit during which depositions, interrogatories, and other forms of discovery are conducted (Black, 2011). Discovery allows both sides to have a clear understanding of the case and may lead to settlement prior to trial. The discovery period is set in a scheduling order, by a judge and is often the longest phase of the legal process (Bate, personal communication, 2012).

5. *Motion for summary judgment:* A request that the court enter judgment without a trial because there is lack of material fact to be decided by the fact-finder, i.e., because the evidence is legally insufficient to support a verdict in the non-movant's favor (Black, 2011). Either party may file the motion for summary judgment after the discovery period has ended (Bate, personal communication, 2012).

6. *Alternative dispute resolution:* A procedure for settling a dispute by means other than litigation, such as arbitration or mediation. (Black, 2011). Before a motion in limine (see next section) can be filed, states require cases that have survived summary judgment to attempt alternative dispute resolution with a mediator specially trained in resolving contentious cases (Bate, personal communication, 2012).

7. *Motion* in limine: A pretrial request to the court that certain inadmissible evidence not be referred to or

offered at trial. A party makes this motion when it believes that mere mention of the evidence during trial would be highly prejudicial and could not be remedied by an instruction to disregard. If, after the motion is granted, the opposing party mentions or attempts to offer the evidence in the jury's presence, a mistrial may be ordered. A ruling in motion *in limine* does not always preserve evidentiary error for appellate purposes. To raise such an error on appeal, a party may be required to formally object when the evidence is actually admitted or excluded during trial (Black, 2011). Motion *in limine* can result in limitation of an expert witness' testimony (Bate, personal communication, 2012).

8. *Jury selection (if applicable):* Selection of the jury occurs prior to the opening statements. A jury is a "group of persons selected according to law and given the power to decide questions of fact and return a verdict in the case submitted to them" (Black, 2011). Many states use the *voir dire* process, involving questioning of potential jurors to identify specific personal feelings or bias regarding the case (Bate, personal communication, 2012).

9. *Opening statements and presentation of case:* After the parties give their opening statements to the jury, the plaintiff presents the facts the case through testimony and exhibits. At the end of the plaintiff's case the defendant will usually move for a directed verdict (or judgment as a matter of law), arguing that the plaintiff has not proven the case and that no reasonable juror could find in favor of the opposing party. If that motion is denied, then the defendant presents the case much like the plaintiff. Again, the plaintiff may move for a directed verdict. If that motion is denied, the plaintiff has the opportunity to question the expert as rebuttal and the defendant may move for another directed verdict. Following the defendant's case, the plaintiff, and

then the defendant, may present additional evidence to rebut new evidence from the opposing party, subject to the discretion of the court (D. Bate, personal communication, 2012).

10. *Closing arguments:* In a trial, a lawyer's final statement to the judge or jury before deliberation begins in which the lawyer requests the judge or jury to consider that evidence and to apply the law in his or her client's favor (Black, 2011).

11. *Jury instructions:* A direction or guideline that a judge gives a jury concerning the law of the case (Black, 2011).

12. *Verdict:* A jury's finding or decision on the factual issues of a case. In a nonjury trial, a judge's resolution settles the issues of a case (Black, 2011).

13. *Motion for judgment, N.O.V. (notwithstanding verdict):* A party's request that the court enter a judgment in its favor despite the jury's contrary verdict because there is no legally sufficient evidentiary basis for a jury to find in favor of the other party (Black, 2011).

14. *Motion for a new trial:* A party's post-judgment request for the court to vacate the judgment and order a new trial for such reasons as factually insufficient evidence, newly discovered evidence, and jury misconduct. In many jurisdictions, this motion is required before a party can raise such a matter on appeal (Black, 2011).

15. *Final judgment order:* A court's last action that settles the rights of the parties and disposes of all issues in controversy, except for the award of costs (and, sometimes, attorney's fees) and enforcement of the judgment (Black, 2011).

16. Appeal: A proceeding undertaken to have a decision reconsidered by a higher authority; especially, the submission of a lower court's or agency's decision to a higher court for review and possible reversal (Black, 2011). Appeals are frequently based on legal issues or amount of damages (excessive or insufficient) (Bate, personal communication, 2012).

References

American Association of Nurse Life Care Planners (AANLCP®), (2012). Standards of practice.

American Nurses Association, (2010). Nursing, scope and standards of practice (2ⁿᵈ ed.). Silver Spring, MD: Nursebooks.org.

American Nurse Association, (2010). Nursing's social policy statement, the essence of the profession. Silver Spring, MD: Nursebooks.org.

Babitsky S and Mangraviti J. (2004). Writing and defending your expert report, the step-by-step guide with models. Falmouth, Massachusets: SEAK, Inc.

Black HC. (2011). *Black's Law Dictionary* (4ᵗʰ pocket edition). St. Paul, MN: West Publishing Company.

Cornell University Law School. (2011, December 1). Federal rules of evidence. Retrieved from http://www.law.cornell.edu/rules/fre/

Cornell University Law School. (2010, December 1). Federal rules of civil procedure. Retrieved from http://www.law.cornell.edu/rules/frcp/#chapter_v (www.law.cornell.edu/rules/fre, www.law.cornell.edu/rules/frcp/#chapter_v.)

Bate D. (personal communication in 2012).
Nofsinger J. (personal communication in 2012).

CHAPTER 3

Disability Rights Laws

April Pettengill, BSN, RN, CRRN, CNLCP, MSCC

Introduction

Numerous federal civil rights laws have been enacted over the years to help ensure that persons with and without disabilities are afforded equal opportunities. In addition to laws that affect the general public there are others that pertain to specific populations, such as the Longshore and Harbor Workers' Compensation Act. While disability rights laws were originally set up to provide protection for disabled persons as part of the Civil Rights Law of 1964, they have benefited the non-disabled population as well. This is notable, for example, in the Americans with Disability Act (ADA), which makes it easier for all citizens to access and traverse public spaces.

Although focus tends to stay on some of the more recent disability rights laws enacted after the Civil Rights Law of 1964, such as the ADA, the Rehabilitation Act of 1973, and the Individual with Disabilities Education Act (IDEA), disability rights acts have been part of US law as early as 1927. This chapter will briefly describe some of the disability rights laws and will focus on those that have the most effect on the practice of nurse life care planning. While we are taught not to consider collateral resources as part of our planning except in very limited and specific instances, in some cases these laws directly affect what is included the life care plan and should be considered when writing a life care plan.

Lesser-Known Disability Laws

While these may not pertain to every life care plan, understanding each act and how it may affect nurse life care planning is important. Examples are discussed below.

Telecommunications Act of 1996

This Act requires that manufactures and providers of telecommunication equipment must ensure that all equipment is accessible and usable by persons with disabilities (FCC, 2011). This is especially important for blind or deaf persons who must use telephones, cell phones, or pagers.

A nurse life care planner could be certain that a person with deafness or blindness would be able to call for help or use telecommunications systems. The person with dual disability, such as traumatic brain injury with loss of vision, may require additional education on how to access these systems and additional support (e.g., equipment, training) for access. The nurse life care planner should have an understanding of these needs to ensure the costs and placement costs are accurate.

The telecommunications device for the deaf (TDD) is an electronic device designed for persons with hearing or speech difficulties. It is a keyboarded device that uses LED or LCD to electronically send messages over phone lines via a relay operator from the hearing-impaired sender to the message recipient. The operator will type the sender's message, which is displayed on the recipient's TDD device. The recipient can dictate the reply to the relay operator, who then sends it to the sender's device. There is no charge to use the phone line or the operator; however, there is a cost to the device of between $150 and $250 for the teletype phone. With the advancement of text messaging, the TDD system may become obsolete. The life care planner should look at the option of using a cell phone with texting capabilities as an option to the TDD system.

Fair Housing Act of 1965, Amended 1988

The Fair Housing Act (FHA), originally enacted in 1965, was amended in 1988 and prohibits discrimination based on race, color, religion, sex, disability, familial status, or national origin. It includes private housing and housing that receives federal assistance (HUD, 2011).

Nurse life care planners will most likely be concerned with the portion of the law that requires housing facilities to make reasonable exceptions in their policies and operations to allow equal housing opportunities to persons with disabilities. A landlord must allow tenants to make reasonable access-related home modifications to private living spaces and common use areas. The landlord is not required to pay for those modifications. In addition, new multifamily housing with four or more units must be built to allow access for disabled persons, including wider doorways to accommodate wheelchair access.

The FHA is important in nurse life care planning for home modifications. If the person is in a rented home and meets the criteria of this act, the landlord may have to allow the disabled person to make necessary accommodations in the tenant's private living area and common areas (such as lobbies, walkways, and playgrounds). It is important to note that the Act specifically states that the landlord does not have to pay for these accommodations and the accommodations must be reasonable. There are stipulations as to which housing units qualify under the FHA but generally the FHA binds any housing of more than four units and receiving federal funding, such as Section 8 housing.

Air Carrier Access Act of 1986
The Air Carrier Access Act of 1986 prohibits discrimination in air travel based upon mental or physical disability. This act pertains to domestic flights and foreign air carriers that use airports in the United States. This act address boarding assistance and accessibility of the aircraft as well newly built or altered facilities (DOT, 2011).

In a life care plan, knowledge of this act would be helpful in planning vacations or treatment that required air travel. It is important to know that airlines are mandated to provide accessibility to air travel to ensure that the person with a disability can travel safely. It is also important to know the

Act's requirements of the airline and the airport, as additional accommodations may need to be made. This information can be found on an airline's webpage or by calling the airline directly.

Voting Accessibility for the Elderly and Handicapped Act (VAEHA)
National Voter Registration Act (NVRA)

Both VAEHA and the NVRA allow measures for persons with disability to be able to exercise their right to vote.

The Acts provide for alternative means for individuals to be able to vote, e.g., for telecommunications device for the deaf (TDD) and TTYs for the blind, and an alternative method of voting, such as mail-in ballots, if the municipality is unable to provide access.

While nurse life care planners may not think of citizenship when developing a life care plan, it is extremely important to many people to be able to exercise their voting rights. The life care planner may want to provide for the cost of transportation to and from the polling site as part of the plan. The NVRA allows for a person to register to vote at home, with the forms to be transported by a state official. This would be important for people who have had to relocate due to disability. If they have moved to a new town, they will need to register to vote in that town.

Civil Rights of Institutionalized Persons Act

The Civil Rights of Institutionalized Persons Act (CRIPA) authorizes the U.S. Attorney General to investigate the conditions of state and locally run institutions, e.g., publicly operated nursing homes, psychiatric institutions, and homes for the developmentally delayed. While the attorney general is not able to investigate single incidents, he or she can bring a civil action against an institution where there are allegations of egregious conditions that subject the residents to "grievous harm" (DOJ, 2011)

This act makes it possible for the nurse life care planner to ensure that facilities are operating without causing harm to the residents. When investigating facilities, the nurse life care planner can refer to the Department of Justice website to determine if a suit has been filed against any institution or agency. It may be important for the nurse life care planner to note if there were egregious conditions at an institution. It may also expose the nurse life care planner to an action for nursing malpractice should an institution that has numerous or egregious conditions be recommended in the life care plan.

Major Disability Rights Law That Impact Life Care Planning
There are three major disability rights laws that can directly affect life care planning. The *Rehabilitation Act of 1973* prohibits discrimination based on disability to any program that receives federal funding. The *Individuals with Disability Education Act (IDEA) of 1975* requires public schools to make available to all eligible children with disabilities a free and appropriate education in the least restrictive environment. The *Americans with Disability Act (ADA) of 1990* prohibits discrimination based on disability in employment, state, and local government, public accommodations, commercial facilities, transportation, and telecommunications.

The Rehabilitation Act of 1973
The Rehabilitation Act of 1973 was developed by Congress to replace the Vocational Rehabilitation Act and to

> extend and revise the authorization of grants to the states for vocational rehabilitation services, with special emphasis on services to those with the most severe handicaps, to expand special federal responsibilities and research and training programs with respect to handicapped individuals, to establish special responsibilities in the Secretary of Health, Education, and Welfare for coordination of all programs with respect to handicapped individuals

within the Department of Health, Education, and Welfare, and for other purposes (America, 1973).

While its main purpose was for vocational rehabilitation, the Act provided funding for research and pilot projects, increased funding for construction and improvement to rehabilitation facilities, develop new medical technologies, expand services to disabled individuals, and evaluate architectural and transportation barriers to disabled individuals.

The Rehabilitation Act lays out the provisions in each of the sections and expansion of the services offered to disabled individuals. It is divided into separate titles addressing specific parts of the Act. *Section 504* of the Rehabilitation Act is of primary concern for nurse life care planners and deals with nondiscrimination under federal grants and programs. This section will be explored in greater depth later in the chapter.

Who qualifies under the Rehabilitation Act is defined. The amended version in 1998 defines disability as

(A) except as noted in subparagraph (B), a physical or mental impairment that constitutes or results in substantial impediment to employment, or (B) for the purposes of Title V, a physical or mental impairment that substantially limits one or more major life activities (RA, 2000).

Major life activities include self-care, mobility, seeing, hearing, speaking, breathing, working, manual tasks, and learning. Examples would include chronic conditions, such as AIDS, alcohol and substance abuse, visual impairment, hearing impairment, attention deficit-hyperactivity disorder, autism, and mental illness.

Section 504 of the Rehabilitation Act

Section 504 of the Rehabilitation Act of 1973 states that no otherwise qualified disabled person in the United States shall be excluded from participation in, denied the benefit of, or be subject to discrimination under any program or activity receiving federal assistance based solely on their disability (RA, 2000). This section applies to education, pertinent to life care planning.

The entities covered under this section include state and local governments or their sub-entities; a college, university, post-secondary institution, or public system of higher education; local educational agencies such as elementary, secondary, or vocational schools; a corporation (must receive federal funding); health care facilities; parks and recreation services or social services; or any other employer that receives federal funding.

Section 504 requires a plan to be implemented to assist the person with a disability. This plan lists specific accommodations required help them to participate in education, employment, and recreation, e.g., assistive technology, a peanut-free area, or extra textbooks.

The 504 plan addresses the barriers to education or employment and puts in place the accommodations necessary for the individual to function on a level plane with their peers. A sample 504 plan template is included in Table 1.

Table 1. Sample 504 plan

AIKEN COUNTY PUBLIC SCHOOLS
Section 504 Accommodation Plan

Student: _____ Date of Meeting:
_____

School: _____ D.O.B: _____ Grade:
_____

Anticipated annual review: _____

The Section 504 Team determines that this student has a
disability, under Section 504.
DISABILITY:

CONCERNS:

**HOW THE DISABILITY/HANDICAP AFFECTS A MAJOR LIFE
ACTIVITY:**

REASONABLE ACCOMMODATIONS THAT ARE NECESSARY:
Accommodation   *Person(s)*
responsible

_____   _____
_____   _____
_____   _____
_____   _____

Used with permission, Aiken County Public School, 2011

The 504 plan is different from an Individualized Educational Plan (IEP), which falls under the Individuals with Disability Education Act (IDEA) and will be discussed later. A comparison of the two is made in Table 2. *One major difference is funding for the accommodations; a 504 plan is funded by the individual entity such as the school system while the IEP is supported by federal funds.* It is important for the life care planner to understand this difference as it may affect the implementation of the 504 plan.

Table 2. Comparison of IDEA and Section 504 (DREDF, 2011)

	IDEA	504 Plan
Purpose	Education Act to provide federal funding to state and local agencies for qualified disabled children	A civil rights law created to prohibit discrimination on the basis of disability in programs that receive federal funding
Free, appropriate public education	Yes, including special education services specially designed at no cost to parents. States are required to provide the recommended services. An IEP is developed which outlines those services	Yes. An appropriate education as compared to students without disabilities even if no special education services are received. A 504 plan is developed which outlines the accommodation which will be provided.
Funding to implement services	IDEA provides for federal funding under Parts B and C.	No. The state and local agencies are required to fund the 504 plan.
Evaluation and placement	A comprehensive multidisciplinary team evaluation is required initially and at least every 3 years but most are performed annually. An IEP meeting is required with the parents prior to implementing the IEP or making any changes. The IEP can provide services in environments other than the school such as home or a special facility (the least restrictive environment).	504 Plan requires notification and not consent for an evaluation. A meeting is not required to make changes. The 504 plan requires that students be educated with their peers to the maximum extent possible.

Keep in mind that some accommodations under the 504 plan may not have financial cost but may affect how the classroom activities are conducted. For example, a 504 plan for a child with ADHD might include extra time to complete tests or work. This provision may mean the rest of the class may need to wait for the child to complete this task before moving on to the next one or that the child is removed from the classroom while the other children move on to the next task. If this continues, however, it reinforces the disabled child's inability to keep up with school.

The nurse life care planner needs to understand how the 504 plan is implemented and whether it will have additional consequences that should be taken into consideration in the plan. The family may have to hire a tutor, at considerable expense, for the child to stay at the same class level as his peers. Another example may be a companion dog trained to keep an autistic child moving in the appropriate direction or away from danger. Neither of these would be covered under the 504 plan but would be an expense borne by the family.

Individuals with Disability Education Act (IDEA)

IDEA, originally enacted in 2000, has been reauthorized as the Individuals with Disability Education Improvement Act of 2004. IDEA provides federal financial assistance to state and local education agencies. A multidisciplinary evaluation is required to determine what specific educational assistance the person with the disability requires. The person cannot be charged for education-related assistance.

Nurse life care planners should be most familiar with Part B, which pertains to children ages three to twenty-one, and Part C, which pertains to children age 0 to 2 (IDEA, 2011).

The multidisciplinary team consists of qualified personnel with professional standards of practice to evaluate the child and determine what services are required. This could be physical, occupational, speech, or vision therapy. It could be counseling or family training, or it could be transportation to and from school. An IEP is developed with input from all of the team members and the parents of the child. Both Part B and Part C require an in-depth, multidisciplinary evaluation and development of IEP.

The multidisciplinary team may consist of physical, occupational, speech, vision therapists, mental health counselors or social workers, audiologists, nurses, mobility specialists, pediatricians, and special educators. Covered services could include, but are not limited to, family training, home visits, physical, occupational, speech therapies, psychological counseling, and service coordination including transition programs for those children moving from Part C to Part B eligibility. Keep in mind that these services must be educationally focused and are not for maintenance of function.

Only children with certain classifications of disabilities are eligible for an IEP. They are those who require significant remediation and assistance and are more likely to work on their own level at their own pace even in an inclusive classroom. These would include children with developmental delay. Each state must have a definition of developmental delay and that definition would determine eligibility for the IEP and services under IDEA. This is important for the nurse life care planner to understand and research to determine if the child meets the criteria. If not, they may be eligible for services under Section 504 of the Rehabilitation Act. States also have the option of serving children at risk for developmental delay but again this is defined by each state.

In addition to the IEP, an *Individual Family Service Plan* (IFSP) may be developed. This is a written document, which explains in detail how the family's and child's needs are to be met. It also documents what the family's resources are and concerns that family has expressed. The IFSP must also outline transition program from early education (Part C) to education

(Part B). The IFSP must outline the environment in which the services will be provided. For example, they may be provided in the family home, childcare setting, or special educational facility. A sample IEP template is included in Table 3.

Table 3. IEP Sample template.

Service, Aid, or Modification	Frequency	Location	Beginning Date	Duration

The nurse life care planner should understand the process and requirements under IDEA. It is important to know what is and is not covered by IDEA. This information is available on the state's webpage or in their information about disability assistance. It should also be outlined in the school's information or policies regarding disabled students. When writing the life care plan, the planner must anticipate any costs that the family will incur for services. The therapies are a typical area of confusion in the life care plan. If the IEP calls for home based early education physical, occupational and speech therapies, those services are typically provided at no cost to the family. There may be additional therapies recommended that are not covered under IDEA because they are not related to education. The child may require private therapy more often than the IEP recommends. The family is responsible for these costs.

Americans with Disability Act

The ADA was originally passed in 1990. The ADA Amended Act (ADAAA) was passed in 2008 and became effective in 2009. The purpose of the ADA was to allow persons with disability protection against social and structural barriers. It protects individuals with physical or mental disabilities from discrimination in the workplace, private businesses, public buildings, or other organizations that operate places of public accommodation. Congress found that persons with disabilities have been precluded from fully participating in all aspects of society because of discrimination (ADA Amended, 2009).

The ADA defines a disability as a physical or mental impairment that substantially limits one or more major life activities, or there is a record of such impairment, or the person is regarded as having impairment (ADA Amended, 2009). Major life activities include activities such as self-care, seeing, hearing, eating, sleeping, walking, standing, lifting, bending, speaking, breathing, and working. The ADA does not apply to disability that is not permanent, e.g., temporary postoperative restrictions.

The ADA provides for accessibility to buildings, federally owned lands, and private businesses. The accommodations set forth in the ADA have become standardized when building a commercial building. Many states also adopted these regulations for private homes to be considered accessible. If a public entity can prove that making accommodation under ADA is an undue burden, they become responsible for providing services to the extent that it is not a burden.

The ADA affects life care planning in the area of employment. An employer can no longer refuse to hire a person due to disability. The employer must have a list of essential job functions. Once the job is offered, the employer can require a post-offer, pre-employment physical to ensure the person meets the essential job functions. The employer is required to make reasonable accommodations, which may include making the work place accessible or a job modification such as adding devices or changing hours. If the employer fails to meet these requirements and discriminates, they may be legally liable. It is important to note that ADA only applies to employers with more than 15 employees for 20 weeks per year.

ADA is important for the life care planner because the provisions it sets forth around barrier-free access are important for planning future care needs for the person. As noted above many municipalities have adopted the ADA guidelines for accessibility to private residences. Therefore it is important to make sure that the contractor who provides a quote or does any accommodation must be aware of the regulations and abide by them.

Employment accommodations need to be addressed in the life care plan if the person is capable of return to work. While the employer should provide reasonable accommodations, they may consider it an undue hardship and therefore will require financial assistance to employ the person. This needs to be considered in the life care plan and addressed accordingly. The ADA, like the Rehabilitation Act, is a civil rights law and provides for accommodation. It does not apply directly to education but becomes important when looking at accessibility of the educational facilities. It does not provide for funding of the accommodations.

The Rehabilitation Act, IDEA, and ADA work together to provide reasonable accommodations for persons with disabilities to perform essential functions in the workplace or the school. In the case of the student, it may be the ability to get from one level of the school to another. This is also true if special education is providing job-coaching services under IEP or vocational rehabilitation is providing job placement under the 504 plan.

Summary
All disability rights laws come together to affect the life care plan. While IDEA provides funding, the ADA, and 504 require accommodations to ensure barrier-free access. Other acts have mandates related to housing, public accommodations and access, travel, and other aspects of daily life. The costs for the accommodations need to be identified and considered in the life care plan. Each plan must be individualized to the specific person and the situation. It is imperative, when appropriate, for the life care planner to evaluate the

educational, home, and work setting to determine if additional accommodations would be beneficial or required.

References

Aiken County Public School. (2011, August 28). Department of special education: 504 forms. Retrieved from http:// www.aiken.k12.sc.us/site/specialprograms/se_index. html#504

Disability Rights Education and Defense Fund. (n.d.). A comparison of ADA, IDEA, and Section 504. Retrieved from http://www.dredf.org/advocacy/comparison.html

Federal Communications Commission. (2011, September 14). Disability rights office. Retrieved from http://www.fcc. gov/cgb/dro

Rehabilitation Act of 1973, Pub. L. No. 93-112, 29 U.S.C. § 701-796I

Rehabilitation Act Amendments of 1973, as amended. (n.d.). Retrieved from www.access-board.gov/enforcement/ Rehab-Act-Text/intro.htm

U.S. Department of Education. (n.d). Building the legacy: IDEA 2004. Retrieved from http://idea.ed.gov

U.S. Department of Education. (2011, September 6). Office of Special Education Rehabilation Services. Retrieved from http://ed.gov/osers

US Department of Justice. (June 15, 2009). Americans with Disability Act of 1990, as amended. Retrieved from http://www.ada.gov/pubs/adastatute08.htm

U.S. Department of Transportation. (June 29, 2011). Aviation consumer protetion and enforcement. Retrieved from http://airconsumer.ost.dot.gov

U.S. Department of Justice. (August 24, 2011). Civil Rights Division. Retrieved from www.Justice.gov/CRT/about/ spl/cripa.php

U.S. Department of Housing and Urban Development. (n.d.). Fair housing/equal opportunity. Retrieved from http:// www.hud.gov/offices/fheo